Manual for Dental Hygienist

Manual for Dental Hygienist

A Complete Guide as per DCI Curriculum

Maj Gen PN Awasthi VSM (Retd)
MDS FICD (Hony)

Formerly
Professor and Head
Department of Dental Surgery
Armed Forces Medical College (AFMC)
Pune, Maharashtra, India

Head, Indian Army Dental Corps
Secretary, Dental Council of India
Advisor, Manav Rachna Dental College
Faridabad, Haryana, India

Foreword
Lt Gen Vimal Arora PVSM (Retd)

JAYPEE

JAYPEE BROTHERS MEDICAL PUBLISHERS
The Health Sciences Publisher
New Delhi | London

Jaypee Brothers Medical Publishers (P) Ltd

Headquarters
EMCA House
23/23-B, Ansari Road, Daryaganj
New Delhi 110 002, India
Landline: +91-11-23272143,
+91-11-23272703
+91-11-23282021, +91-11-23245672
E-mail: jaypee@jaypeebrothers.com

Corporate Office
Jaypee Brothers Medical Publishers (P) Ltd.
4838/24, Ansari Road, Daryaganj
New Delhi 110 002, India
Phone: +91-11-43574357
Fax: +91-11-43574314
E-mail: jaypee@jaypeebrothers.com

Overseas Office
JP Medical Ltd.
83, Victoria Street, London
SW1H 0HW (UK)
Phone: +44-20 3170 8910
E-mail: info@jpmedpub.com

EU GPSR Authorised Representative
Logos Europe, 9 rue Nicolas Poussin
17000, La Rochelle, France
Phone: +33 (0) 6 67 93 73 78
E-mail: Contact@logoseurope.eu

Website: www.jaypeebrothers.com
Website: www.jaypeedigital.com

Inquiries for bulk sales may be solicited at: jaypee@jaypeebrothers.com

Manual for Dental Hygienist: A Complete Guide as per DCI Curriculum

First Edition: 2018, Reprint: **2025**

ISBN: 978-93-5270-228-2

Printed in India

Dedicated to

The Indian Army Dental Corps—
"My source of inspiration".

Foreword

It is indeed a privilege to write a foreword for a person so immensely accomplished and distinguished as the author of this book, Maj Gen PN Awasthi. He was the transforming force behind the Army Dental Corps whose vision and emphasis on achieving the highest rank of Lt Gen for the Corps was the aim of his life and who could give a credibility to the Corps in his short but highly fruitful tenure as the Head of the Army Dental Corps. He has been laying foundation on which the profession has excelled over a period of time and even now he is laying the same foundation for a structured and organized training for the dental support staff; the 'Dental Hygienists' without whom the profession of dentistry is not complete.

The contents of the book speak volumes about the author's ingenuity and dedicated approach to cover the topics in a most simple and lucid manner and the topics have been narrated very simply which makes the book an interesting reading and keeps the reader engrossed with the contents. The author has put the essence of his 50 plus years of clinical and academic experience in the writing of this book which will be a storehouse of knowledge for the generations to come.

The *Manual for Dental Hygienist* starts with the very basic lessons which are the essential foundation stones for the advanced learning of the complexities of understanding the periodontal disease and its presentation in the oral cavity. The chapters also cover detailed information on generating awareness, motivation for prevention and also the therapeutic measures both surgical and medical for the treatment of dental disease. The scenario of Oral Health Care in India has undergone a massive change and the role of the dental hygienist has become an integral part of the overall treatment. With over 87% prevalence of the gum disease amongst the Indian population, there is never going to be any dearth of work for the dental hygienists provided, they are proficient in their work, possess the necessary soft skills and have expertise in the most recent trends in the delivery of dental services to the masses.

As a humble professional, I recognize the immense work put in towards writing this book by Maj Gen PN Awasthi and wish to compliment him for this exceptional work. I earnestly hope that the readers will find it informative and easy to understand.

Lt Gen Vimal Arora (Retd)
MDS, FDS RCPS (Glasgow), FRSM (London)
PVSM, AVSM, VSM & Bar, OSRE (Oman)

Formerly
Director General Dental Services, Army Dental Corps
Member of Dental Council and Hony Dental Surgeon to President of India

Preface

Regulation of the profession of Dentistry in India was enacted by Dentist Act 16 of 1948 on 29th March 1948, and Dental Council of India (DCI) was constituted. Besides profession of dentistry, two other para dental diploma courses were also constituted, i.e. Dental Hygienist and Dental Mechanic.

Another para dental diploma course notified by Ministry of Health and Family Welfare, Government of India in 2007 is Dental Operating Room Assistant (DORA) course. The qualifying criteria for the para dental diploma courses is 12th (10+2) with Science and English.

These courses can only be started in a dental college with the prior permission of the respective State Government and subsequently by the Ministry of Health and Family Welfare, Government of India on the recommendations of DCI.

Though the dental surgeons are the nucleus of the profession, the para dental personnel are the vital links between the patient and the dentist to augment the resources and to meet the vast need of oral health care of the people.

In India, the Dental Hygienist course was pioneered by the Army in 1955 to meet the oral hygiene needs of the soldiers who have to be kept in perfect oral health status at all the time.

The author while heading as Professor in the Department of Dental Surgery at Armed Forces Medical College (AFMC), Pune, Maharashtra prepared dental hygienist notes as it was observed that in the absence of a dedicated textbook on the lines of DCI regulations; dental hygienist trainees are finding difficulties in grasping the course contents in English as most of them are from the rural backgrounds who were not very affluent in English language. Dental hygienist regulations according to DCI are appended at the end of book.

The present manual is the modification of those notes with substantial improvements in the text which includes recent advancements in oral health care and code of ethics for dental hygienist. All chapters have been written in a very simplified, concise pattern so that the contents can be easily grasped by the trainees and the trainers.

Among the three para dental diploma courses, Dental Hygienist is the only course where dental hygienist is directly involved in providing oral health prophylaxis treatment to the patient and dental health education of the community and the school children.

In some advance countries including East European countries, dental hygienist training is further modified to provide class I dental fillings, topical applications of fluorides, jaw impressions and temporary analgesics, dressings, etc. After obtaining laid down credits, they are permitted to pursue dental graduate courses like DDS and DMD.

The need of the hour is to update dental hygienist training so that skilled dental hygienist cadre spreads throughout the country and meets the preventive dental health needs of all, specially the villagers and the underprivileged population.

This first attempt, I hope will go a long way in improving the competencies of our dental hygienist to the international standards which at present are far superior than the existing Indian standards.

Maj Gen PN Awasthi **VSM** (Retd)

Acknowledgments

I take this opportunity to thank all those who have helped me in preparing this manual, Brig BP Khattak (Retd.), Col SK Ojha (Retd.), Dr Anil Chaudhary, Dr Kapil Arora, Brig S Roy, Brig NK Singla, and many others. My special thank goes to Dr Sangeeta Dhir, editor, IP Journal for her valuable suggestions and my Secretary Ms Anita Arora for typing the manuscript.

Finally, I would like to put on records my sincere thanks to Shri Jitendar P Vij (Group Chairman), Mr Ankit Vij (Group President), Ms Ritu Sharma (Director-Content Strategy), Ms Samina Khan (Executive Assistant to Director-Content Strategy), Dr Ambika Kapoor (Development Editor), Ms Seema Dogra (Cover Visualizer), Mr Rajesh Sharma (Production Coordinator), Ms Geeta Rani Barik (Proofreader), Mr Nitesh Jain (Graphic Designer) and Mr Raj Kumar (DTP Operator) of M/s Jaypee Brothers Medical Publishers (P) Ltd, New Delhi, India, for their encouragement to write this manual. M/s Jaypee Brothers have truly standardized the medical literature at an affordable cost without compromising the quality contents. Their support will ever remain laudable in the entire Medical/Dental fraternity not only in India but in its neigboring countries as well.

Acknowledgments

Contents

SECTION 1: HUMAN ANATOMY

SECTION 2: GENERAL AND DENTAL PHYSIOLOGY AND HISTOLOGY

SECTION 3: GENERAL AND DENTAL PHARMACOLOGY

SECTION 4: PATHOLOGY AND MICROBIOLOGY: GENERAL AND DENTAL

SECTION 5: DENTAL RADIOLOGY

SECTION 6: GINGIVAL AND PERIODONTAL DISEASES: CLASSIFICATION AND MANAGEMENT

Plate 1

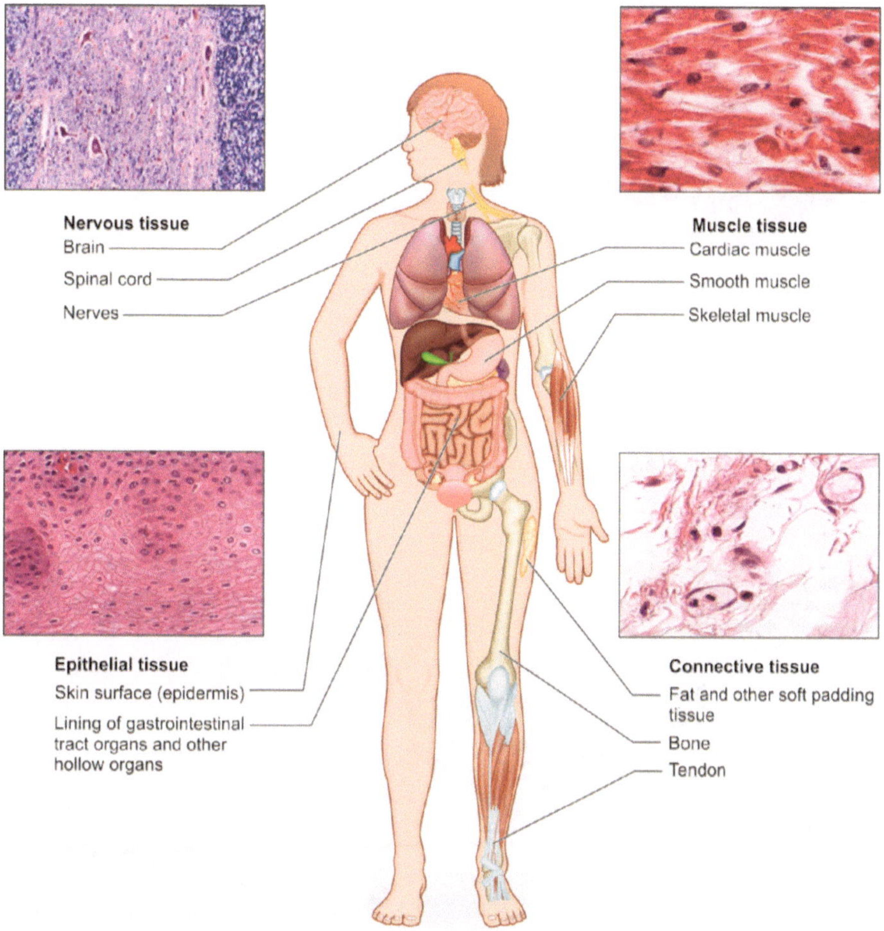

Fig. 1.2: Classification of four basic types of tissues

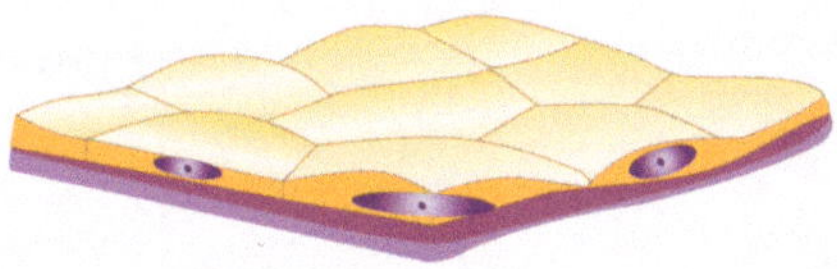

Description: Single layer of flattened cells with disc-shaped central nuclei and sparse cytoplasm; the simplest of the epithelia.

Function: Allows passage of materials by diffusion and filtration in sites where protection is not important; secretes lubricating substances in serosae.

Location: Kidney glomeruli, air sacs of lungs, lining of heart, blood vessels, and lymphatic vessels, and lining of ventral body cavity.

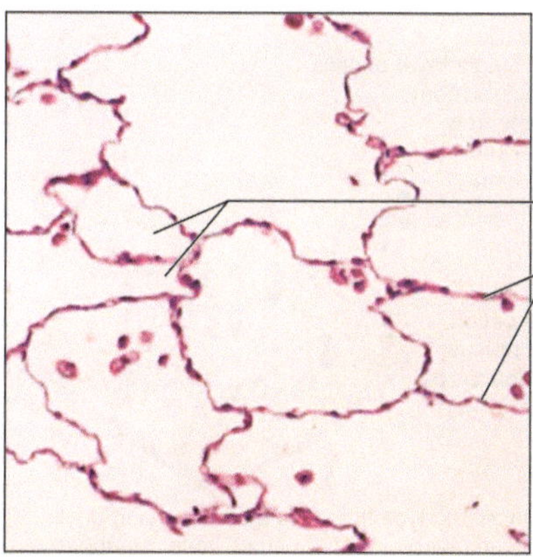

Fig. 1.4A: Simple squamous epithelium in alveolar wall

Plate 2

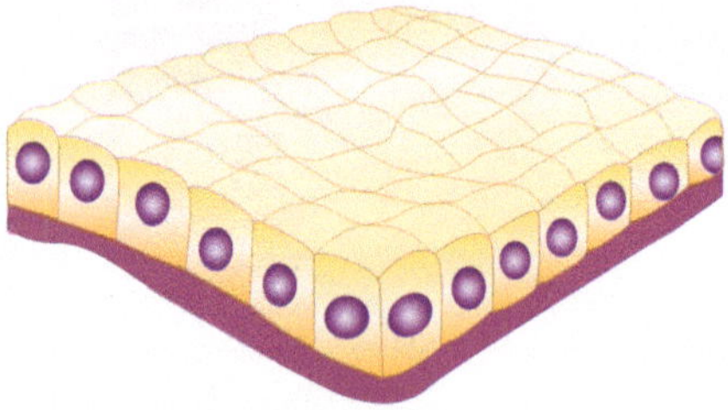

Description: Single layer of cube like cells with large, spherical central nuclei.

Function: Secretion and absorption.

Location: Kidney tubules, ducts and secretory portions of small glands, and ovary surface.

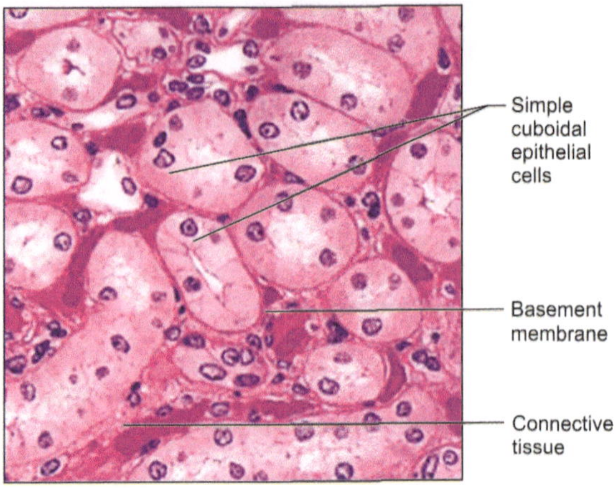

Fig. 1.4B: Simple cuboidal epithelium in kidney tubules

Description: Single layer of tall cells with round to oval nuclei; some cells bear cilia; layer may contain mucus-glands (goblet cells).

Function: Absorption; secretion of mucus, enzymes, and other substances; ciliated type propels mucus (or reproductive cells) by ciliary action.

Location: Nonciliated type lines most of the digestive tract (stomach to anal canal), gallbladder, and excretory ducts of some glands; ciliated variety lines small bronchi, uterine tubes, and some regions of the uterus.

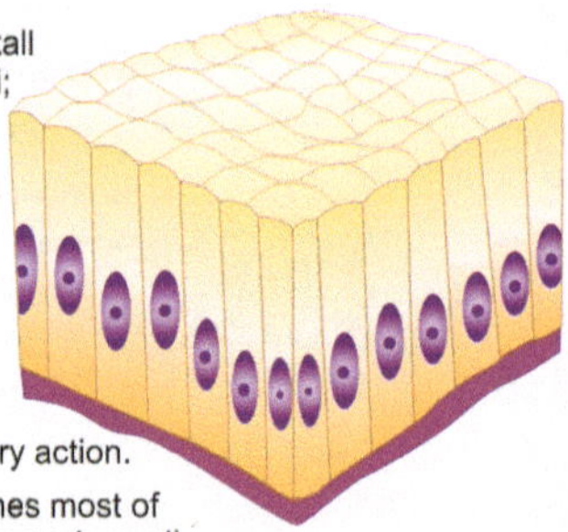

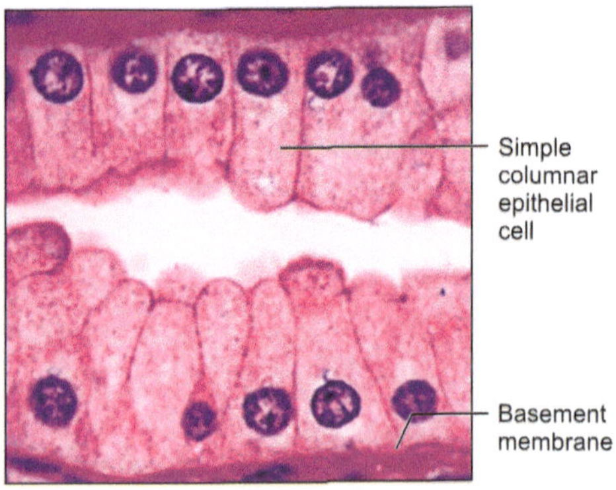

Fig. 1.4C: Simple columnar epithelium in stomach mucosa

Description: Single layer of cells of differing heights, some not reaching the free surface; nuclei seen at different levels; may contain goblet cells and bear cilia.

Function: Secretion, particularly of mucus; propulsion of mucus by ciliary action.

Location: Nonciliated type in male's spermcarrying ducts and ducts of large glands; ciliated variety lines the upper respiratory tract.

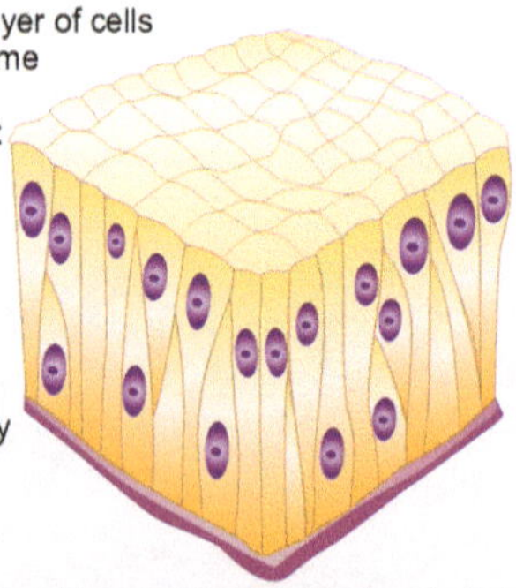

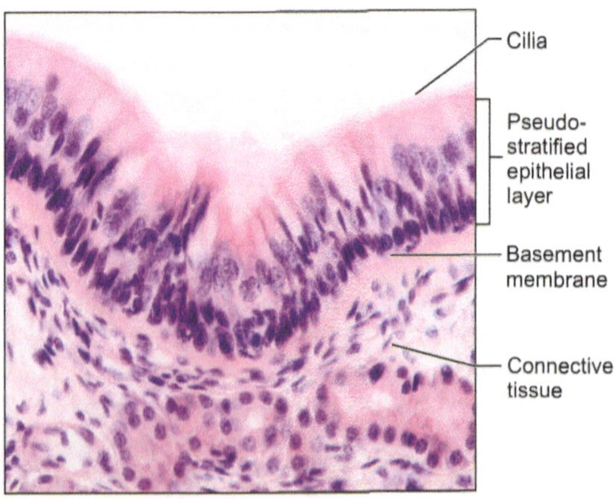

Fig. 1.4D: Pseudostratified columnar epithelium in human trachea

Plate 3

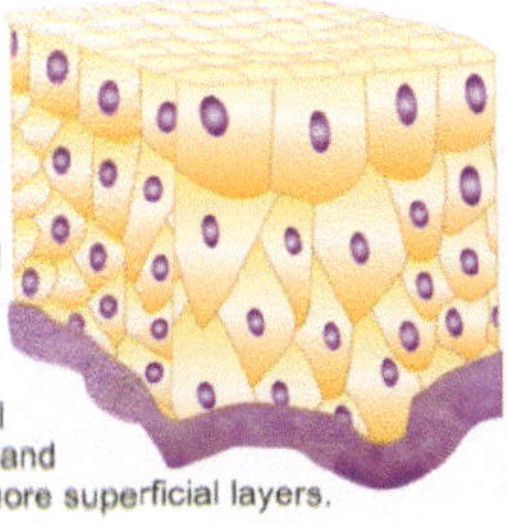

Description: Thick membrane composed of several cell layers; basal cells are cuboidal or columnar and metabolically active; surface cells are flattened (squamous); in the keratinized type, the surface cells are full of keratin and dead; basal cells are active in mitosis and produce the cells of the more superficial layers.

Function: Protects underlying tissues in areas subjected to abrasion.

Location: Nonkeratinized type forms the moist linings of the esophagus,mouth, and vagina; keratinized variety forms the epidermis of the skin, a dry membrane.

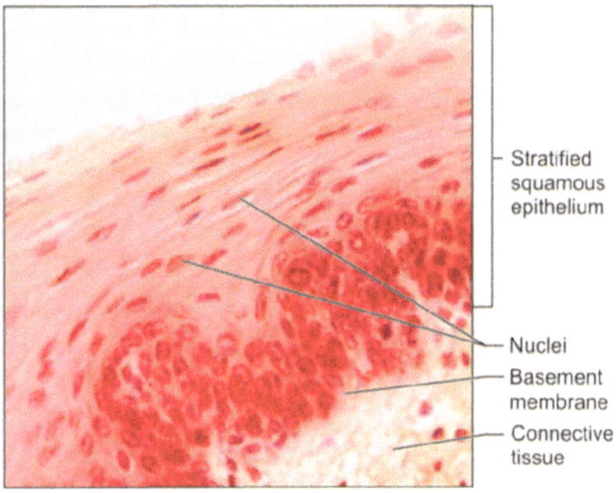

Fig. 1.4E: Stratified squamous epithelium in esophagus

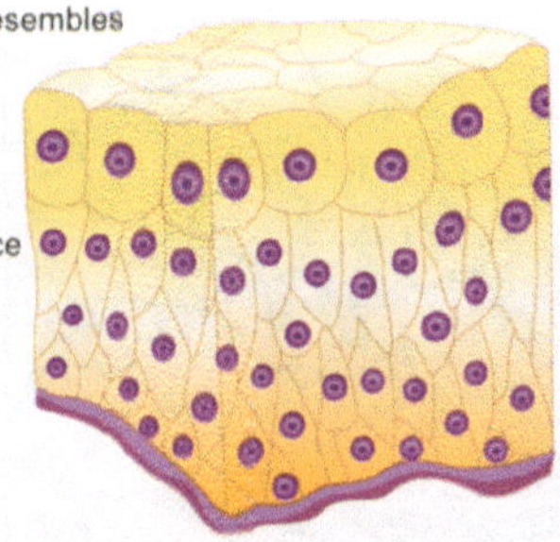

Description: Resembles both stratified squamous and stratified cuboidal; basal cells cuboidal or columnar; surface cells dome-shaped or squamous-like, depending on degree of organ stretch.

Function: Stretches readily and permits distension of urinary organ by contained urine.

Location: Lines the ureters, bladder, and part of the urethra.

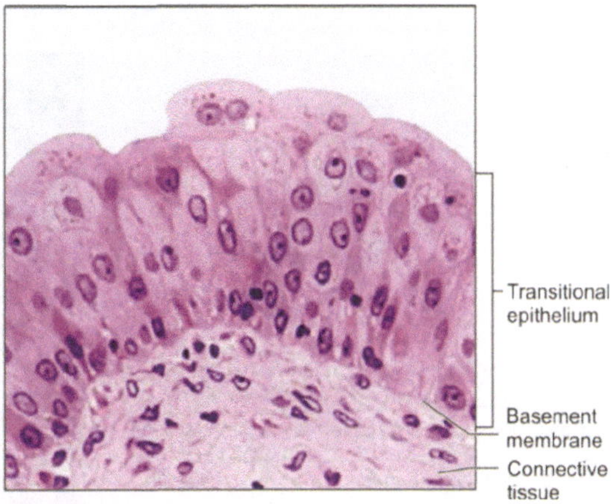

Fig. 1.4F: Transitional epithelium in bladder

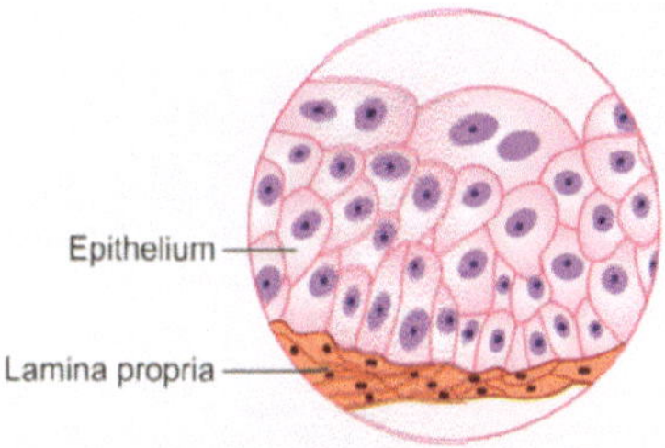

Description: Gel-like matrix with all three fiber types cells: fibroblasts, macrophages, mast cells, and some white blood cells.

Function: Wraps and cushions organs; its macrophages phagocytize bacteria; plays important role in inflammation; holds and conveys tissue fluid.

Location: Widely distributed under epithelia of body, e.g; forms lamina propria of mucous membranes; packages organs; surrounds capillaries.

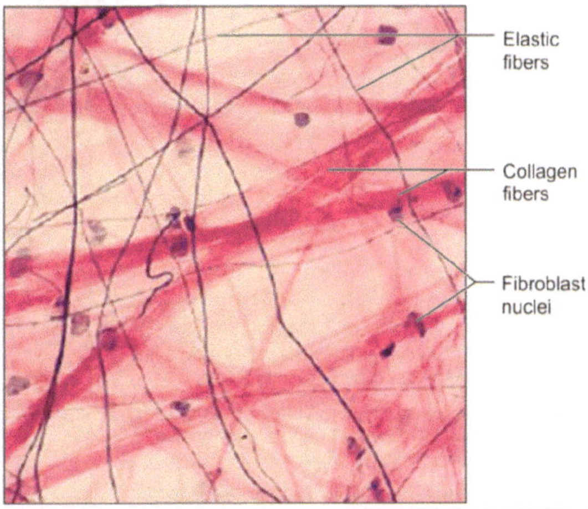

Fig. 1.5B: Areolar tissue

Plate 4

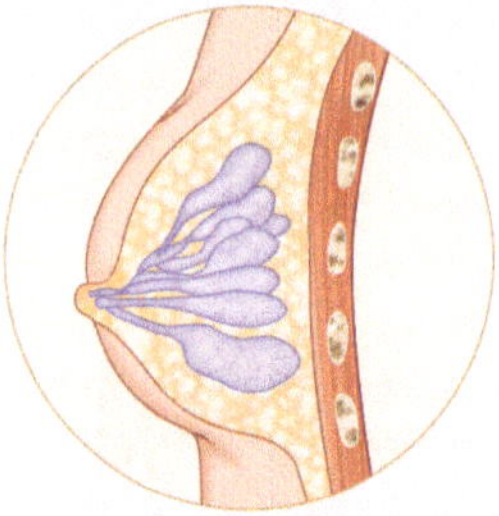

Description: Matrix as in areolar but very sparse; closely packed adipocytes, or fat cells, have nucleus pushed to the side by large fat droplet.

Function: Provides reserve food fuel; insulates against heat loss; supports and protects organs.

Location: Under skin, around kidneys and eyeballs; within abdomen; in breasts.

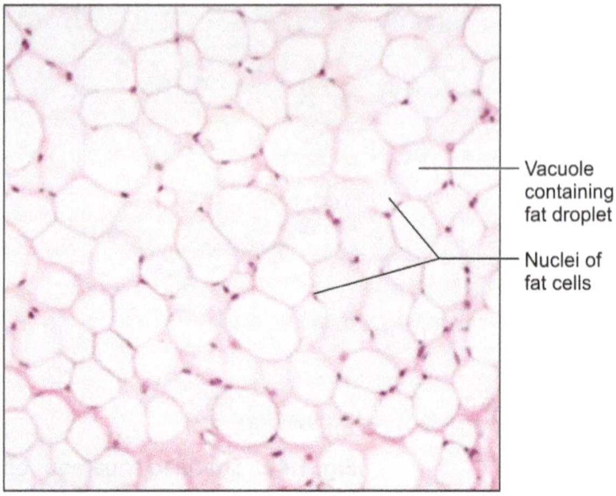

Fig. 1.5C: Adipose tissue

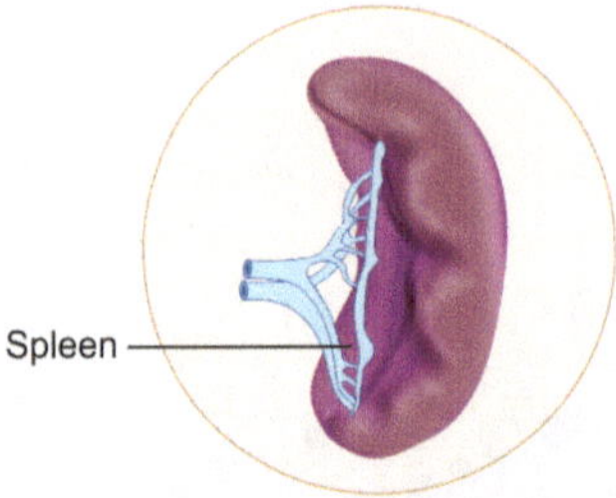

Description: Network of reticular fibers in a typical loose ground substance; reticular cells lie on the network.

Function: Fibers form a soft internal skeleton (stroma) that supports other cell types including white blood cells, mast cells, and macrophages.

Location: Lymphoid organs (lymph nodes, bone marrow, and spleen).

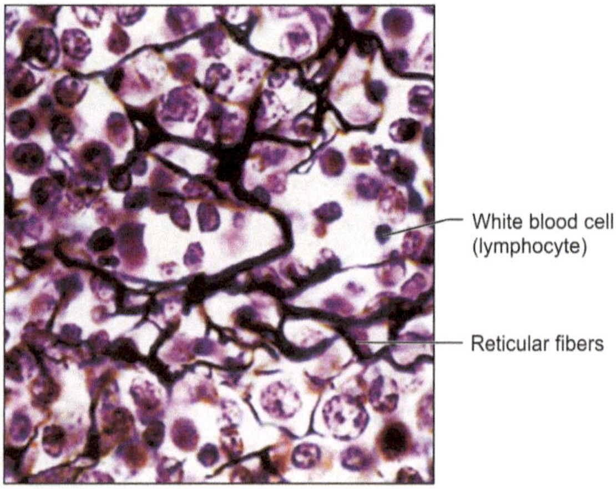

Fig. 1.5D: Reticular tissue

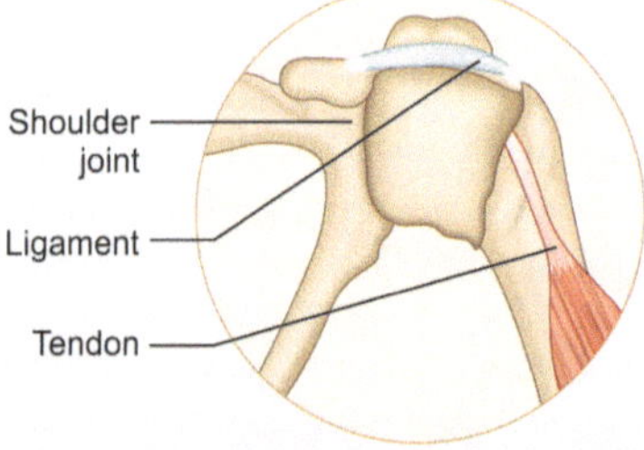

Description: Primarily parallel collagen fibers; a few elastin fibers; major cell type is the fibroblast.

Function: Attaches muscles to bones or to muscles, attaches bones to bones; withstands great tensile stress when pulling force is applied in one direction.

Location: Tendons, most ligaments, aponeuroses.

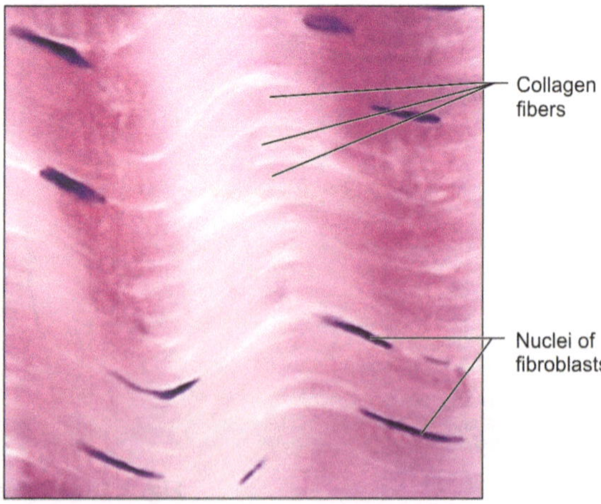

Fig. 1.5E: Dense regular connective tissue

Plate 5

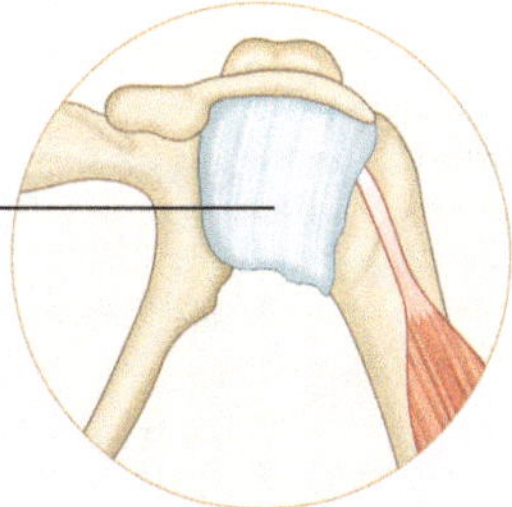

Description: Primarily irregularly arranged collagen fibers; some elastic fibers; major cell type is the fibroblast.

Function: Able to withstand tension exerted in many directions; provides structural strength.

Location: Dermis of the skin; submucosa of digestive tract; fibrous capsules of organs and of joints.

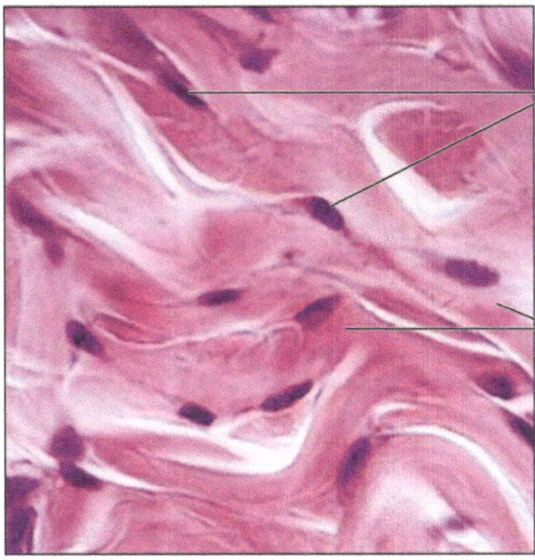

Fig. 1.5F: Dense irregular connective tissue

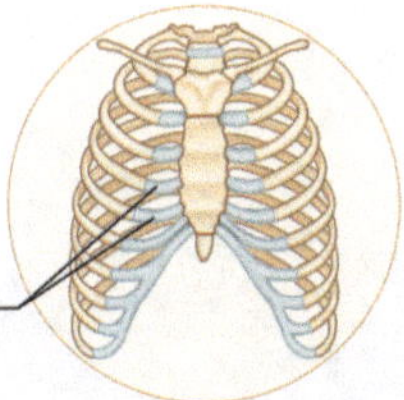

Description: Amorphous but firm matrix; collagen fibers form an imperceptible network; chondroblasts produce the matrix and when mature (chondrocytes) lie in lacunae.

Function: Supports and reinforces; has resilient cushioning properties; resists compressive stress.

Location: Forms most of the embryonic skeleton; covers the ends of long bones in joint cavities; forms costal cartilages of the ribs; cartilages of the nose, trachea, and larynx.

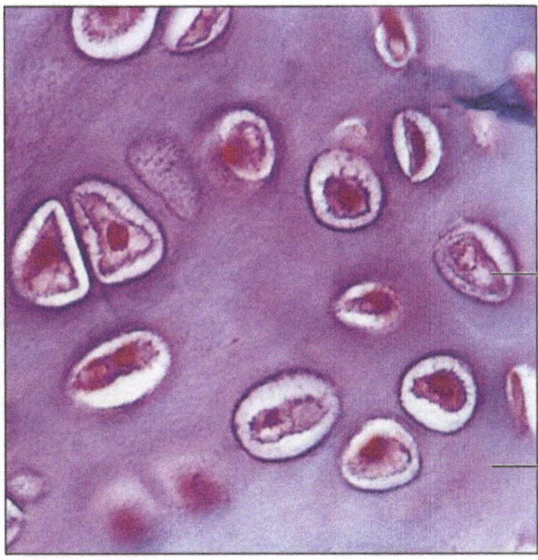

Fig. 1.6: Hyaline cartilage

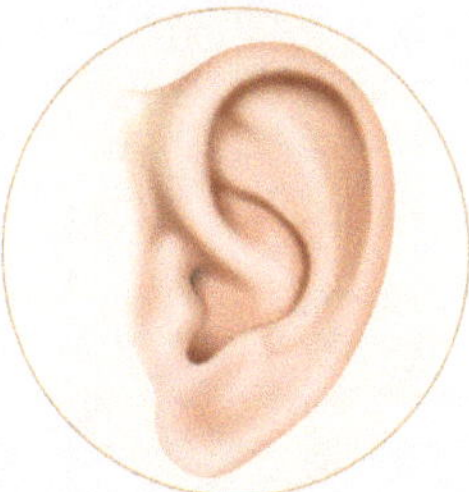

Description: Similar to hyaline cartilage, but more elastic fibers in matrix.

Function: Maintains the shape of a structure while allowing great flexibility.

Location: Supports the external ear (pinna); epiglottis.

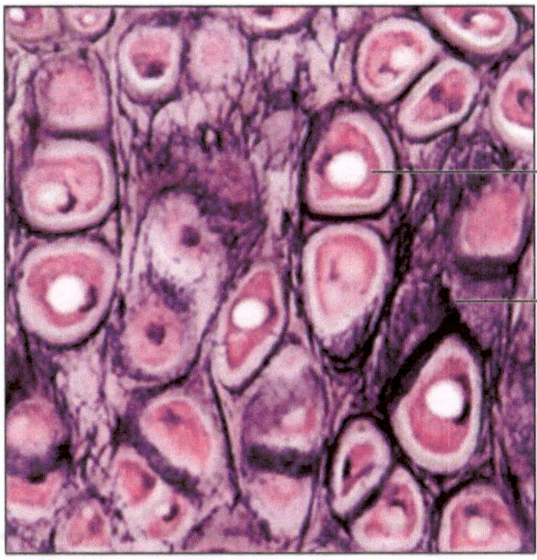

Fig. 1.7: Elastic cartilage

Plate 6

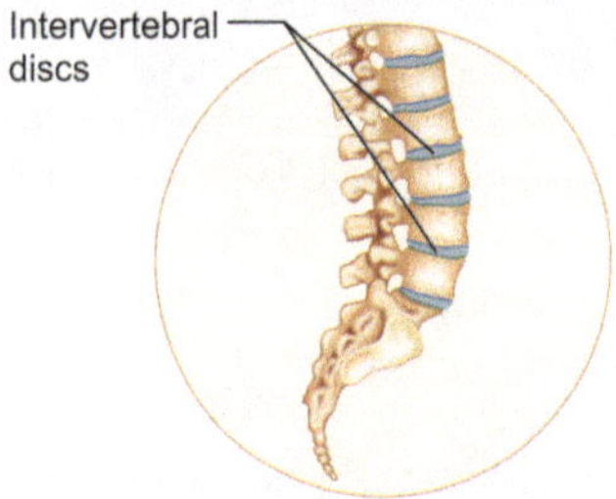

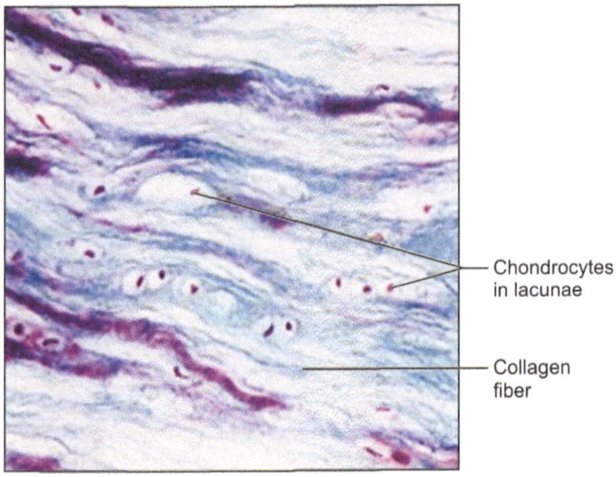

Description: Matrix similar to but less firm than that in hyaline cartilage; thick collagen fibers predominate.

Function: Tensile strength with the ability to absorb compressive shock.

Location: Intervertebral discs; pubic symphysis; discs of knee joint.

Fig. 1.8: Fibrocartilage

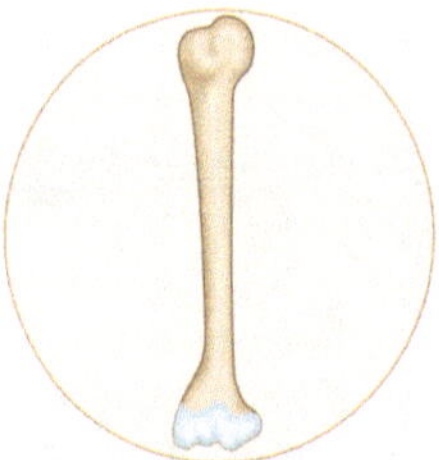

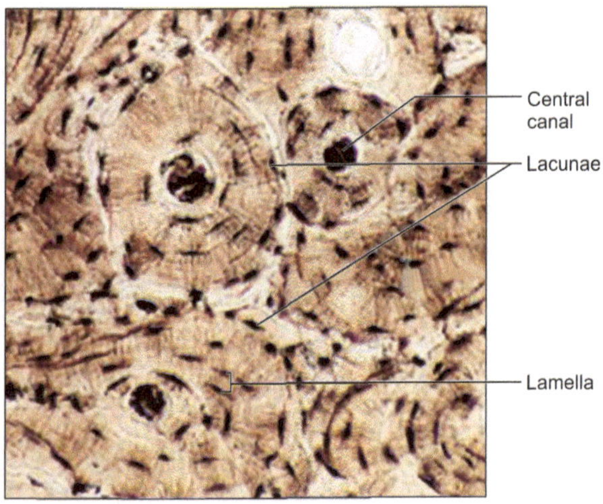

Description: Hard, calcified matrix containing many collagen fibers; osteocytes lie in lacunae, very well-vascularized.

Function: Bone supports and protects (by enclosing); provides levers for the muscles to act on; stores calcium and other minerals and fat; marrow inside bones is the site for blood cell formation (hematopoiesis).

Location: Bone

Fig. 1.9: Bone or osseous tissue

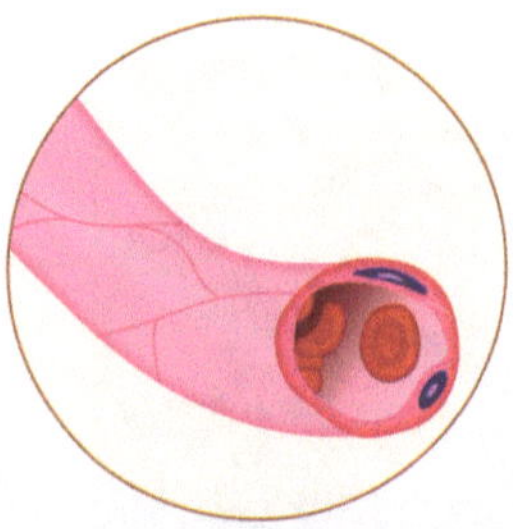

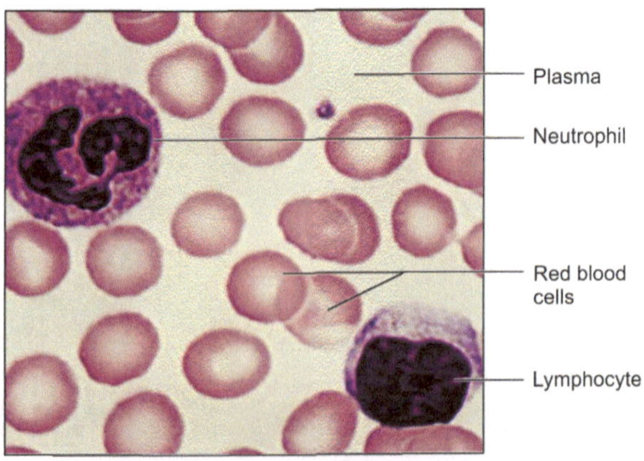

Description: Red and white blood cells in a fluid matrix (plasma).

Function: Transport of respiratory gases, nutrients, wastes, and other substances.

Location: Contained within blood vessels.

Fig. 1.11: Blood smear showing various types of blood cells

Plate 7

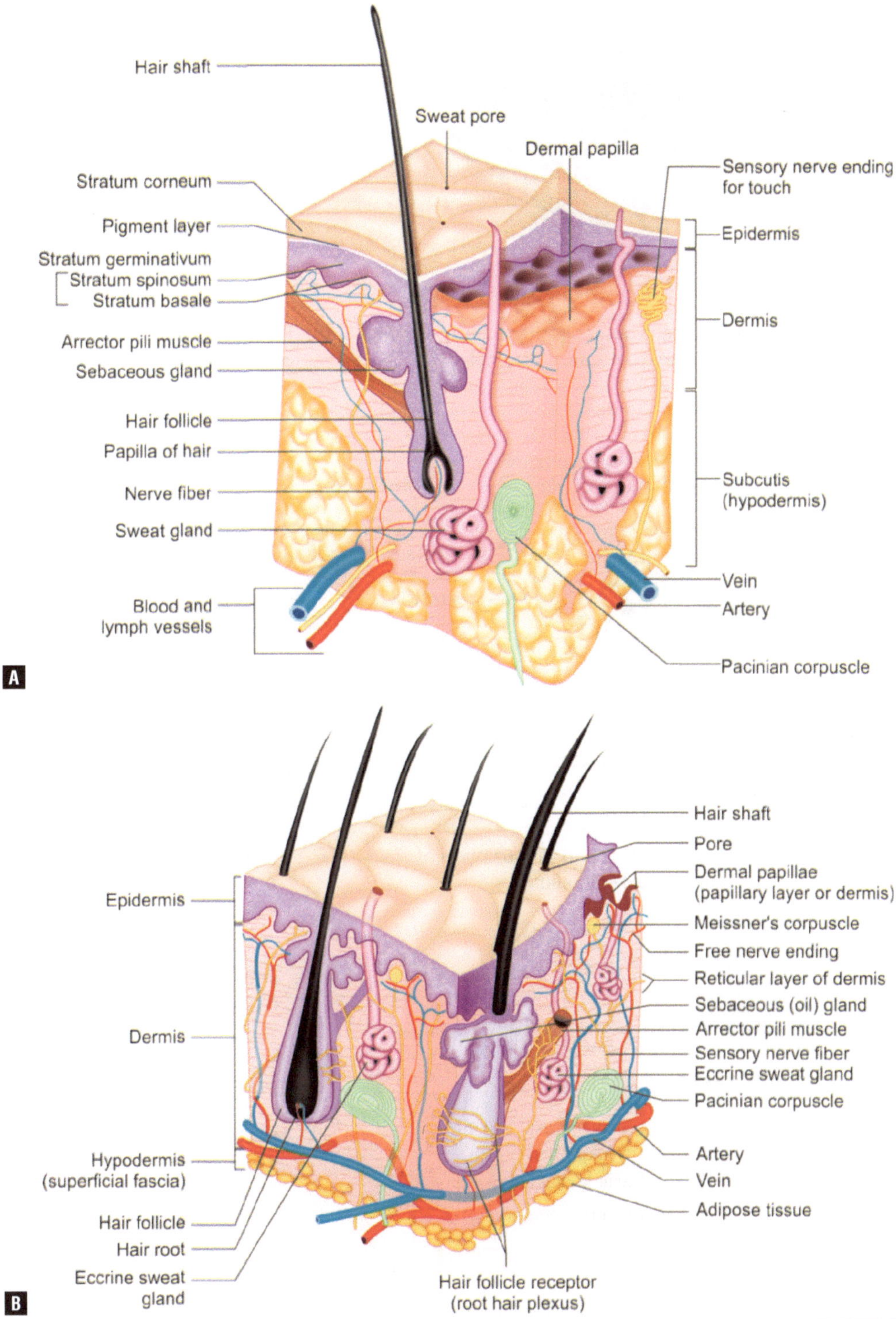

Figs 1.13A and B: Structure of skin

Plate 8

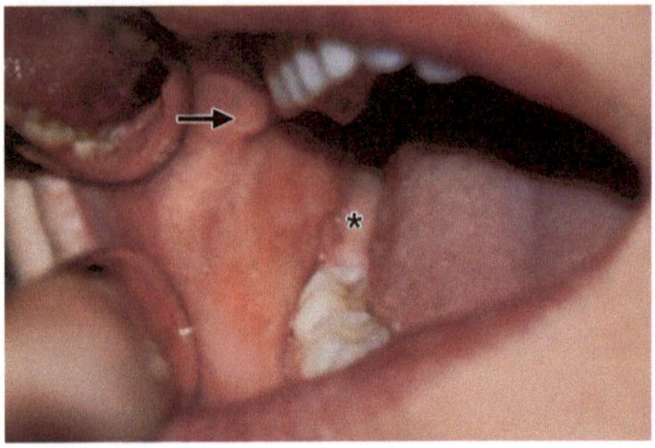

Fig. 2.5: Opening of Stensen's duct opposite second upper molar (arrow). Asterisk indicates retromolar trigone

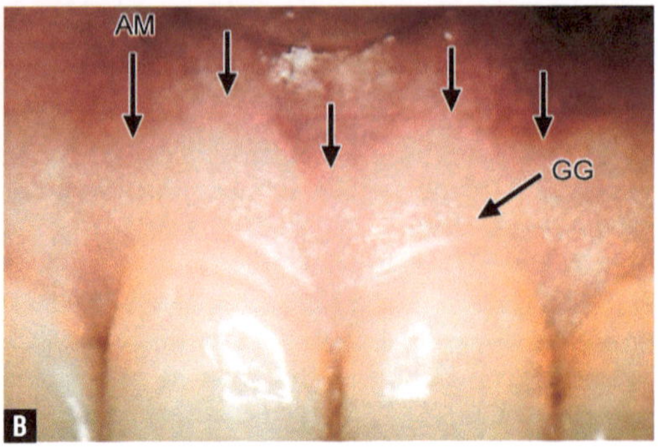

Fig. 5.3B: Tapered contours and pointed interdental gingiva

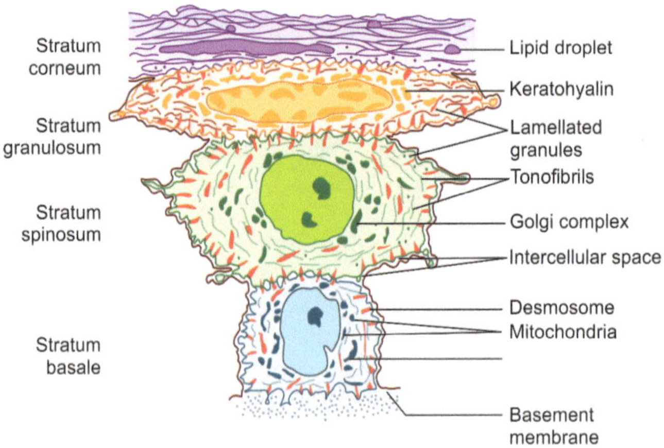

Fig. 5.5: Different types of cells in various layers of oral keratinized epithelium

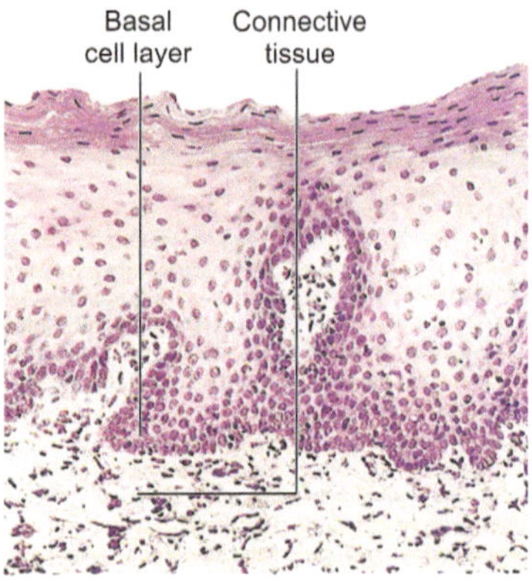

Fig. 5.6: Histological view of oral epithelium and underlying connective tissue

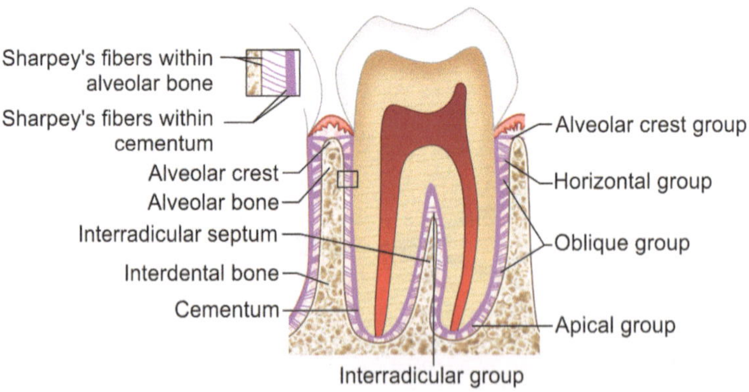

Fig. 5.10: Principal groups of periodontal ligament fibers and their terminal portion

Plate 9

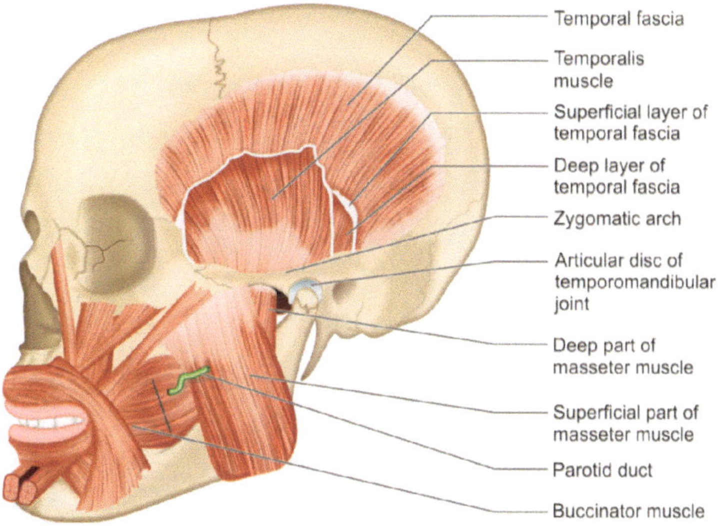

Fig. 8.1: Muscles involved in mastication

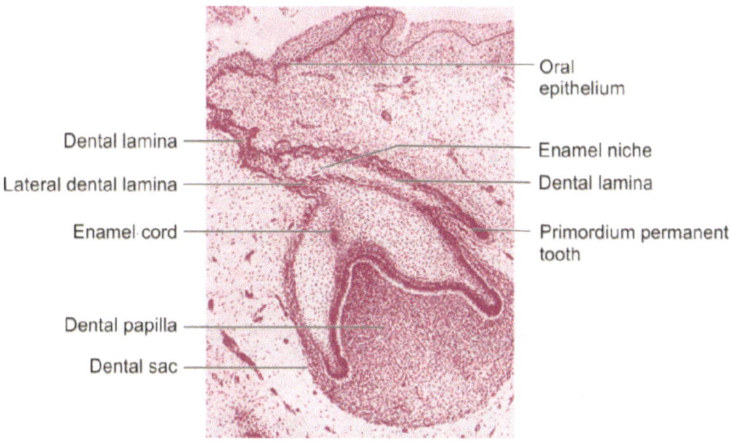

Fig. 13.1: Labiolingual section of tooth bud showing different parts

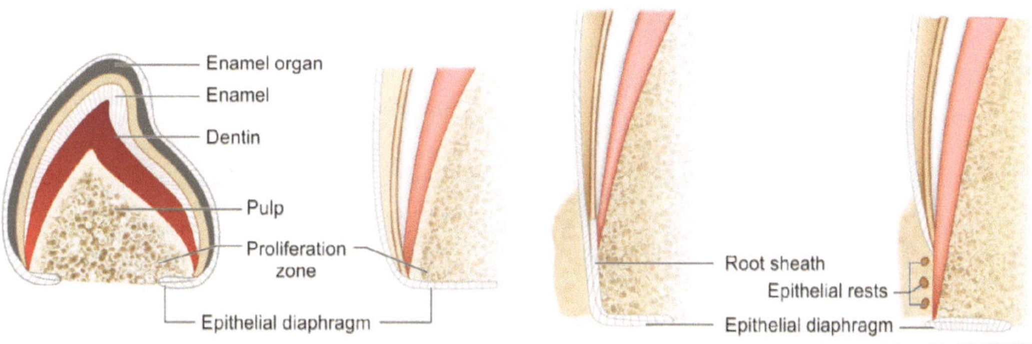

Fig. 13.2: Development of root

Plate 10

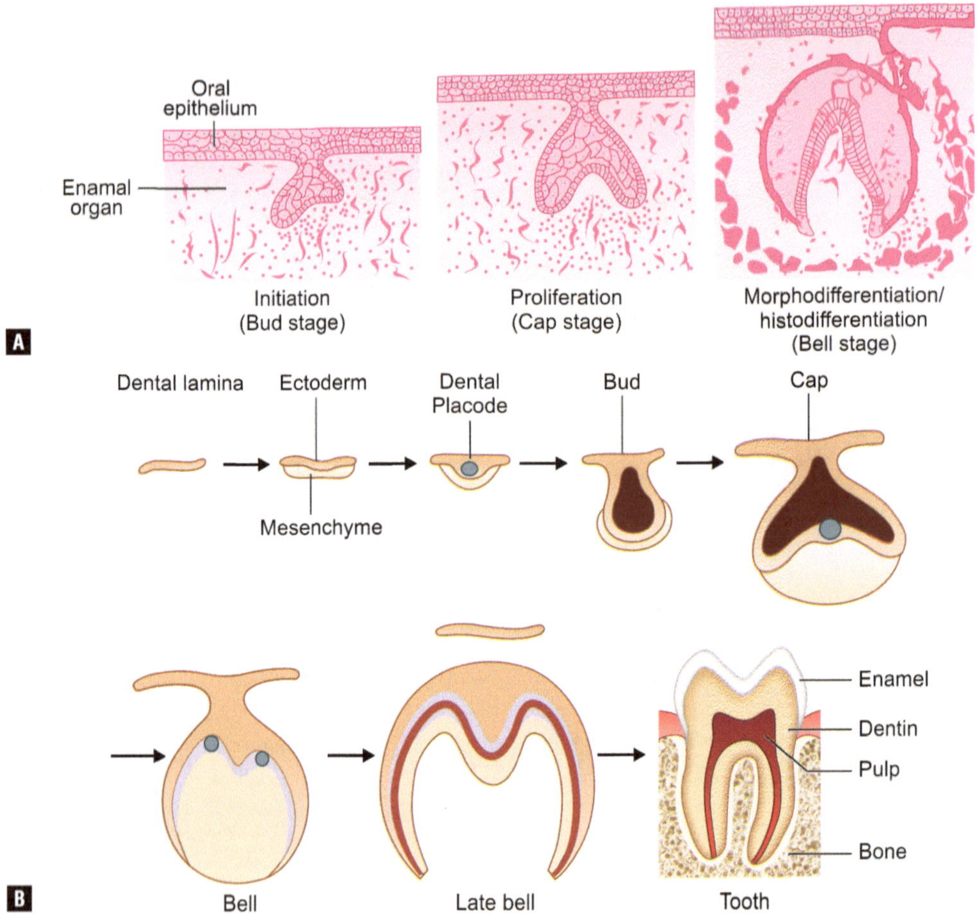

Figs 13.3A and B: Stages in tooth growth

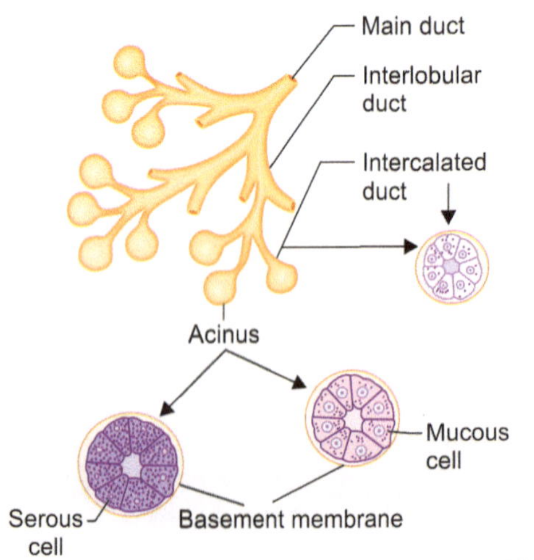

Fig. 15.2: Structure of salivary gland duct system

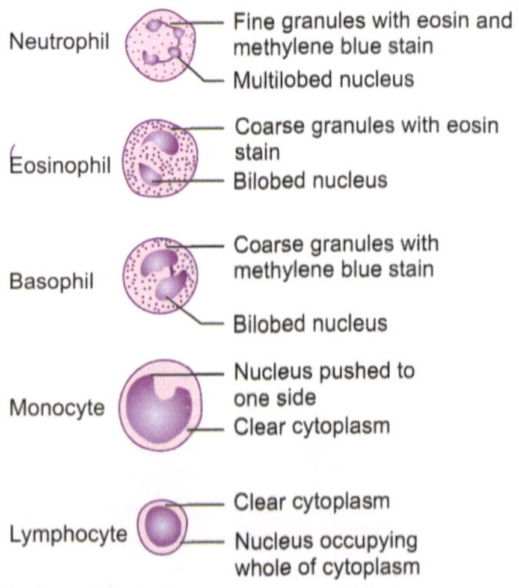

Fig. 17.2: Different types of white blood cells

Plate 11

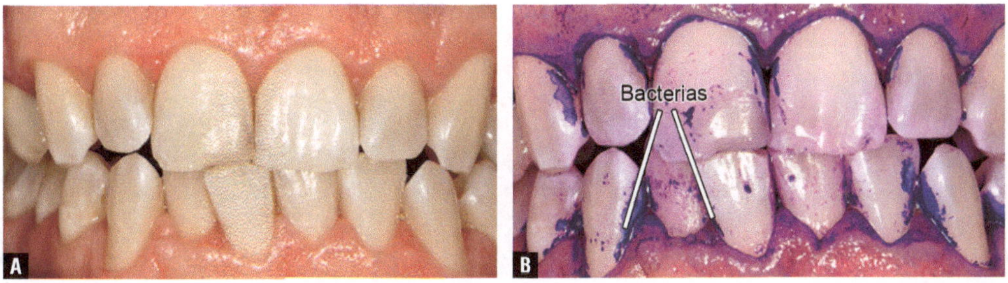

Figs 27.1A and B: (A) Bacteria invisible to naked eye; (B) Bacteria visible after applications of disclosing agent

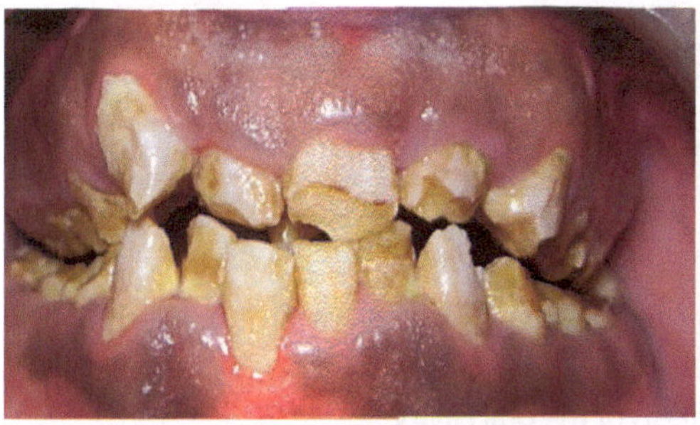

Fig. 34.5: Amelogenesis imperfecta

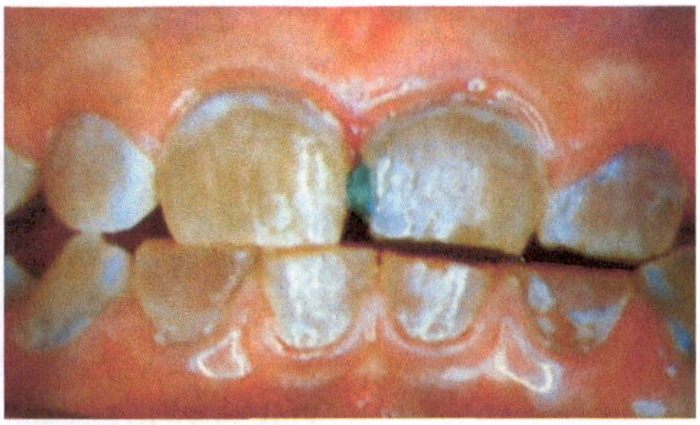

Fig. 34.6: Dentinogenesis imperfecta type I

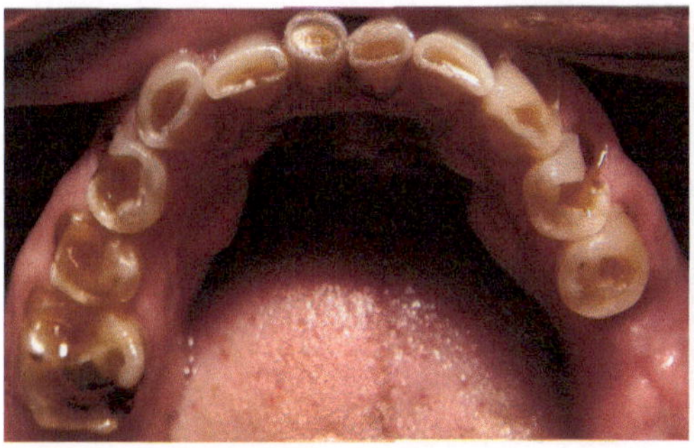

Fig. 36.1: Attrition

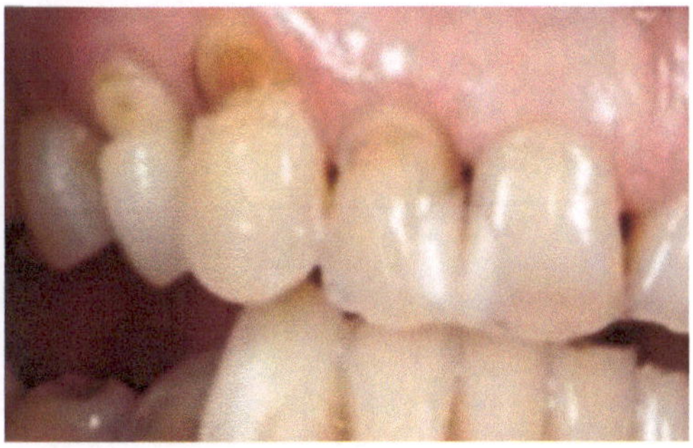

Fig. 36.3: Abrasion

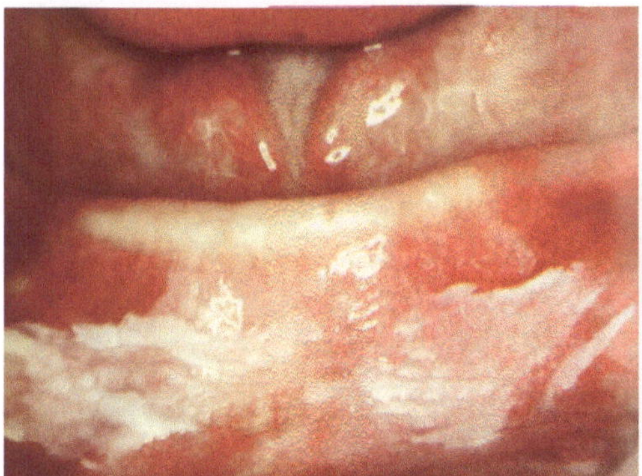

Fig. 39.1: Leukoplakia

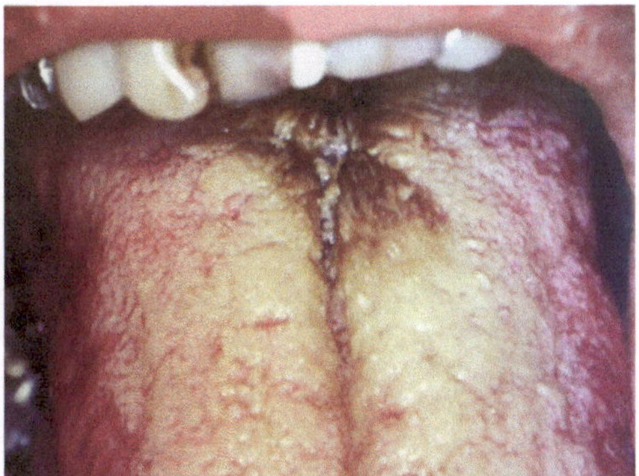

Fig. 39.2: Black hairy tongue

Plate 12

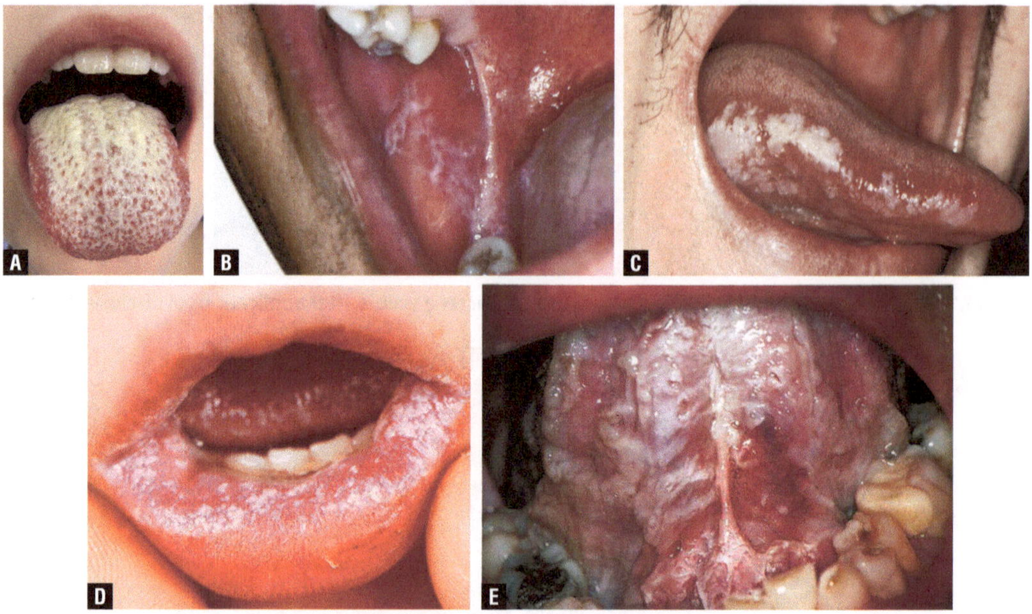

Figs 39.4A to E: Candidiasis of the oral cavity

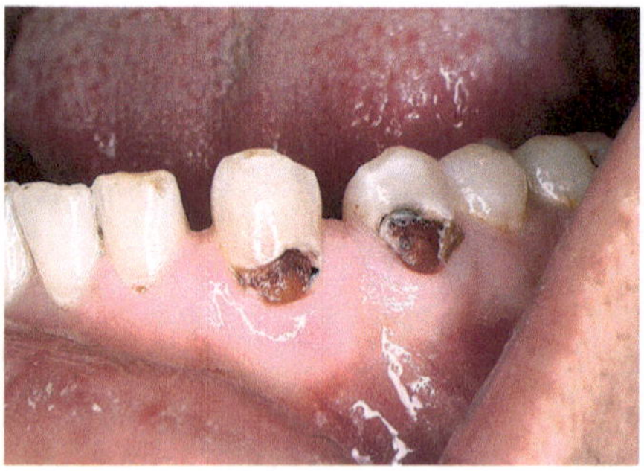

Fig. 41.1: Smooth surface caries

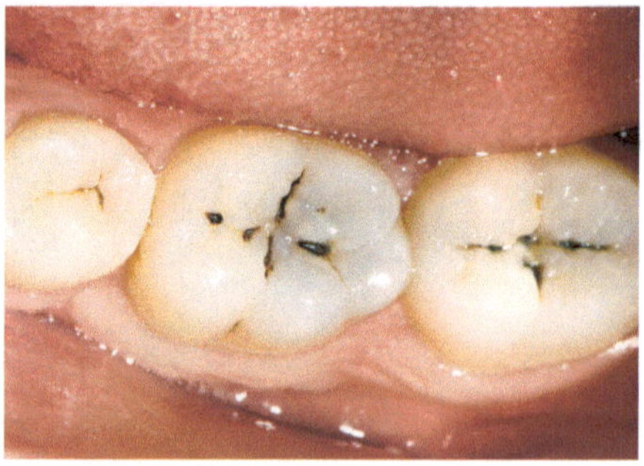

Fig. 41.2: Pit and fissure caries

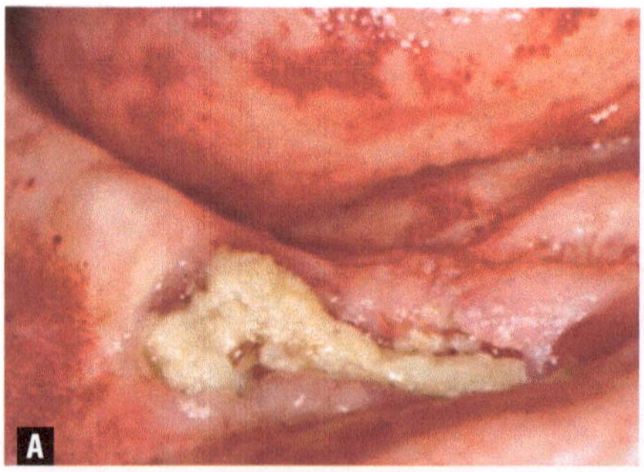

Figs 47.1A: Prolonged exposures of bone intraorally

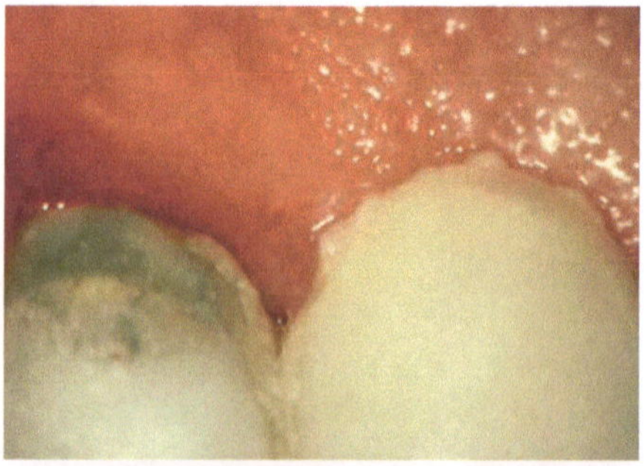

Fig. 48.1: Plaque-induced gingivitis

Plate 13

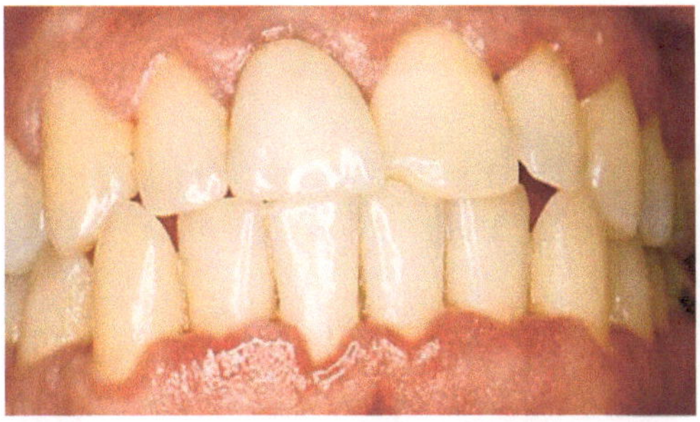

Fig. 48.2: Acute necrotizing ulcerative gingivitis

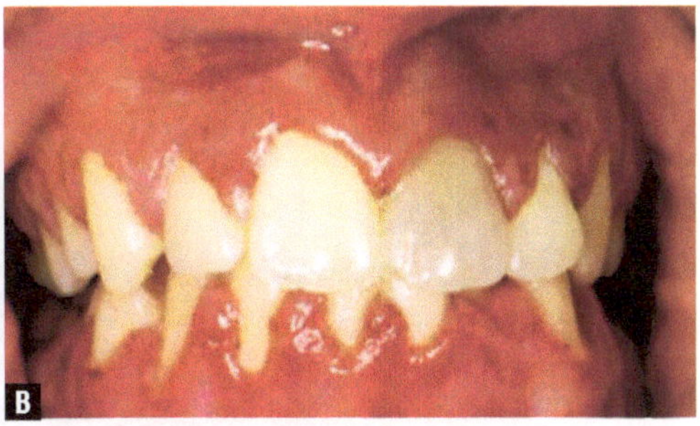

Fig. 48.3B: Acute herpetic gingivostomatitis

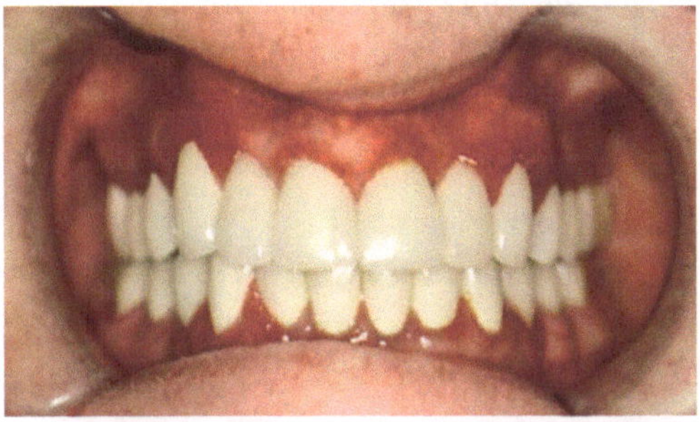

Fig. 48.4: Desquamative gingivitis

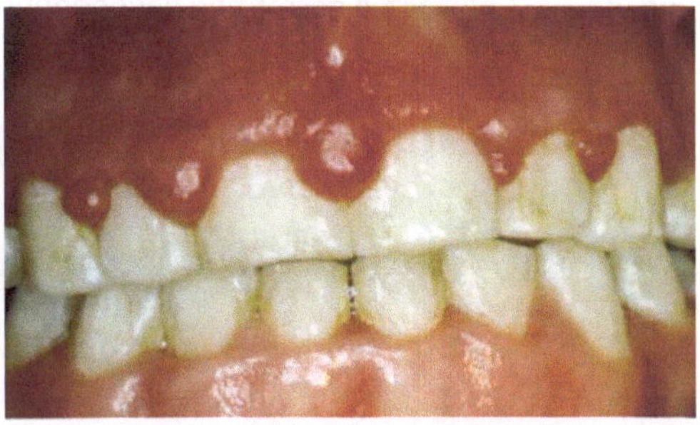

Fig. 48.5: Inflammatory enlargement

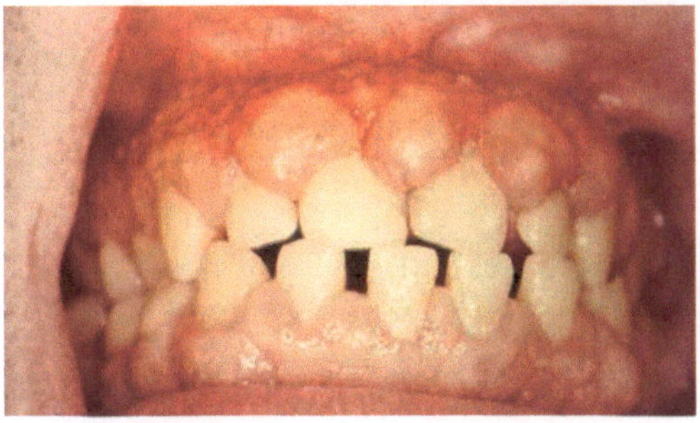

Fig. 48.6: Phenytoin-associated enlargement

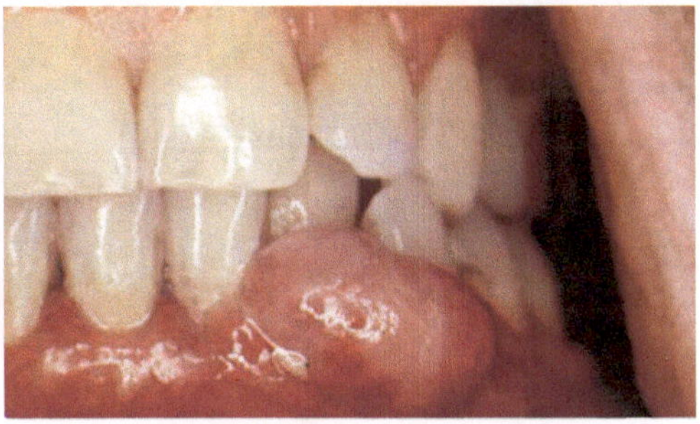

Fig. 48.7: Giant cell granuloma

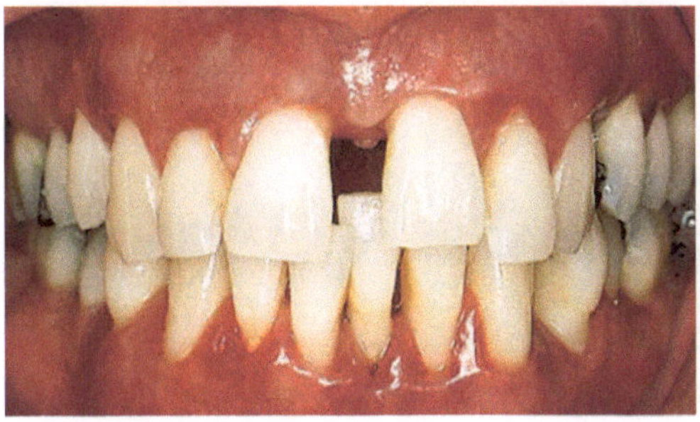

Fig. 48.8: Chronic generalized periodontitis

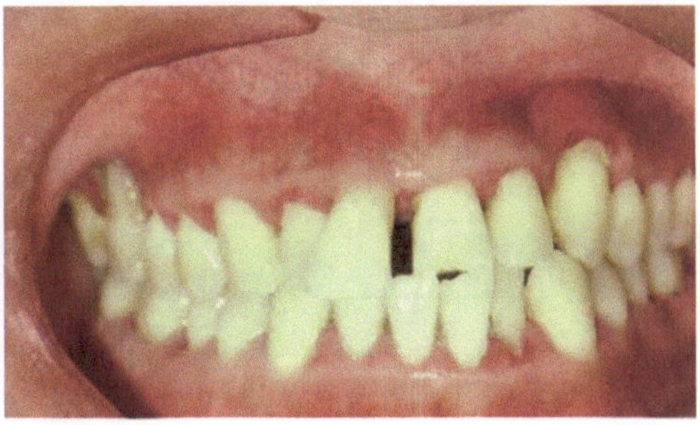

Fig. 48.9: A 21-year-old male with aggressive periodontitis

Plate 14

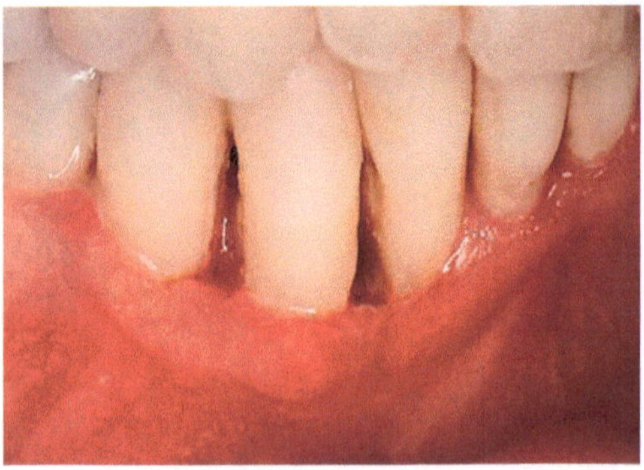

Fig. 48.10: Generalized necrotizing periodontitis

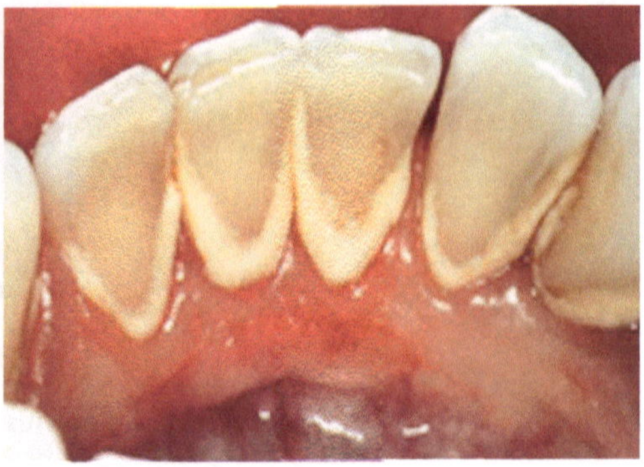

Fig. 48.13: Supragingival calculus

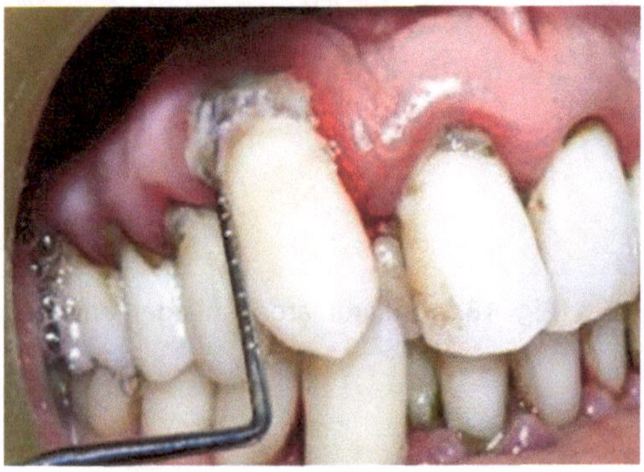

Fig. 48.14: Subgingival calculus

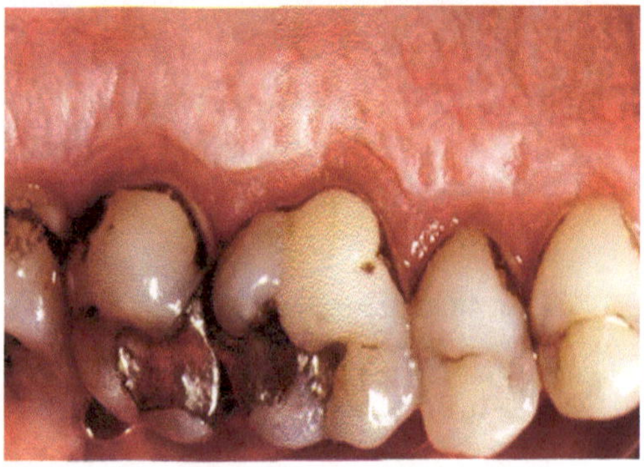

Fig. 48.15: Tobacco stains

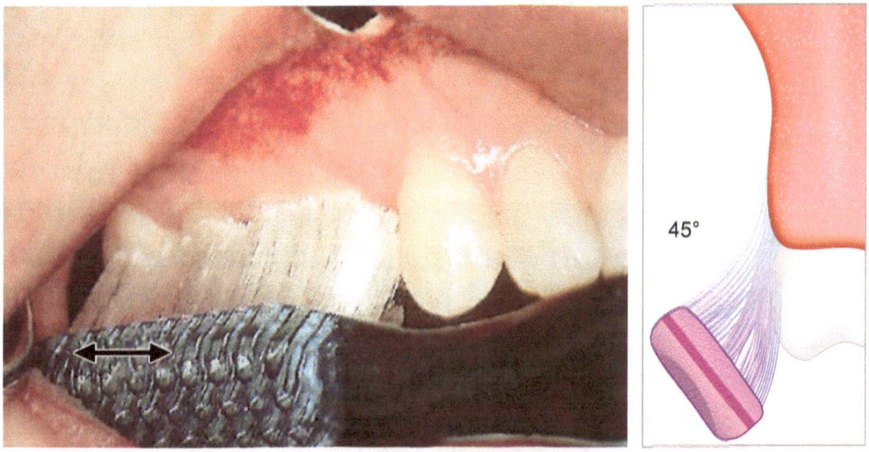

Fig. 49.17: Brushing the outer surfaces of the upper posterior teeth at an angle of 45°

Plate 15

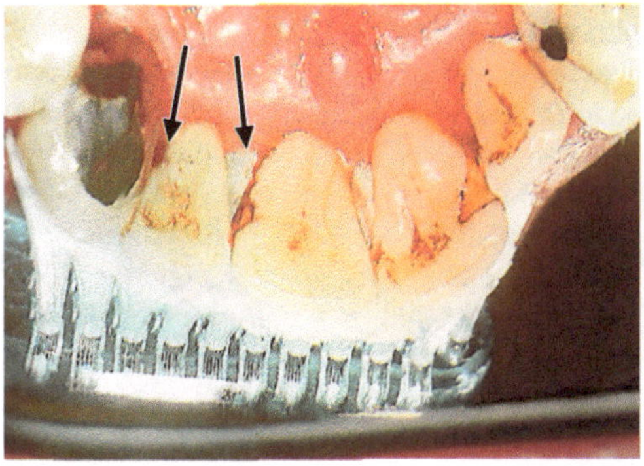

Fig. 49.18: Brushing the outer surfaces of the upper anterior teeth

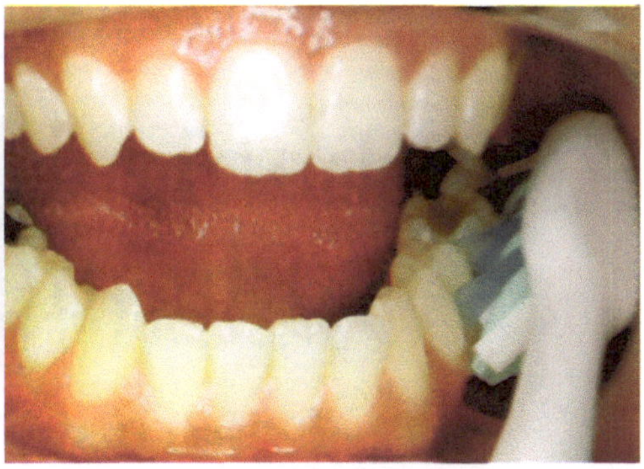

Fig. 49.19: Brushing the outer surfaces of the lower posterior teeth

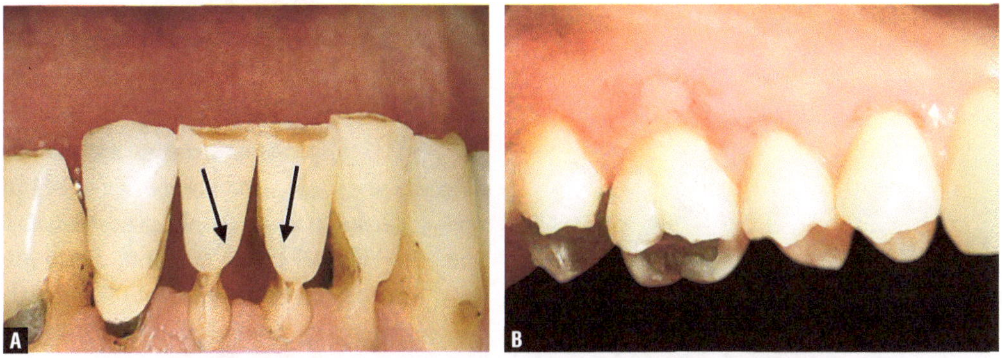

Figs 49.22A and B: (A) Damage to teeth and (B) adjacent soft tissue due to excessive scrubbing technique

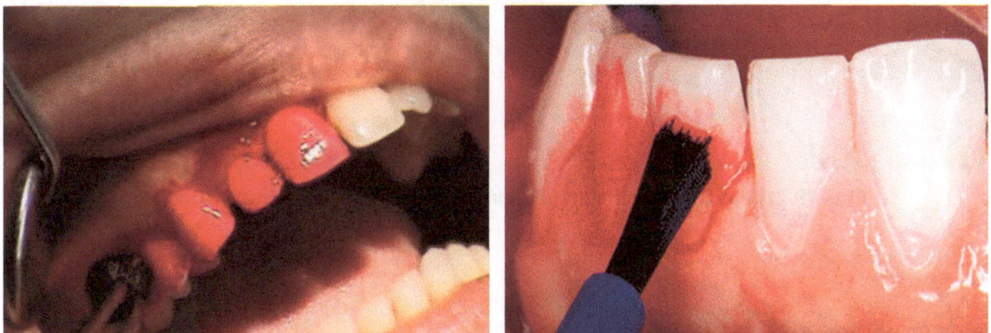

Figs 49.23A and B: Disclosing solution used to identify plaque for patient education

Plate 16

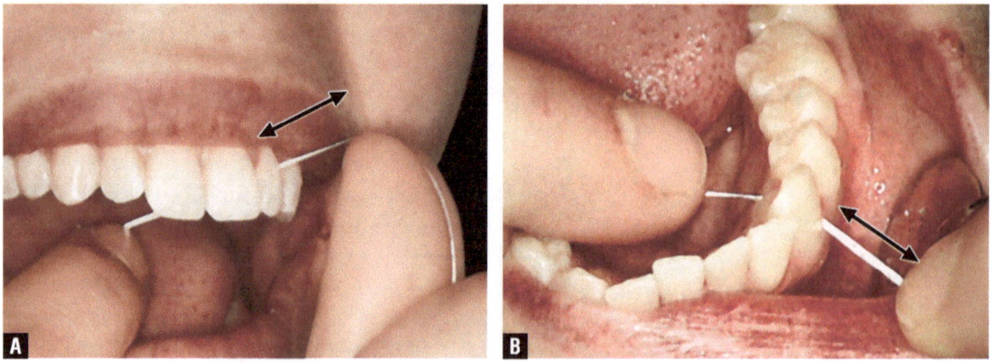

Figs 49.27A and B: Use of floss to clean interdental areas

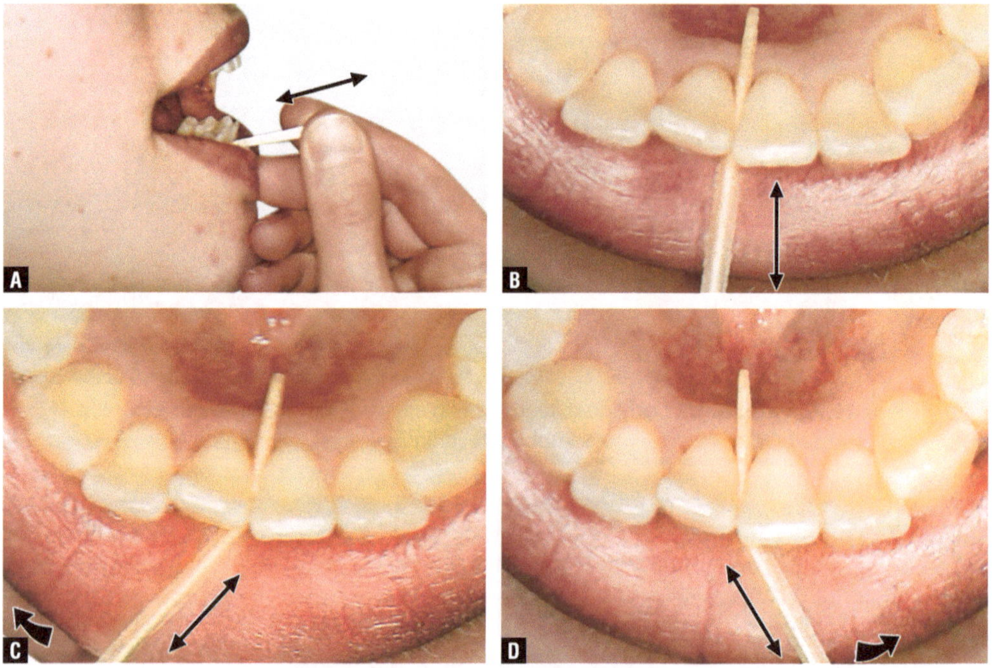

Figs 49.28A to D: Note the angulation and method of applying a wood stick

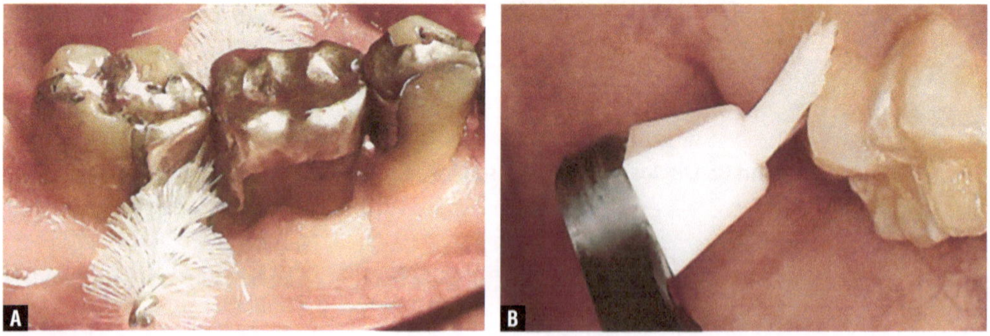

Figs 49.30A and B: (A) Bottlebrush type of interdental cleaner; (B) Unitufted brush for inaccessible areas

SECTION

1

Human Anatomy

SECTION OUTLINE

- Tissues in Human Body
- Oral Cavity
- Anatomy of Jaws
- Human Dentition: Primary and Permanent Teeth
- Periodontal Anatomy: Clinical and Histological Characteristics
- Blood and Nerve Supply of Teeth and Associated Structures
- Cranial Nerves: Trigeminal and Facial Nerve
- Muscles of Mastication
- Muscles of Facial Expressions
- Occlusion and Malocclusion
- Alveolar Process
- Temporomandibular Joint

Tissues in Human Body

CHAPTER 1

INTRODUCTION

Cells are the smallest units of life. Cell is defined as the structural and functional unit of the living body. Clusters of cells are formed according to the comparable structure and function, which in turn leads to the formation of tissues in complex organisms. These tissues act as a unit and aid in various functioning of the organs which are essential to maintain biological life.

The current chapter sheds light on histology, the study of various tissues found in the human body along with its composition and function.

The structure of the cell contains (Fig. 1.1):

- Cell membrane
- Nucleus
- Cytoplasm containing different organelles.

CLASSIFICATION OF TISSUES

The human body is made up of four basic types of tissues depending on their composition and function; namely epithelium, connective, muscular, and nervous tissues (Fig. 1.2).

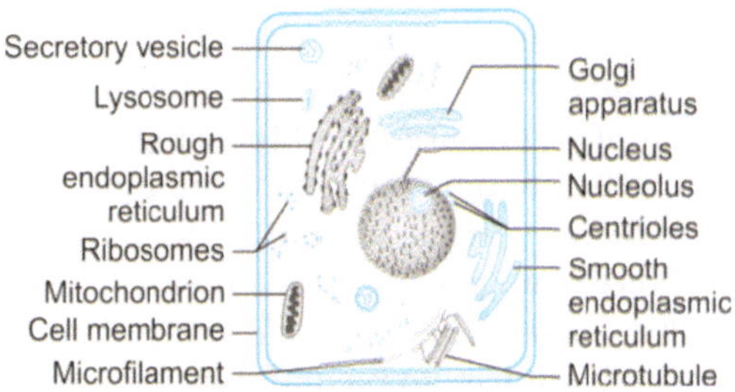

Fig. 1.1: Structure of the cell

The different function of each tissue is as follows:

- *Epithelium:* Lines and covers surfaces
- *Connective tissue:* Protects, supports, and binds together
- *Muscular tissue:* Produces movement
- *Nervous tissue:* Receive stimuli and conduct impulses.

EPITHELIUM

It forms the covering of surface of the body and aids in protection, adsorption, excretion, secretion, filtration, and sensory reception. However, it is important to consider the following points, which are as follows:

- Arrangement of epithelium is done to make one surface free and one surface attached, known as apical surface and basal surface, respectively
- Cells in epithelium are arranged either side by side or atop each other to form sheets of cells which in turn are held together by specialized junctions
- Basement membrane is formed by the attachment of epithelium to a layer of connective tissue at the basal surface. This adhesive layer is basically composed of secretions from the epithelial cells and the connective tissue cells
- Epithelium does not have its own blood supply

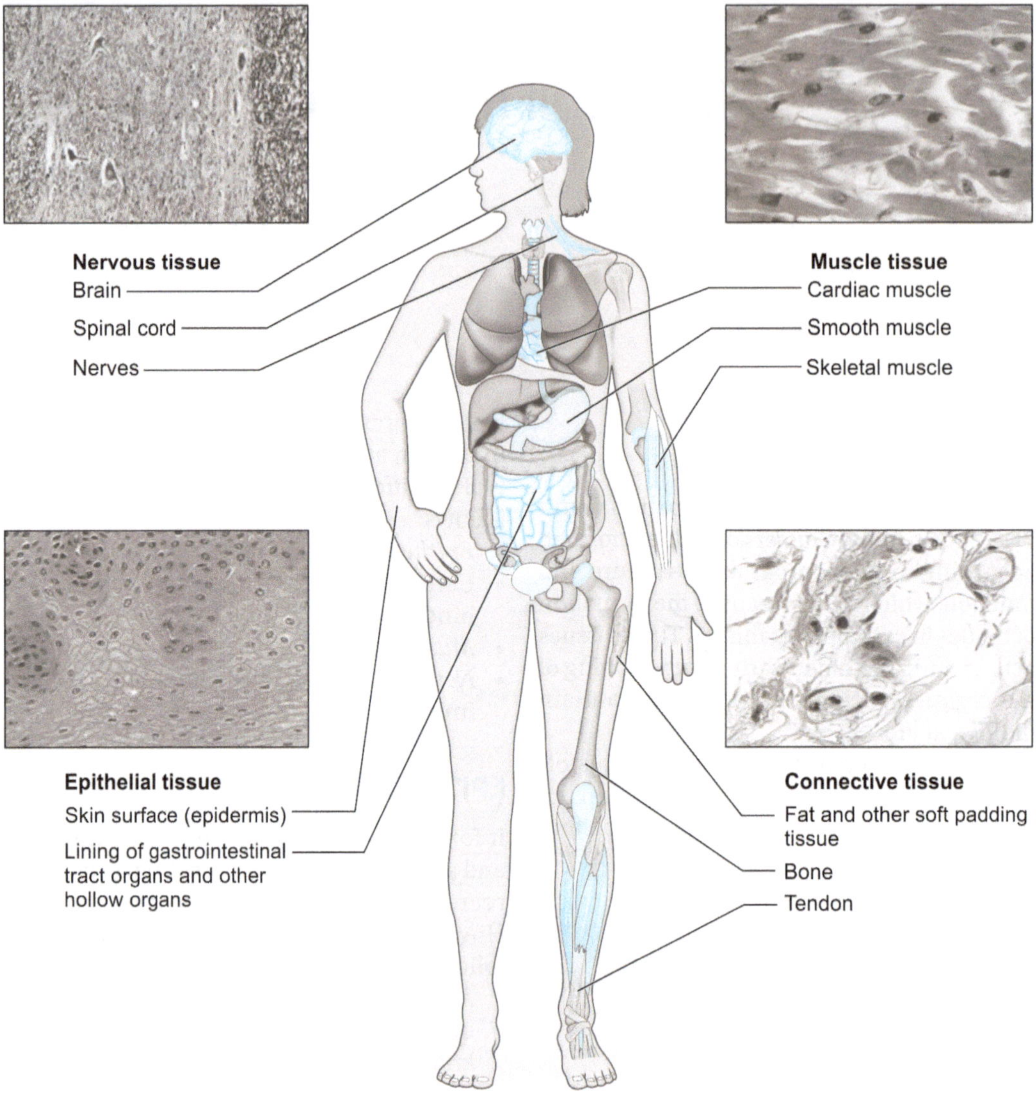

Fig. 1.2: Classification of four basic types of tissues *(For color version, see Plate 1)*

- However, cells of epithelium can be regenerated, if properly nourished.

Classification

Depending upon the basis of shape of the cells and the arrangement of the cells within the tissue, the epithelium is divided (Figs 1.3A and B). Generally, the arrangement of the cells is stated first, then the shape which is followed by epithelium to complete the naming, e.g. simple squamous epithelium.

According to the arrangement of the cells:

- *Simple:* Cells are found in a single layer attached to the basement membrane
- *Stratified:* Cells are found in two or more layers arranged atop each other
- *Pseudostratified:* A single layer of cells which appears to be multiple layers due

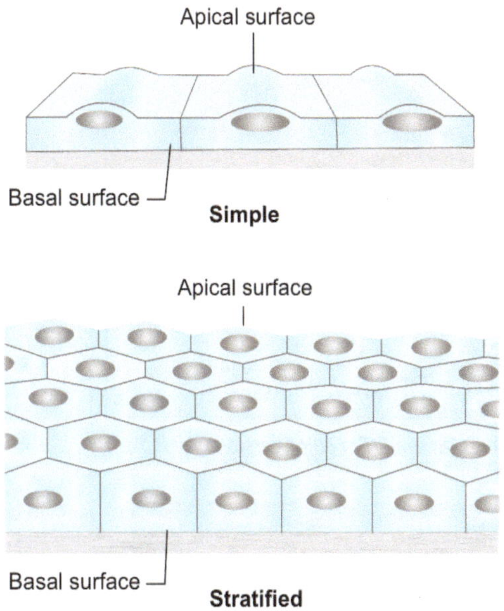

Fig. 1.3A: Classification of epithelium on the basis of arrangement of cells

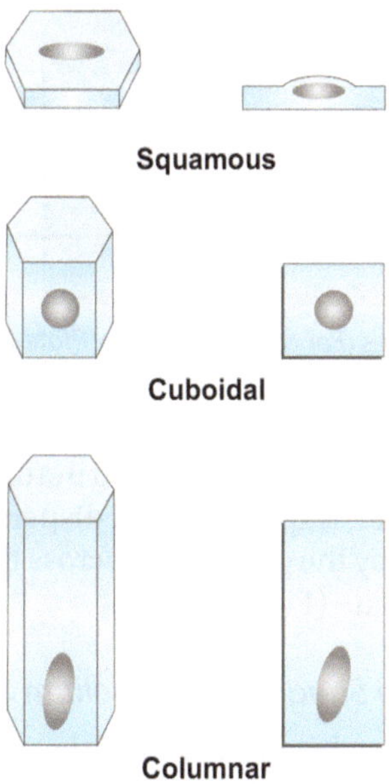

Fig. 1.3B: Classification of epithelium on the basis of shape of cells

to difference in height and location of the nuclei in the cells

- *Transitional:* Cells are round in shape and can slide across one another to allow stretching.

According to the shape:

- *Squamous:* Flat, thin, scale-like cells
- *Cuboidal:* Cells have a basic cube shape in which the cell's height and width are about equal
- *Columnar:* Tall, rectangular or column-shaped cells which are basically taller in comparison to their width.

Distinguished Features

- *Cilia (singular: cilium, Latin: eyelash):* These are hair-like appendages which attaches to the apical surface of cells to produce movement
- *Goblet cells*: Specialized cells secrete mucus for lubrication and protect the surface of an organ
- *Villi (singular: villus, Latin: shaggy hair):* Some organ exhibits finger-like projections that arise from the epithelial layer to increase the surface area for faster and more efficient adsorption
- *Microvilli:* Small projections that arise from the cell's surface also help in enhancing surface area for absorption. Based on their bushy appearance, they are sometimes called as brush border of an organ.

Simple Squamous Epithelium

Simple squamous epithelium, single layer of flattened cells lines small air sacs of lungs called alveoli (Fig. 1.4A). One surface of epithelium faces an open space to the inside of the air sac, known as lumen and the cell surface facing it is the apical surface.

Simple Cuboidal Epithelium

Simple cuboidal epithelium lines kidney tubules and appears as dispersed thick-walled circular structures, when seen in the histological cross section (Fig. 1.4B).

Simple Columnar Epithelium

Simple columnar epithelium covers the lining of the intestine. The lining extends

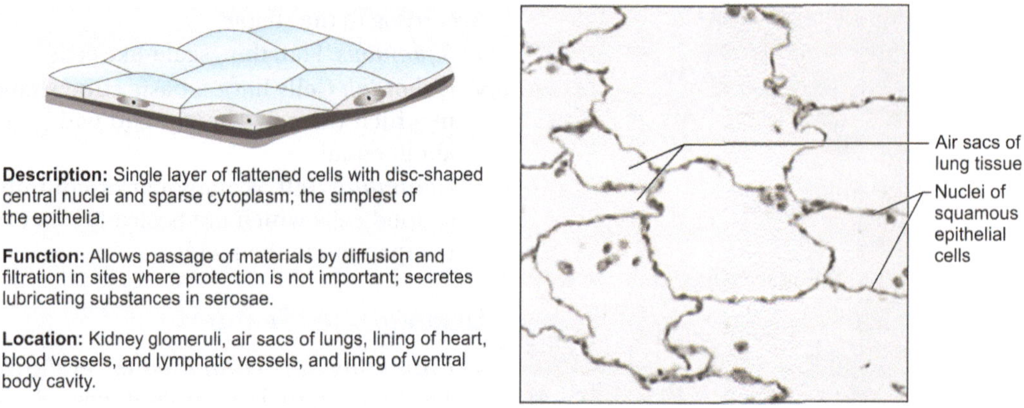

Fig. 1.4A: Simple squamous epithelium in alveolar wall *(For color version, see Plate 1)*

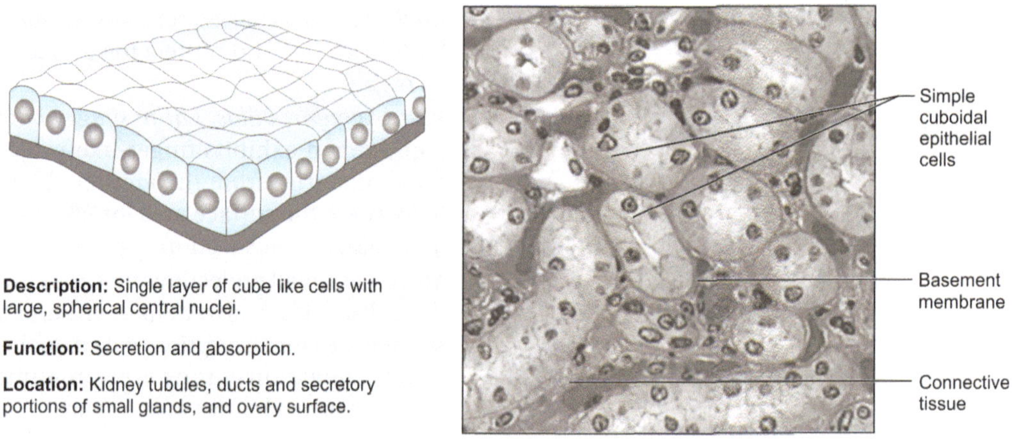

Fig. 1.4B: Simple cuboidal epithelium in kidney tubules *(For color version, see Plate 2)*

into the lumen and is usually seen as finger-like projections called villi. These villi aids in enhancing the absorption of the intestine by increasing the surface area. On cross section, along with large rectangular cells, clear-looking goblet cells are also found which secretes mucus for protection of the intestinal lining (Fig. 1.4C).

Pseudostratified Columnar Epithelium

This type of epithelium is typified by irregularly shaped cells which mark the lining of trachea. The nuclei of the cells are seen scattered in different spots within the cells, which provide the tissue its false-layered appearance. In addition, it is covered with numerous tiny hair-like structures called cilia, which trap debris and dispense mucus secreted by the goblet cells across the surface of the tissue (Fig. 1.4D).

Stratified Squamous Epithelium

Epidermis, the outer layer of skin constitutes multiple layers of flattened cells. However, these cells get flattened and subsequently die as the cells are pushed higher. The death of the cell is attributed to the depletion of nutrients from the sources present in the connective tissue. These, in turn, form the outer dead layers of the epidermis (Fig. 1.4E).

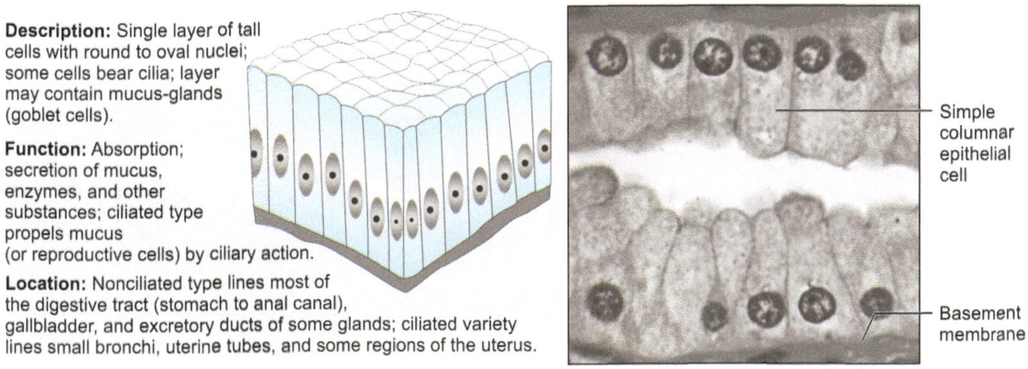

Fig. 1.4C: Simple columnar epithelium in stomach mucosa *(For color version, see Plate 2)*

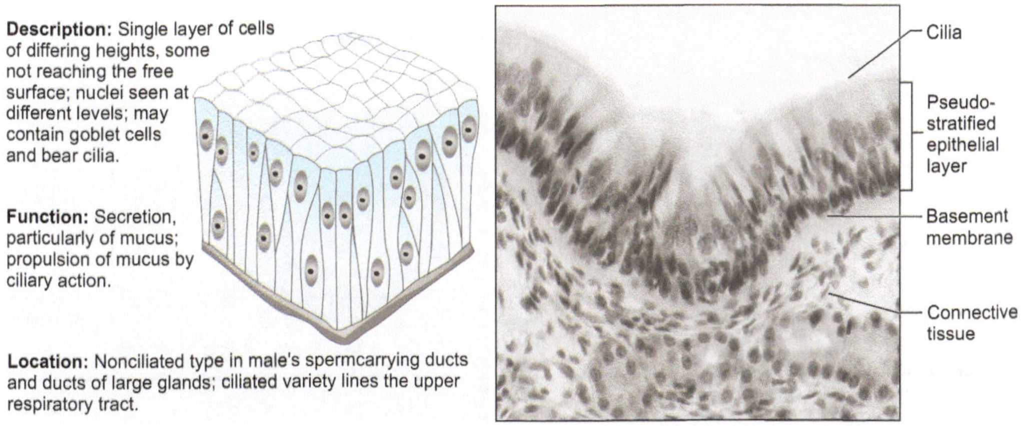

Fig. 1.4D: Pseudostratified columnar epithelium in human trachea *(For color version, see Plate 2)*

Transitional Epithelium

This type of epithelium resembles a combination of cuboidal and columnar shaped cells. This is seen in the inner lining of the bladder in which tissue can stretch and distend without causing perforations in the wall lining (Fig. 1.4F).

CONNECTIVE TISSUE

It is the most extensively scattered tissue type present in the human body. It helps in protecting, supporting and binding together parts of the body.

The following section throws some light on the chief characteristics of connective tissue:

- Though connective tissue is extremely vascularized, some tissues such as tendons, ligaments, and cartilages are less vascular in nature
- It is composed of various types of specialized cells
- It encompasses a huge amount of non-living material known as the matrix in the form of ground substance and fibers, which in turn are formed and secreted by the cells of the specific connective tissues.

Description: Thick membrane composed of several cell layers; basal cells are cuboidal or columnar and metabolically active; surface cells are flattened (squamous); in the keratinized type, the surface cells are full of keratin and dead; basal cells are active in mitosis and produce the cells of the more superficial layers.

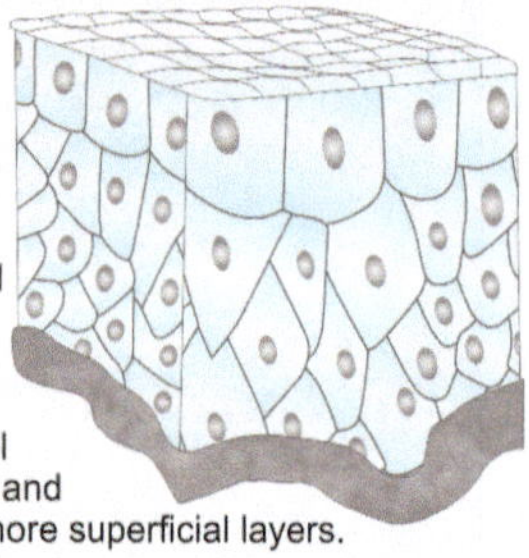

Function: Protects underlying tissues in areas subjected to abrasion.

Location: Nonkeratinized type forms the moist linings of the esophagus,mouth, and vagina; keratinized variety forms the epidermis of the skin, a dry membrane.

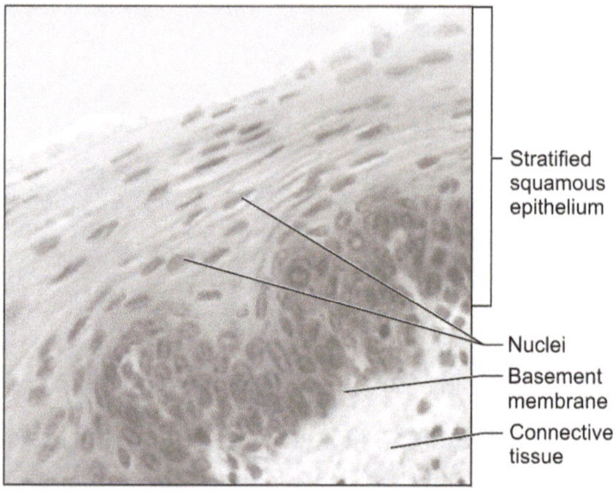

Fig. 1.4E: Stratified squamous epithelium in esophagus *(For color version, see Plate 3)*

Description: Resembles both stratified squamous and stratified cuboidal; basal cells cuboidal or columnar; surface cells dome-shaped or squamous-like, depending on degree of organ stretch.

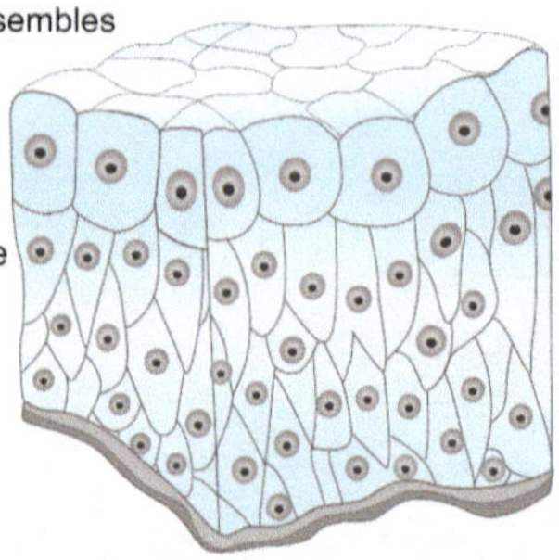

Function: Stretches readily and permits distension of urinary organ by contained urine.

Location: Lines the ureters, bladder, and part of the urethra.

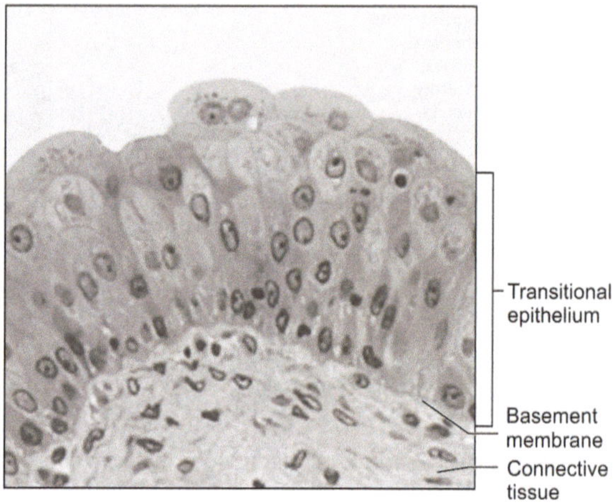

Fig. 1.4F: Transitional epithelium in bladder *(For color version, see Plate 3)*

Classification

There are four types of connective tissues found in the human body (Fig. 1.5A):

- Connective tissue proper
  - Loose connective tissue
    - ◊ Areolar
    - ◊ Adipose
    - ◊ Reticular.
  - Dense connective tissue
    - ◊ Dense regular
    - ◊ Dense irregular.
- Supporting connective tissue
  - Cartilage
    - ◊ Elastic
    - ◊ Hyaline
    - ◊ Fibrocartilage.
  - Bone
- Fluid connective tissue
  - Blood
  - Lymph.

Areolar Tissue

It is a loose type of connective tissue which constitutes intermixing of fibers and cells. It shows a very diffuse arrangement (Fig. 1.5B). The cells appearing as dark spots within the tissue are known as fibroblasts (fibro: fiber, blast: to create). The prime function of these

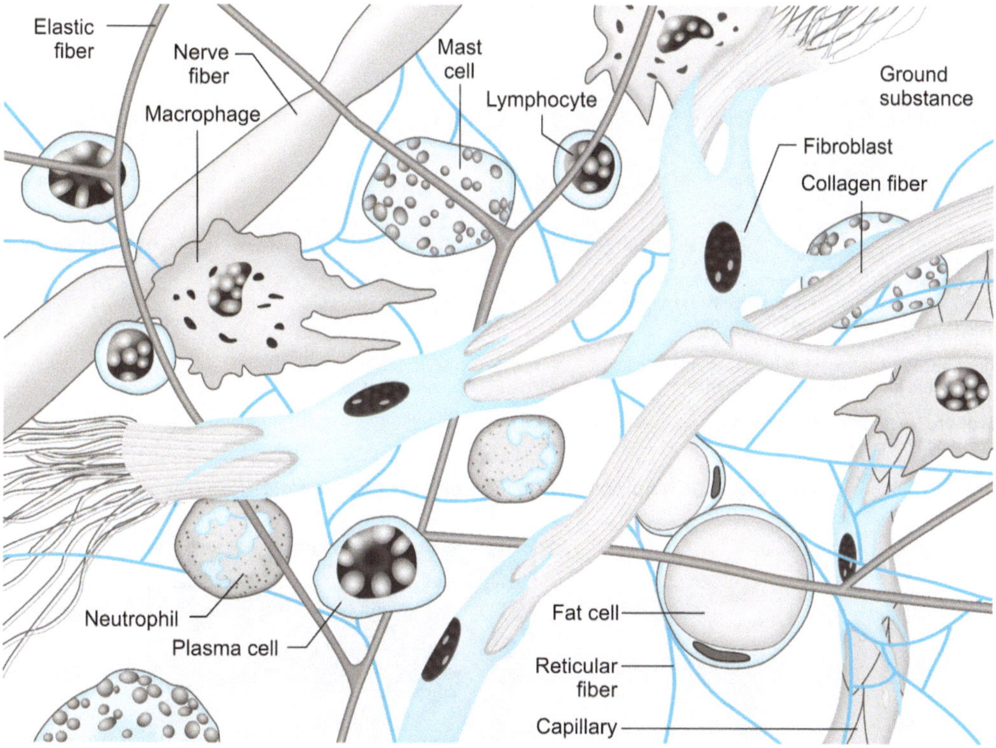

Fig. 1.5A: Network of connective tissues

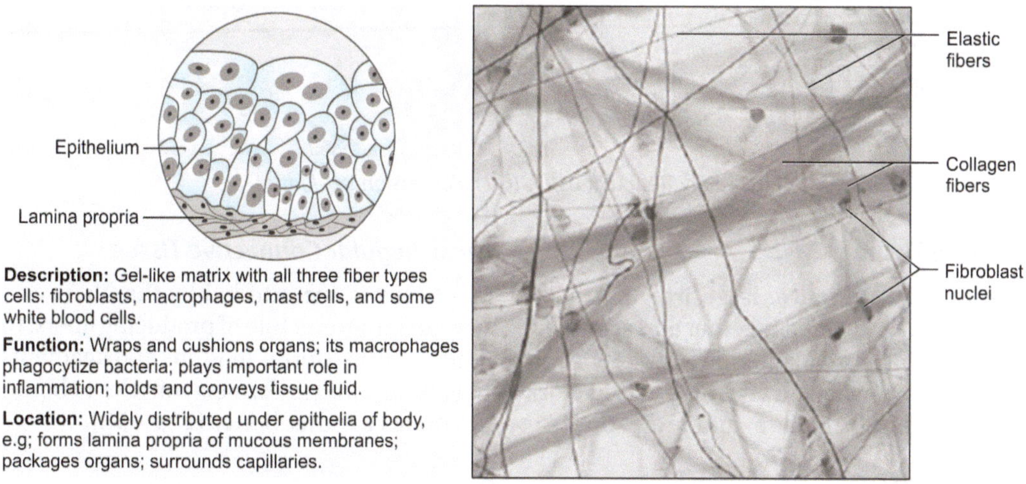

Description: Gel-like matrix with all three fiber types cells: fibroblasts, macrophages, mast cells, and some white blood cells.

Function: Wraps and cushions organs; its macrophages phagocytize bacteria; plays important role in inflammation; holds and conveys tissue fluid.

Location: Widely distributed under epithelia of body, e.g; forms lamina propria of mucous membranes; packages organs; surrounds capillaries.

Fig. 1.5B: Areolar tissue *(For color version, see Plate 3)*

cells is to secrete the fibers. The larger fibers which appear pink in color and small black fibers are called collagen fibers and elastic fibers, respectively. Both these fibers and the rest of the substance collectively surround the cells, known as matrix.

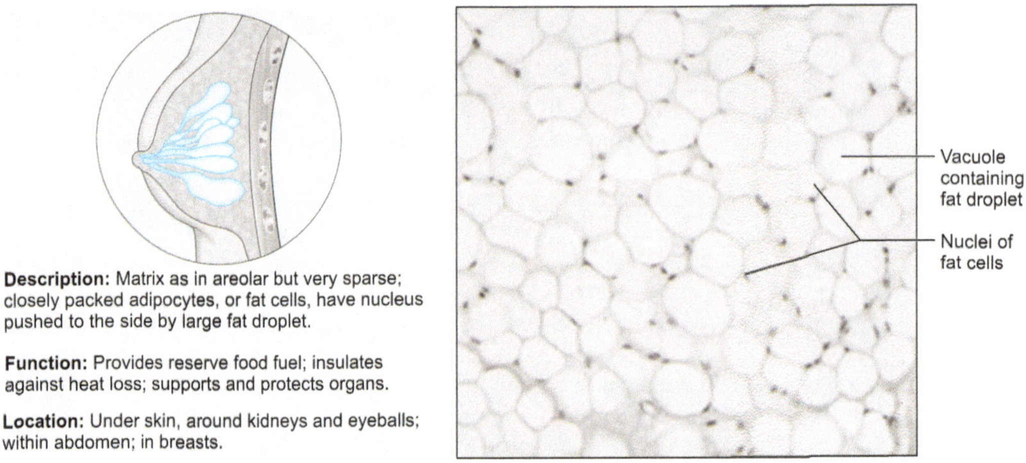

Fig. 1.5C: Adipose tissue *(For color version, see Plate 4)*

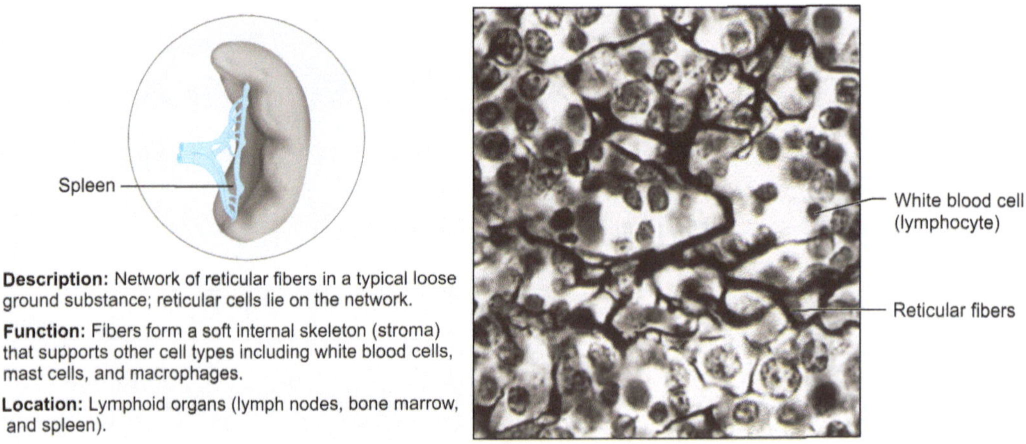

Fig. 1.5D: Reticular tissue *(For color version, see Plate 4)*

Adipose Tissue

These tissues present as large, irregular, bubble-like cells clustered together and scattered in a matrix alike areolar tissue (Fig. 1.5C). The cells are occupied with fat which acts as storage of energy, insulation, and protection.

Reticular Tissue

These fibers aid in supporting the cells of a soft internal skeleton like spleen, lymph nodes, and bone marrow (Fig. 1.5D).

Dense Regular Connective Tissue

This tissue is surrounded by the fibers and plays an important role of producing fibers. In addition, it also forms tendons and ligaments that are required to connect muscles to bones and bones to other bones (Fig. 1.5E).

Dense Irregular Connective Tissue

Dermis, the middle layer of the skin constitutes this type of tissue. Though composition is homogenous as of dense regular tissue, its

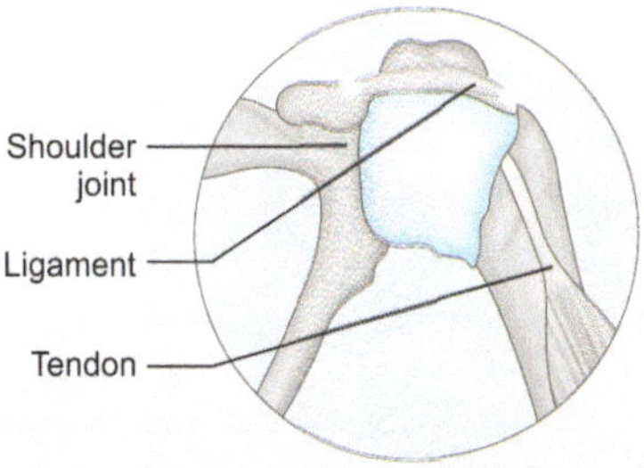

Description: Primarily parallel collagen fibers; a few elastin fibers; major cell type is the fibroblast.

Function: Attaches muscles to bones or to muscles, attaches bones to bones; withstands great tensile stress when pulling force is applied in one direction.

Location: Tendons, most ligaments, aponeuroses.

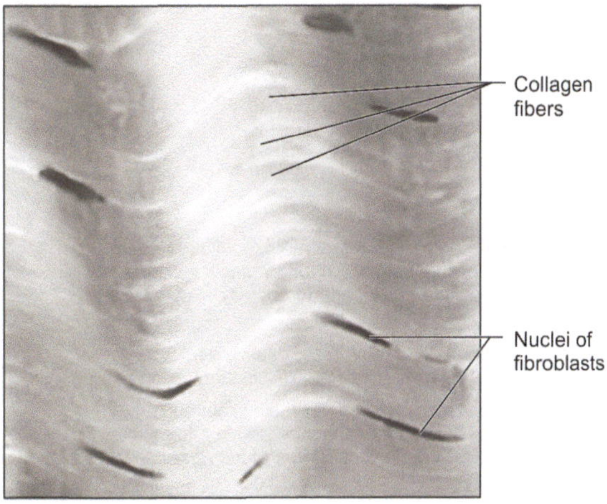

Fig. 1.5E: Dense regular connective tissue *(For color version, see Plate 4)*

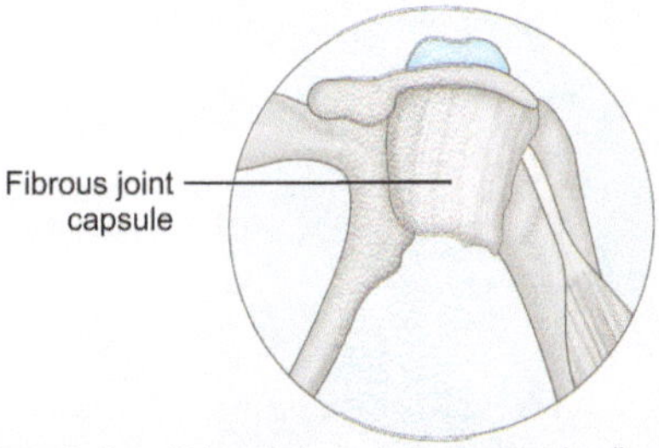

Description: Primarily irregularly arranged collagen fibers; some elastic fibers; major cell type is the fibroblast.

Function: Able to withstand tension exerted in many directions; provides structural strength.

Location: Dermis of the skin; submucosa of digestive tract; fibrous capsules of organs and of joints.

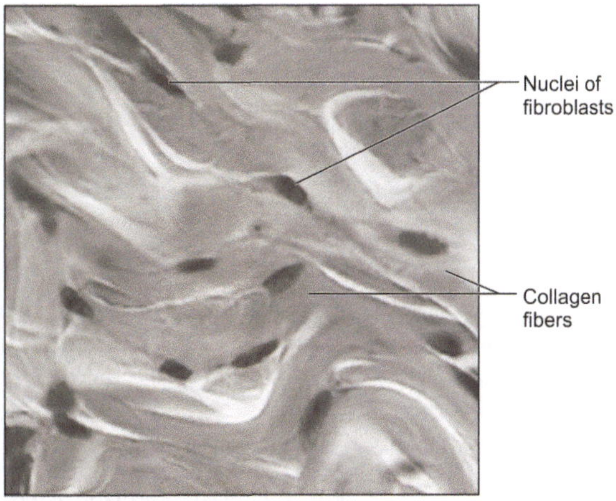

Fig. 1.5F: Dense irregular connective tissue *(For color version, see Plate 5)*

constituents are not arranged appropriately as compared to dense regular tissue (Fig. 1.5F).

Hyaline Cartilage

The lining below trachea is composed of rings of hyaline cartilage which are immersed in the organ in order to offer structure and support. The cartilage on cross section shows smooth, amorphous matrix containing collagen fibers with cells embedded within it. This matrix is produced by the cells known as chondrocytes which are contained within tiny chambers called lacunae or little lakes (Fig. 1.6).

Elastic Cartilage

The tissue that needs more stretching and maintenance of shape contains elastic fibers within the matrix of the tissue (Fig. 1.7). This type of tissue is present majorly in the structure of the external ear.

Fibrocartilage

Its arrangement is comparable to hyaline cartilage and forms the intervertebral discs in the spinal column, the pubic symphysis, and in the discs of the knee. It differs from hyaline cartilage in its rigidity, as it is less firm

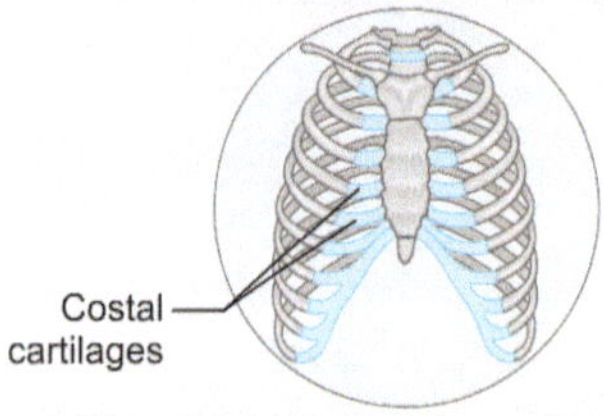

Description: Amorphous but firm matrix; collagen fibers form an imperceptible network; chondroblasts produce the matrix and when mature (chondrocytes) lie in lacunae.

Function: Supports and reinforces; has resilient cushioning properties; resists compressive stress.

Location: Forms most of the embryonic skeleton; covers the ends of long bones in joint cavities; forms costal cartilages of the ribs; cartilages of the nose, trachea, and larynx.

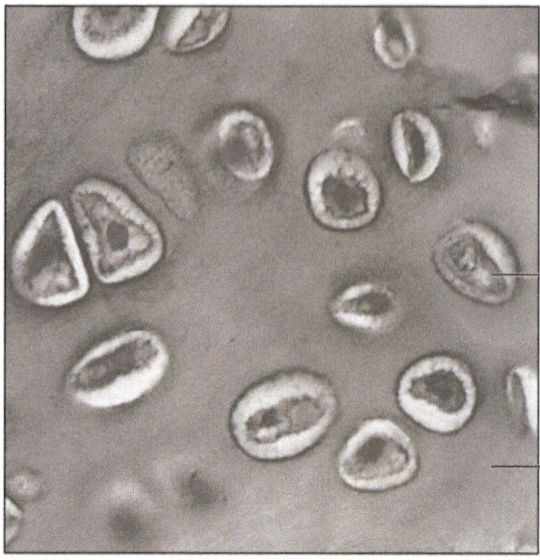

Fig. 1.6: Hyaline cartilage *(For color version, see Plate 5)*

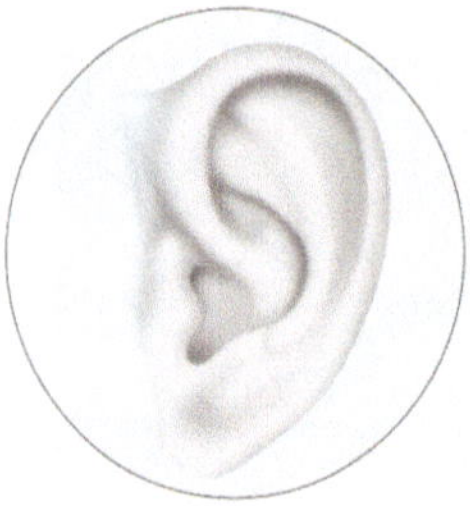

Description: Similar to hyaline cartilage, but more elastic fibers in matrix.

Function: Maintains the shape of a structure while allowing great flexibility.

Location: Supports the external ear (pinna); epiglottis.

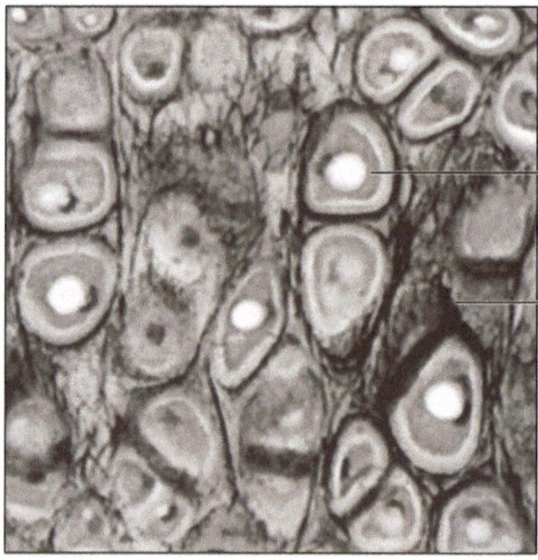

Fig. 1.7: Elastic cartilage *(For color version, see Plate 5)*

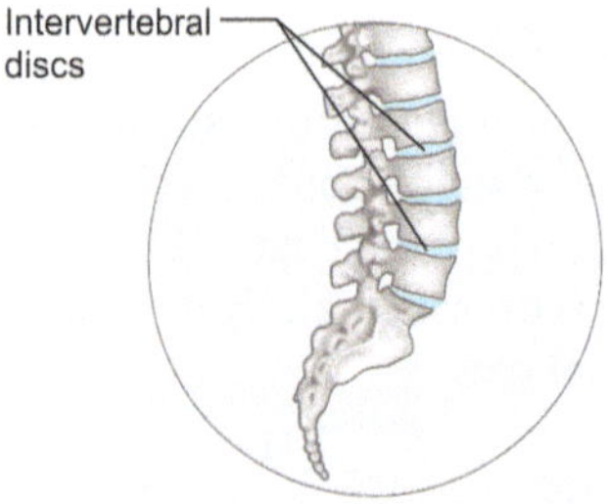

Description: Matrix similar to but less firm than that in hyaline cartilage; thick collagen fibers predominate.

Function: Tensile strength with the ability to absorb compressive shock.

Location: Intervertebral discs; pubic symphysis; discs of knee joint.

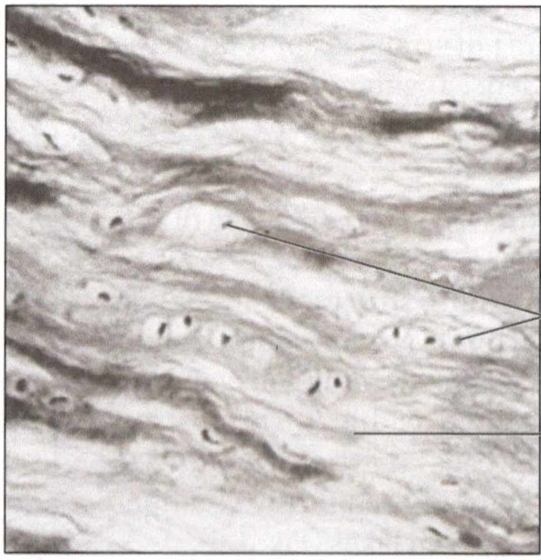

Fig. 1.8: Fibrocartilage *(For color version, see Plate 6)*

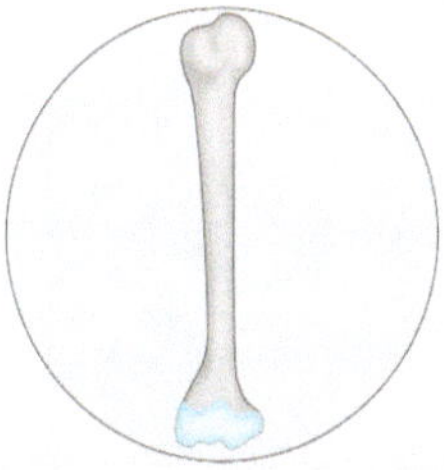

Description: Hard, calcified matrix containing many collagen fibers; osteocytes lie in lacunae, very well-vascularized.

Function: Bone supports and protects (by enclosing); provides levers for the muscles to act on; stores calcium and other minerals and fat; marrow inside bones is the site for blood cell formation (hematopoiesis).

Location: Bone

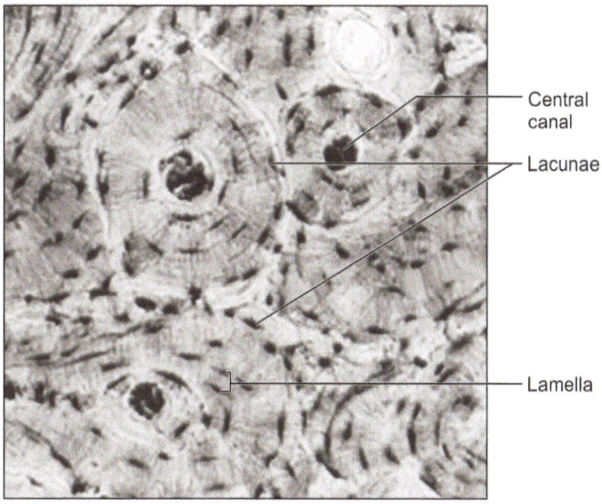

Fig. 1.9: Bone or osseous tissue *(For color version, see Plate 6)*

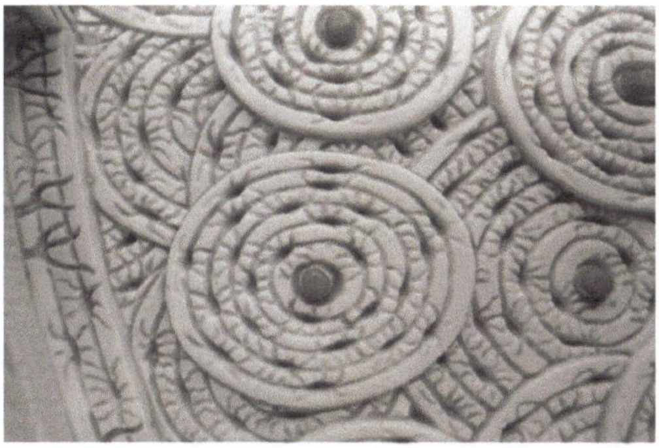

Fig. 1.10: Lacunae in bone tissue

and exhibits more number of collagen fibers (Fig. 1.8). The cells found are also known as chondrocytes which are found in the lacunae.

Bone (Osseous) Tissue

Bone tissue is organized in concentric ring structures called osteons in center of which lies a Haversian canal (Fig. 1.9A). This canal contains blood vessels and provides nutrition to the cells within the tissue.

Moreover, this canal is surrounded by rings of bone tissue called lamellae which contain chambers as lacunae (Fig. 1.10). These lacunae in turn possess tiny channels called as canaliculi which permit the interaction of the cells with the blood supply. The cells embedded in the tissue are known as osteocytes (osteo: bone, cyte: cell).

Blood

Blood is wrongly not considered as a tissue due to its liquid state, yet it fulfills all the requirements of being a connective tissue. It contains chiefly two types of cells; red blood cells (erythrocytes) and white blood cells (leukocytes).

In addition, tiny fragments of cells called platelets are also seen in this tissue (Fig. 1.11). Along with these cells, matrix also known as plasma is present which is made up of water, salts, gases, and proteins (nonliving materials).

Lymph

It is a thin opalescent fluid originating in organs and tissues of the body that circulates through the lymphatic vessels and is filtered by the lymph nodes. It fight infection, and in which are formed blood cells that is lymphocytes, monocytes, and plasma cells (Figs 1.12A and B).

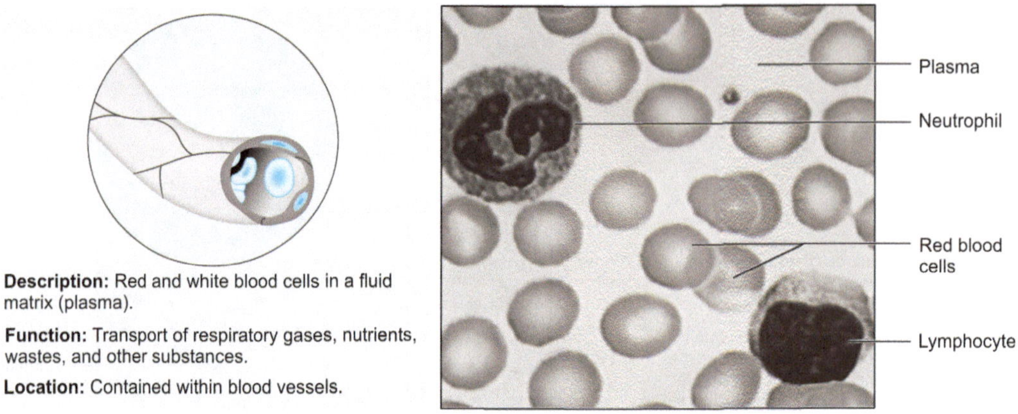

Fig. 1.11: Blood smear showing various types of blood cells *(For color version, see Plate 6)*

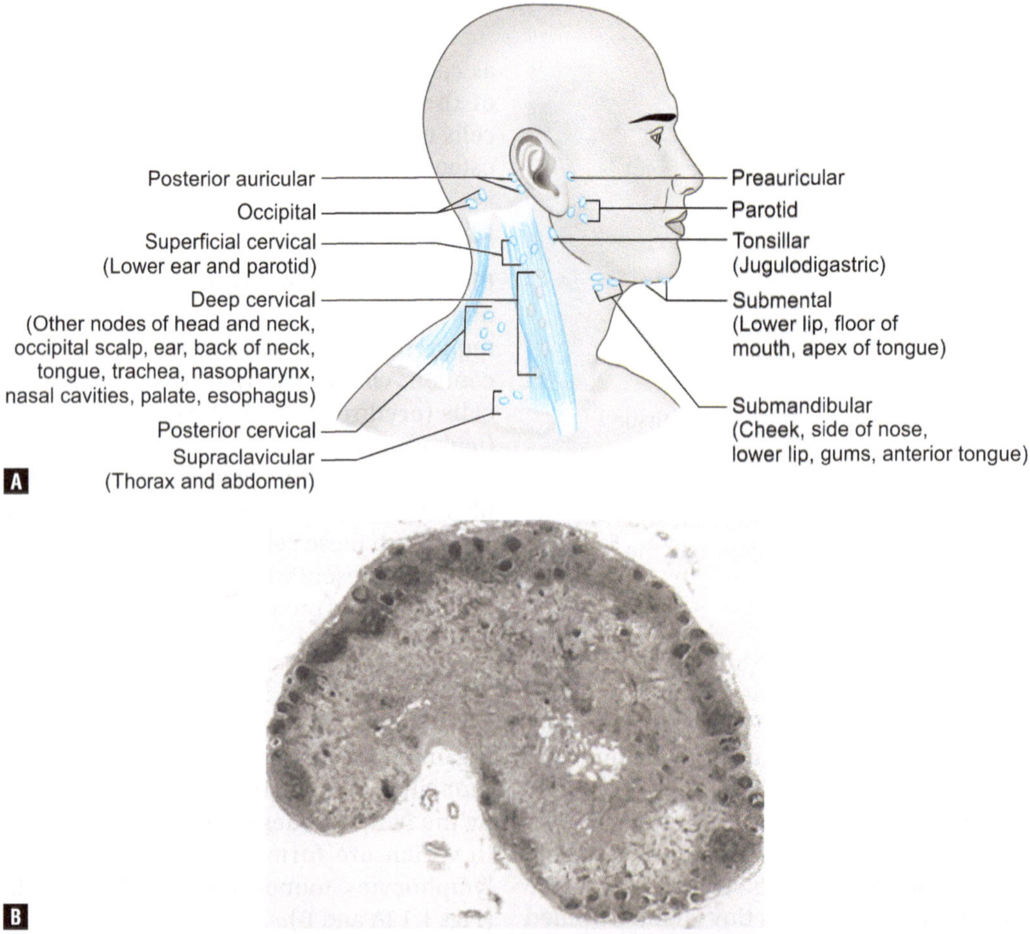

Figs 1.12A and B: Lymph nodes of head and neck (A) Anatomical locations; (B) Histology

Lymphatic system is a vast, complex network of capillaries, thin vessels, ducts, nodes and organs that help to protect and maintain the internal fluid environment of the entire body.

THE INTEGUMENT

The skin or integument is the main organ which protects the body externally. Besides protection, it plays a vital role in providing insulation, temperature regulation and tactility (sense of touch). It also aids in the formation of vitamin D, essential for proper functioning of the body.

Composition

The skin is composed of three distinctive layers namely; epidermis, dermis and hypodermis.

Epidermis

It is the outer layer which is formed of keratinized stratified squamous epithelium, which is arranged into five layers called strata (singular: stratum), which are shown in Figs 1.13A and B)

- Stratum corneum, which is the outermost layer of flattened, dead cells
- Stratum lucidum, thin translucent layer present only in thick areas of the skin
- Stratum granulosum is named because of its richness of granules. The cells begin to die in the upper boundary of this layer
- Stratum spinosum is one of the thicker layers of dermis with potential of fast division of cells
- Stratum basale is the lowest layer of the skin which is attached to the dermis to form basement membrane. In this layer, cells continuously divide to create new cells.

Dermis

It is the middle layer and is formed from dense irregular connective tissue.

Dermal papillae, projections or ridges arise from the dermis and offer attachment points for the epidermis.

Hypodermis

It is the innermost or subcutaneous layer which is composed of adipose tissue.

Various Structures and Functions

The distinctive structures and functions of skin are as follows:

- Gland structures
  - *Eccrine gland:* It secretes sweat which is the combination of water, salts, and urea and helps in cooling down the temperature of the body
  - *Sebaceous gland:* It secretes sebum or oil which aids in keeping the skin soft and pliable.
- Nervous structures
  - *Free nerve endings:* These are positioned near dermal papillae and are related with pain sensation
  - *Meissner's corpuscle:* These touch receptors are positioned near dermal papillae and are associated with tactility
  - *Pacinian corpuscle:* These pressure receptors are situated deep within dermis at the boundary of the dermis and hypodermis.
- Muscle structures
  - *Arrector pili:* These are the muscle that pulls up hair follicle causing goose flesh or goose bumps.
- Appendages
  - Hair shaft
  - Hair follicle.

NERVOUS TISSUE

Neurons are the smallest functional units of the nervous system. Each neuron is composed of a cell body and two types of processes: axon and dendrites (Fig. 1.14). The function of the neurons is reflected in the number and types of processes arising from the cell body.

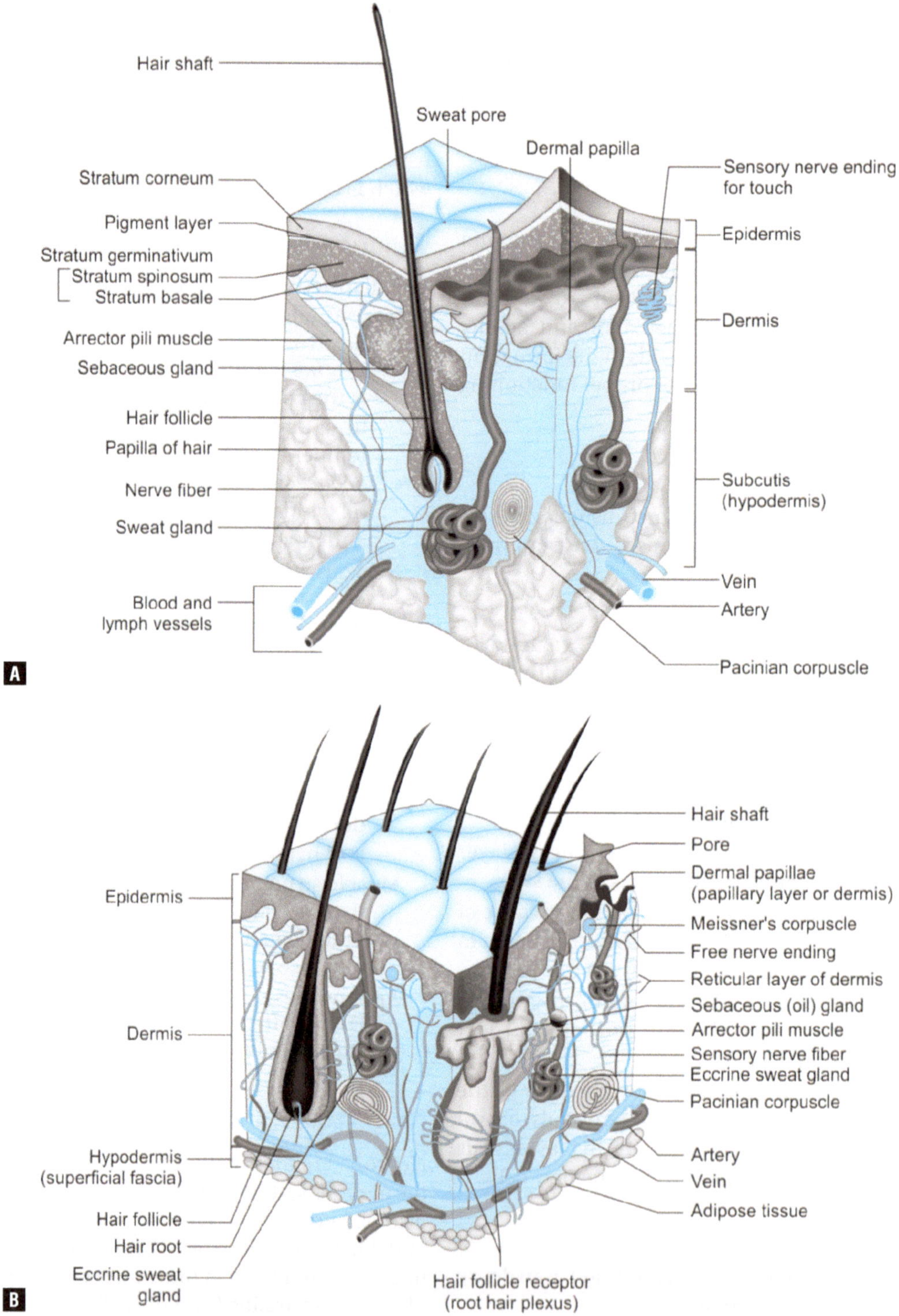

Figs 1.13A and B: Structure of skin *(For color version, see Plate 7)*

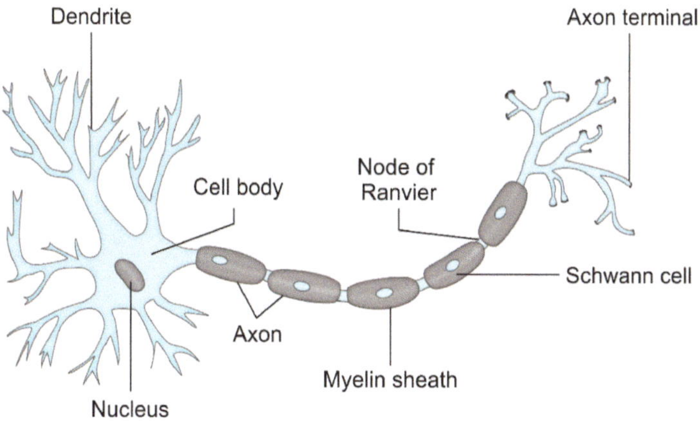

Fig. 1.14: Structure of a typical neuron

Axon

It conducts impulses to other neurons or cells. Neurons have only one axon. The cell membranes of myelin cell predominantly contain fat which gives brain's white matter its fatty appearance.

Dendrite

It conducts impulses from synapse to the cell body. Depending on its function, a neuron may have multiple dendrites. Dendrites may undergo complex arborization to increase their surface area.

CHAPTER 2

Oral Cavity

INTRODUCTION

The entrance of the digestive system is mouth or oral cavity (Figs 2.1A and B). It is divided into two parts:

1. The vestibule is the area between the teeth, lips and cheeks. The oral vestibule is bounded externally by the lips, cheeks and mucosa, and internally by the alveolar processes and the teeth and gums.
2. The oral cavity proper, which is the inner larger part.

ORAL CAVITY PROPER

The temperature of the oral cavity is about 37°C or 98.6°F. Its lining is composed of stratified squamous epithelium and its oral smears are used for chromosomal studies. The oral cavity comprises of two parts, namely the vestibule and the oral cavity proper. Both these parts interact only through a gap between the last molars and the ramus of the mandible, when the teeth are in contact.

The vestibule is the cleft between the lips and cheeks, externally, and the gums and teeth internally. On the contrary, oral cavity proper is surrounded by alveolar arches, teeth and gums, and palate and tongue. Posteriorly, it connects to oropharynx by an opening known as the faucial isthmus, between the palatoglossal arches. Besides, a median fold of mucous membrane termed as frenulum attaches the inferior surface of the tongue to the floor of the mouth.

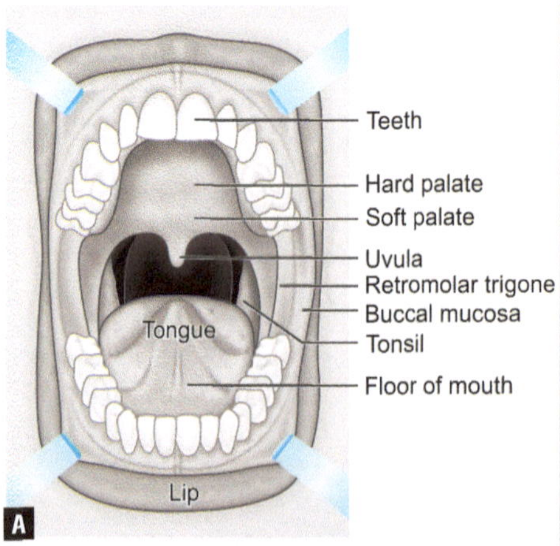

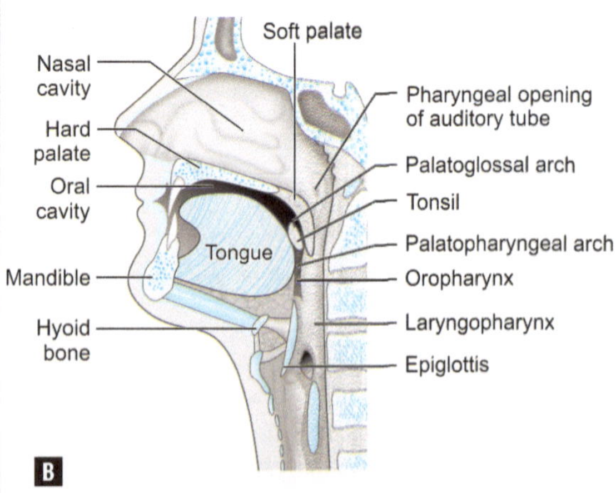

Figs 2.1A and B: (A) Oral cavity proper; (B) Sagittal section of oral cavity

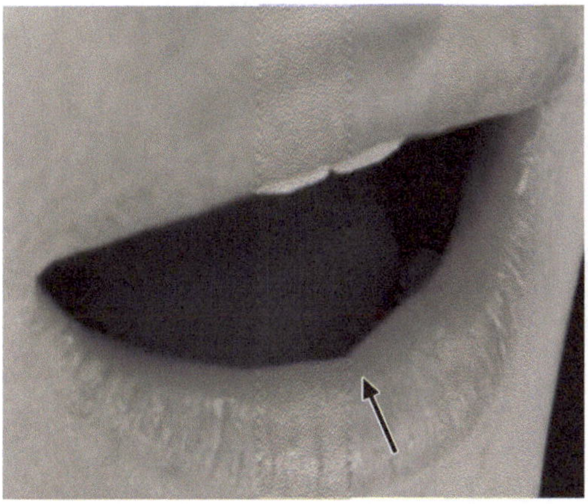

Fig. 2.2: Lips. Arrow indicates red line, which separates dry vermilion from wet vermilion

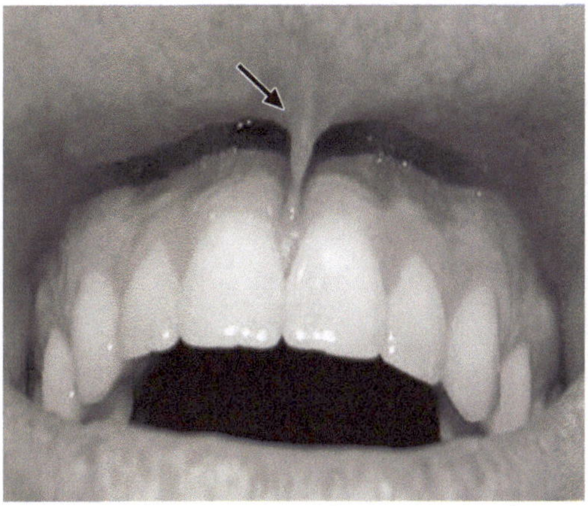

Fig. 2.3: Upper vestibule (upper lip everted). Arrow indicates upper labial frenulum

The parotid gland opens opposite to the maxillary second molar whereas the submandibular duct opens on an elevation on the sides of the frenulum known as sublingual papilla. Laterally, the sublingual gland opens as sublingual ducts in the sublingual fold.

Lips

Labial commissures at the corners of the mouth join longer upper lip and shorter lower lip. Moreover, nasolabial fold separates the lips from the cheeks. Lips have two vermilion borders, one is interior (pale and wet) and another is outer border (darker and dry). These two are separated from each other by the red line. In addition, a white line on outside is also present which is cutaneous part of the lip (Fig. 2.2).

Cheeks (Mucosa)

Cheek is considered as a musculomembranous structure. It is surrounded superiorly and inferiorly by the upper and lower vestibules, anteriorly by the labial commissure, and posteriorly by the retromolar trigone and the intermaxillary commissure. The inner surface of each lip is connected in the middle line to the corresponding gum by a fold of mucous membrane, the labial frenulum.

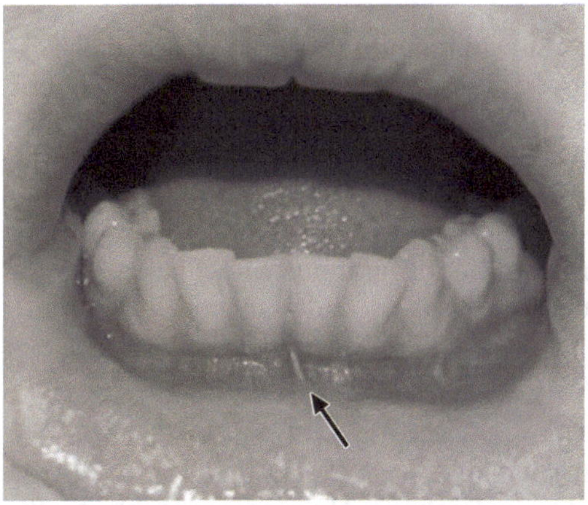

Fig. 2.4: Lower vestibule (lower lip everted). Arrow indicates lower labial frenulum

A fold of mucous membrane called as labial frenulum joins the inner surface of each lip in the middle line to the corresponding gum. Moreover, the upper labial frenulum (Fig. 2.3) is larger than the lower labial frenulum (Fig. 2.4).

The retrocommissural region is situated between the labial commissure and the opening of Stensen's duct (Fig. 2.5). Stensen's duct, the drainage duct of the parotid gland runs through the buccinator muscle. This region gets transversed by a horizontal, marginally elevated streak called the linea alba or occlusal line (Fig. 2.6).

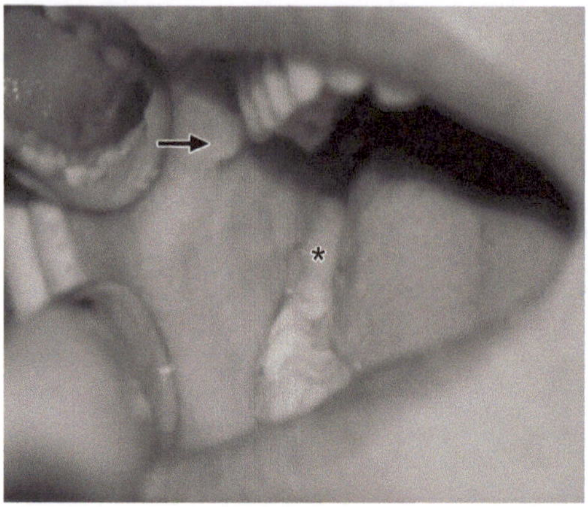

Fig. 2.5: Opening of Stensen's duct opposite second upper molar (arrow). Asterisk indicates retromolar trigone *(For color version, see Plate 8)*

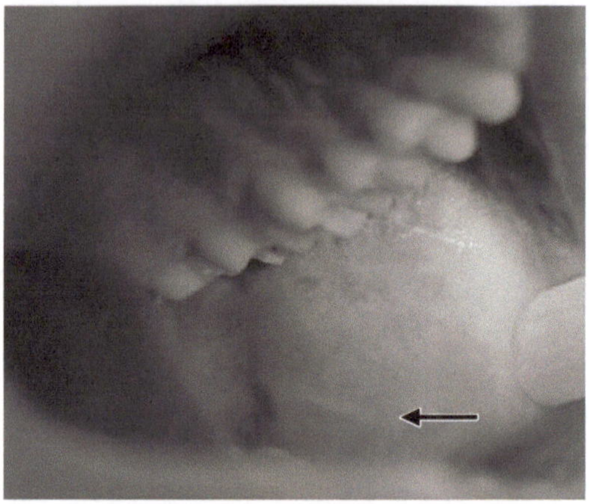

Fig. 2.6: Linea alba (arrow)

Buccinator muscle, the muscle of facial expression forms the framework of the cheek and is covered by the masseter muscle. Cheek is covered by buccal fat pad which forms the cheek contour by filling in the depression. Besides, other muscles which play an important role in the formation of the cheek are zygomaticus, risorius, and platysma.

Gums and Alveolar Process

The gingiva or gum, a fibroepithelial mucosal tissue envelops the teeth and surrounds the alveolar jaw bone. Alveolar process, the tooth-bearing area of the jaws, is made up of a dense outer cortex termed as the cortical plate and looser inner trabecular or medullary bone. The area of cortical bone lining the dental socket or alveolus is known as lamina dura.

Retromolar Trigone

Retromolar trigone is the portion of mucosa which is positioned behind the third molar and overlaps the anterior ramus of the mandible (Fig. 2.5). It is a small triangular-shaped subsite of the mouth, whose base is posterior to the last mandibular molar. The apex of the triangle is in continuation with the tuberosity of the maxilla behind the last maxillary molar. Laterally, it is confined by the gingival buccal sulcus and medially by the anterior tonsillar pillar.

Teeth

Teeth, the calcified structures play a pivotal role in mastication. Tooth is composed of two parts. One is crown, the exposed portion above the gumline, and another is root, which is surrounded within the alveolar bone.

Deciduous teeth, also known as primary or temporary teeth, are the first to erupt in the mouth which is gradually replaced by the permanent or adult dentition.

There are 20 deciduous teeth consisting of 8 molars, 4 canines or cuspids, and 8 incisors. The permanent dentition is comprised of 32 teeth in which 12 are molars including 4 wisdom teeth or third molar, 8 premolars or bicuspids, 4 canines, and 8 incisors.

Incisors have a thin occlusal edge with flat crown and a single root with cutting food as its prime function. Canines have a pointed shape and single long roots and they aid in piercing and tearing food.

The occlusal or masticatory surface of molars and premolars is typified by pointed structures referred as cusps. Premolars usually have 1 or 2 cusps and 1 or 2 roots. Molars usually have 4–5 cusps and 2–3 roots with variations in shape. The main role of molars and premolars is to grind and crush food.

Hard Palate

The palate, horseshoe-shaped, domed roof of the oral cavity is divided into two parts, namely hard and soft palate. The hard palate is concave in shape and it separates the oral cavity from the nasal cavities. The soft palate belongs to the oropharynx and separates it from the nasopharynx. The concavity of the palate is filled by tongue at its rest position. The hard palate is further classified into primary and secondary palates. A small depression called as incisive fossa with opening of incisive foramen behind the central incisors separates the primary palate from secondary palate (Fig. 2.7).

Soft Palate

Soft palate, the mobile posterior third of the palate marks the opening of the oropharynx resulting in the formation of an incomplete septum between the mouth and the pharynx. It is presented as median raphe and is in continuation with the roof of the mouth and the mucous membrane of the nasal floor (Fig. 2.7).

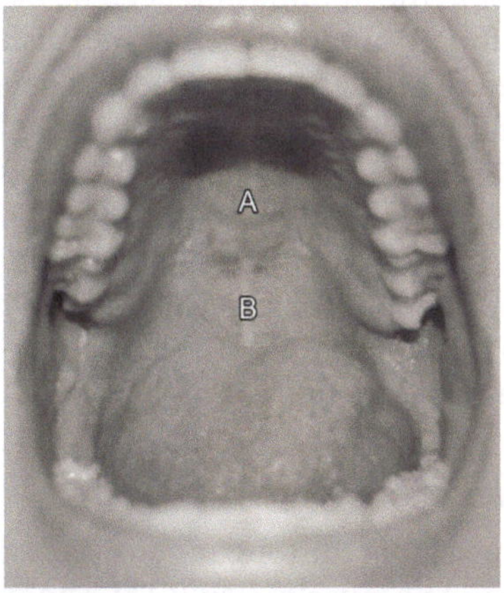

Fig. 2.7: Hard and soft palate. Point A indicates median raphe of hard palate; Point B indicates median raphe of soft palate

At relax position, the anterior surface and posterior surface of soft palate is concave and convex, respectively. The anterior aponeurotic portion is attached to the posterior border of the hard palate. The posterior muscular portion that suspends between the mouth and pharynx is known as the palatine velum or velopharynx.

The velum is extended by a median free process known as uvula and two bilateral processes referred as the palatoglossal and palatopharyngeal arches or pillars. The palatoglossal arch joins the soft palate to the tongue while palatopharyngeal arch joins the soft palate to the pharynx. Palatoglossal and palatopharyngeal arches, along with tongue also, marks the boundary of palatine tonsils which are situated in the tonsillar sinuses or fossae of the oropharynx. The space between the cavity of the mouth and the oropharynx is presented as fauces. Superiorly, these fauces are bounded by the soft palate, inferiorly by the root of the tongue, and laterally by the pillars of the fauces.

Cavity Proper of the Mouth

The mouth proper is surrounded in front and at the sides by the gums and teeth. It communicates with pharynx posteriorly through isthmus of the fauces.

The floor of the oral cavity is formed by tongue, mucous membrane and mylohyoid muscle. The floor joins the tongue with the inner surface of the mandible. However, the roof is vault shaped and is formed by both hard and soft palate. Moreover, mouth proper is also the site of the openings of ducts of submandibular and sublingual glands.

Floor of Mouth

Floor of the mouth appears like a quadrangular pyramid with a posterior base. Base of the oral cavity is formed from the floor of the mouth. It is separated superficially into three zones namely, the anterior floor of the mouth located anterior to the lingual frenulum and the two

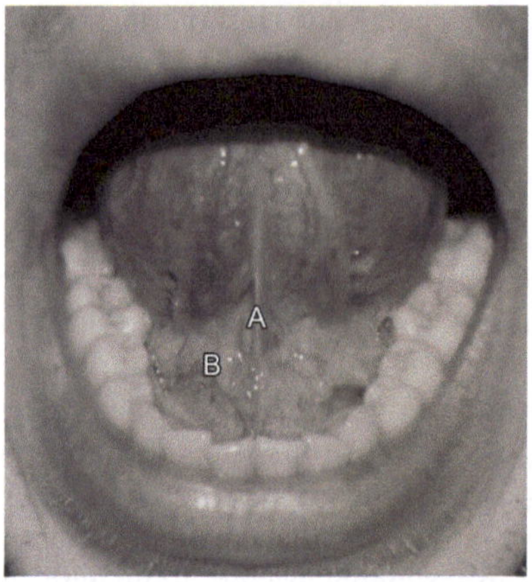

Fig. 2.8: Floor of mouth. Point A indicates lingual frenulum; Point B indicates sublingual papillae

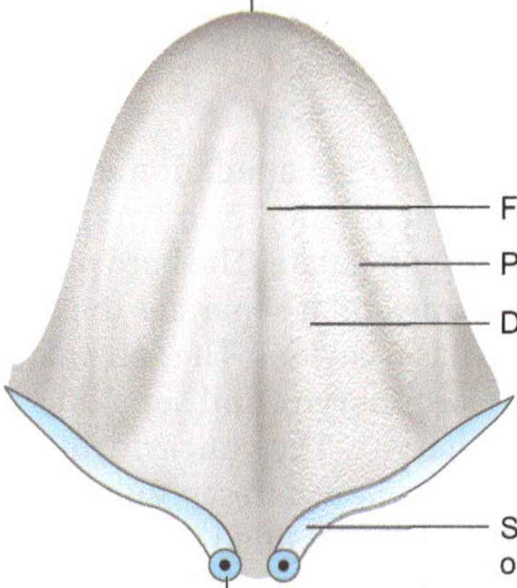

Fig. 2.9: Ventral surface of tongue

sublingual folds located between the lateral tongue and the mandibular gingiva.

Both sides of the frenulum possess sublingual papillae which are also termed as caruncles or folds. These are located in the anterior part of the floor of mouth when the tip of the tongue is raised (Fig. 2.8).

The excretory duct of the submandibular gland, i.e. Wharton's duct runs in the floor of the mouth along the medial border of the sublingual gland and opens at the surface of the mouth at paramedian sublingual caruncle. The sublingual glands exhibit multiple small ducts which open directly into the floor of the mouth (Fig. 2.9).

Tongue

Tongue, a movable muscular organ covers the major part of the mouth and part of the oropharynx. Its prime function includes pushing food into the oropharynx during swallowing and creating words during speaking. Besides, it also helps in mastication, taste and maintaining oral hygiene.

The dorsal surface of the tongue (Fig-2.10) is divided into an anterior horizontal and a posterior vertical part. The first part is in contact with the palate and the second faces the pharynx. The first is designated as palatine surface and the second as pharyngeal surface of the tongue. The palatine surface is situated in front of the terminal sulcus and caries lingual papillae (filiform and fungi form. Filiform papillae are densely arranged and irregularly between the fungi form papillae). Immediately in front of the terminal sulcus are the circumvallate papillae arranged in a "V" shaped line with the largest papillae near or in the midline and decreasing in size laterally and anteriorly. They are mushroom-shaped structures surrounded by a deeply cut circular trough or furrow. The wall of these troughs contains taste buds. Taste buds are also seen on the slope of fungi form papillae. The posterior part of the lateral border of the tongue contains the foliate papillae. They are sharp low folds. They are also the site of the numerous taste buds.

Muscles of the Tongue

The muscles of the tongue consist of extrinsic and intrinsic muscles (Fig. 2.11). The extrinsic muscles originate from the skeleton and spread into the body of the tongue. The later

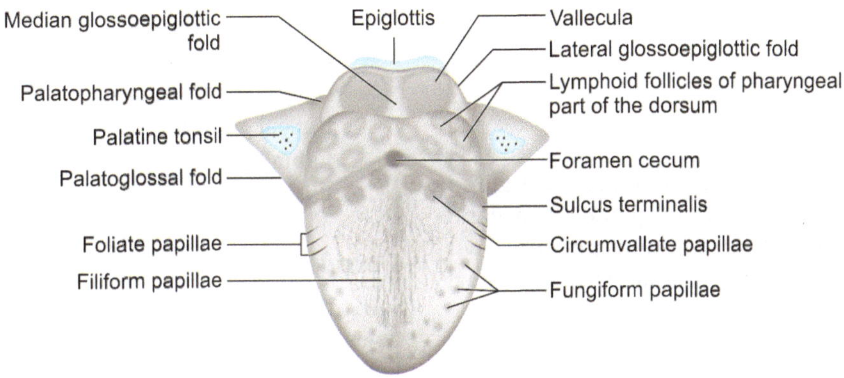

Fig. 2.10: Dorsum of tongue

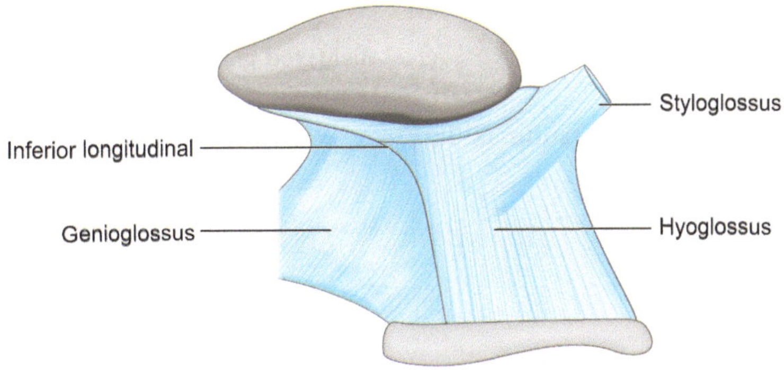

Fig. 2.11: Muscles of tongue

are confined to the tongue itself. The extrinsic muscles are described as follows:

- *Styloglossus muscle:* It arises from the anterior surface of the styloid process, sometime with a few bundles from the stylomandibular ligament. They enter the tongue at about the base of the palatoglossal arch. Nerve supply by the hypoglossal nerve. Action is retraction of the tongue
- *Hyoglossus muscle:* It originates from the upper border of the greater horn of the hyoid bone and adjacent part of the body. Nerve supply by hypoglossal nerve and action is protraction of the tongue
- *Genioglossus muscle:* It arises from the mental tubercle or spine on the inner surface of the chin. Nerve supply by hypoglossal nerve and action is protraction
- *Palatoglossus muscle:* It arises from the palatine aponeurosis and inserts broadly across the tongue. The action is to elevate the posterior aspect of the tongue. The nerve supply is by the vagal nerve.

The intrinsic muscles are divided into longitudinal, transversal and vertical muscles.

- *The longitudinal group:* They are divided into an upper and lower group. They are situated close to the upper and lower borders of the styloglossus muscle
- *The transverse group:* They arises from the lingual septum
- *The vertical group:* This group may exist close to the lateral borders of the body of the tongue where they stretch between the upper and lower surfaces.

The action of the intrinsic muscles is to change the shape of the tongue. Their function combined with that of the extrinsic muscles is responsible for the great mobility and versatility of the tongue.

Function of the tongue:
- Speech
- Swallowing
- Cleansing
- Mastication.

Oral cavity contains major salivary glands which are paired exocrine glands. The glands which secrete their secretions into oral cavity are parotid, submandibular or submaxillary, and sublingual glands.

Salivary Glands

These glands are meant for the production of saliva. The different salivary glands present in humans are:
- Major salivary glands
  - Parotid gland
  - Submandibular gland (submaxillary gland)
  - Sublingual glands.
- Minor salivary glands
  - Lingual serous glands
  - Lingual mucus glands
  - Buccal glands
  - Labial glands
  - Palatal glands.

Classification

Salivary glands can be classified into three types based on the types of secretion.
1. Serous glands—Secretes thin and watery saliva.
2. Mucus glands—secretes thick and viscous saliva.
3. Mixed glands—secretes both serous and mucous saliva.

CHAPTER 3

Anatomy of Jaws

INTRODUCTION

The human body has two jaws—an upper and a lower jaw. They are called maxilla and mandible. The jaws form the oral cavity which is at the entrance of the digestive canal. The inside of the mouth is covered by mucous membrane, and forms the protective covering. The masticatory mechanism is formed by the teeth of upper and lower jaws, temporomandibular joints, the muscles of mastication, and the muscles of cheeks, lips and tongue.

MAXILLA

It contributes a large share in the formation of middle third of the facial skeleton. Maxilla is a spongy bone which is well adapted to sustain the stresses of mastication. It is two in number. It consists of a central pyramidal body which is hollowed by maxillary sinus (Figs 3.1A and B).

The anterior surface of the body of maxilla presents:

- Nasal notch medially
- Anterior nasal spine
- Infraorbital foramen, 1 cm below the infraorbital margin transmitting infraorbital nerve and vessels
- Incisive fossa above the incisor teeth
- Canine fossa lateral to the canine eminence.

In addition to this, four processes of maxilla are also seen:

1. *Frontal process:* It is directed upwards, and articulates anteriorly with nasal bone and posteriorly with lacrimal bone.

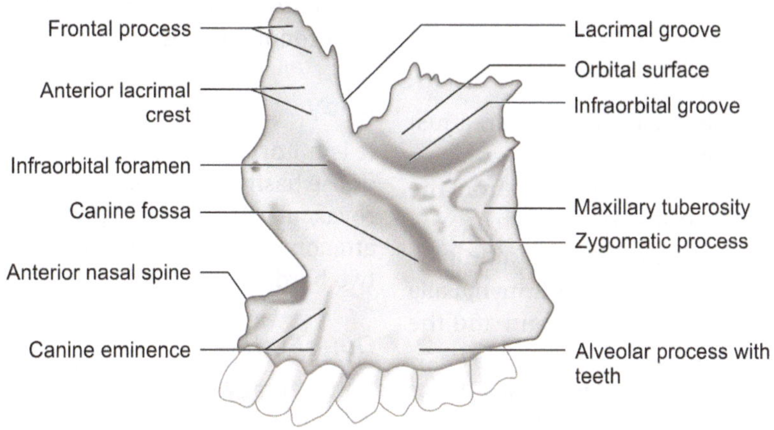

Fig. 3.1A: Lateral aspect of maxilla

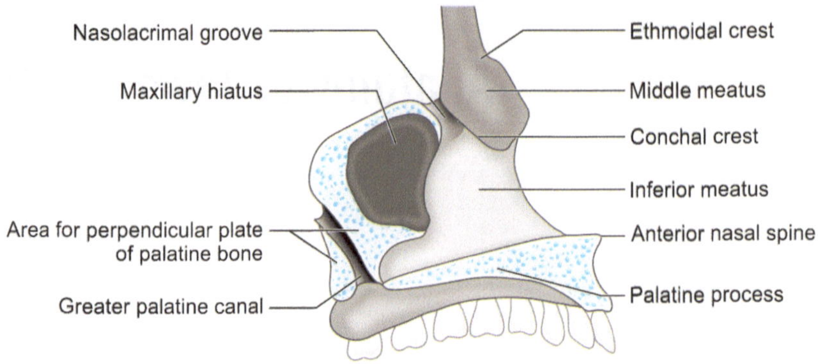

Fig. 3.1B: Medial aspect of maxilla

2. *Zygomatic process*: This process of maxilla is short but stout and articulates with the zygomatic bone.
3. *Palatine process*: This is a horizontal plate at the junction between the body and the alveolar process. Posteriorly, the palatine process unites with the horizontal plate of palatine bone. The posterior part of hard plate is continuous with soft palate.
4. *Alveolar process:* It forms the maxillary dental arch which is comprised of eight cavities containing maxillary teeth. It is an inferior extension of the maxilla which is porous in nature.

The superior surface of maxilla forms floor of the bony socket of orbit and medial surface of the body forms the lateral boundary of the nasal cavity.

Attachments

- Incisive muscle arises from an area just below the foregoing muscle
- Nasalis and depressor septi arise from the surface bordering the nasal notch
- Levator anguli oris arises from canine fossa
- Levator labii superioris arises from maxilla between the infraorbital margin and the infraorbital foramen
- Levator labii superioris alaeque nasi arises from the frontal process of maxilla in front of the orbicularis oculi
- Medial palpebral ligament, to the frontal process of maxilla between the frontal and maxillary origins of the foregoing muscle
- Orbital part of orbicularis oculi arises from the frontal process of maxilla and nasal part of frontal bone.

Among nerve and blood supply, nerve supply is by infraorbital, greater palatine and the incisive branches, while the blood supply is from branches of maxillary artery.

MANDIBLE

It is the largest and strongest bone of the face. The mandible has two parts:

1. *Body*: Containing alveolar process holding teeth.
2. *Ramus*: Containing condylar process and coronoid process.

Body

It is a horizontal U-shaped body having a dense basilar portion that contains the neurovascular bundle and provides for muscle attachments. The body has two surfaces and two borders.

Outer Surface

It presents symphysis menti, a median part ridge in the upper part indicating the linear fusion of the two halves. Mental protuberances

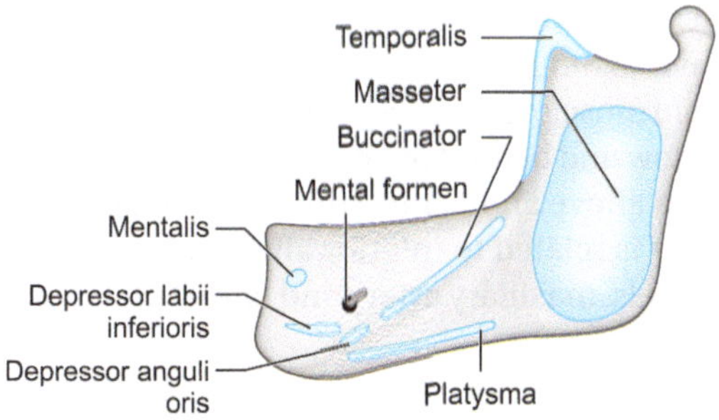

Fig. 3.2: Outer surface of the mandible

or chin is a median triangular projection in the lower part with mental tubercles at the inferolateral angles. It is characteristic of the human jaw. Mental foramen lies below the interval between the premolar teeth. It transmits mental nerve and vessel which is directed backwards and upwards (Fig. 3.2).

An oblique line is the continuation of the sharp anterior border of the ramus of the mandible which is directed downwards and forward towards the mental tubercle. It gives origin to buccinator muscle as far forwards as the anterior of the first molar tooth. In front of this depressor labii inferioris and depressor anguli oris arise from the line below the mental foramen. Incisive fossa between the two incisor teeth gives origin to mentalis and mental slips of orbicularis oris muscle. Above the line of the muscle origin, the surface is covered by mucous membrane of the vestibule.

Inner Surface

It presents mylohyoid line, a prominent oblique ridge, running obliquely downwards below the third molar tooth to the median area below the genial tubercle. It gives origin to mylohyoid muscle, superior constriction muscle of the pharynx from above the posterior end of mylohyoid line.

Lingual nerve is related directly to the above two muscles. Pterygomandibular raphe is attached immediately behind the third molar. Below the mylohyoid line, the surface is slightly hallowed out to form the submandibular fossa, which lodges submandibular salivary glands. Above the mylohyoid line anteriorly, there is sublingual fossa which lodges sublingual salivary glands (Fig. 3.3).

The posterior surface of symphysis menti above the mylohyoid line is marked by genital tubercle. The upper genial tubercle gives origin to genioglossus and the lower genial tubercle to geniohyoid. The mylohyoid groove of the ramus extends to the body below the posterior end of mylohyoid line. Digastric fossa is an oval depression which is situated bilaterally near the midline below the mylohyoid line, which

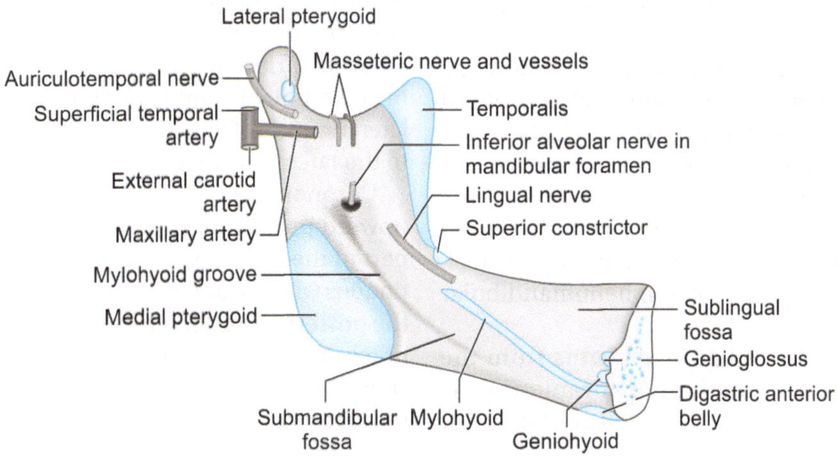

Fig. 3.3: Inner surface of the mandible

gives origin to the digastric muscle. To the whole length of the lower border, the investing layer of deep cervical fascia is attached, but it is interrupted at the anterior border of masseter by the facial vessels and mandibular branch of facial nerve. Still superficially near the outer surface, platysma is inserted into the lower border.

Borders

Alveolar process forms the upper border of the body of the mandible. It bears 16 sockets for permanent teeth. Periodontal membrane is attached to the cavity of the socket. After loss of a tooth during life, the alveolar bone atrophies and bottom of the socket fills up with new bone. Presence of deep socket in the macerated bone indicates loss of a tooth after death.

Ramus

It is quadrilateral in shape and has two surfaces and four borders.

Two Surfaces

It comprises of lateral surface and medial surface.

Lateral surface is flat and obliquely ridged. Whole of this surface except the posterosuperior part, where it is covered by parotid glands, provides insertion to masseter muscle. Medial surface presents mandibular foramen a little above its center at the level of occlusal surface of teeth. It leads to mandibular canal and admits the inferior alveolar nerve and vessels. Mandibular canal opens out at the mental foramen. A sharp projection is situated at the anterior margin of the mandibular canal. It provides attachment of sphenomandibular ligament.

The mylohyoid groove begins from the lower part of mandibular foramen, runs downwards and forwards, and gradually lost in the submandibular fossa. The groove lodges mylohyoid nerve and vessels. Medial pterygoid muscle is inserted on the roughened area below and behind the mylohyoid groove. The area above and behind the mandibular foramen is related to inferior alveolar nerve and vessels, maxillary artery and lateral pterygoid muscle.

Four Borders

The four borders of ramus are as follows namely; upper,lower, anterior and posterior.

Upper border of the ramus is thin and curved to form the mandibular notch which is crossed by masseteric nerve and vessels. Lower border is backward continuation of the base of mandible; it ends behind at the angle of the mandible. Anterior border is thin. This border and adjoining medial surface provide insertion to the lower fibers of temporalis muscle and tendon. Posterior border is thick; it is related to parotid gland.

Condylar and Coronoid Processes

Condylar process is a strong upward projection from the posterosuperior part of the ramus itself. The upper end is expanded from side to side to form the head. It is covered by fibro cartilage and articulates with temporal bone to form the temporomandibular joint. The constriction below the head is the neck. Its anterior surface presents pterygoid fovea for the insertion of lateral pterygoid muscle. The lateral surface of the neck provides attachment to the lateral ligament.

Coronoid process is a flattened triangular upward projection from the anterosuperior part of the ramus. Its anterior border is continuous with the anterior border of ramus, and the posterior border bounds the mandibular notch. The lateral surface is covered by masseter. The medial surface, upper and anterior margins provide insertion to temporalis.

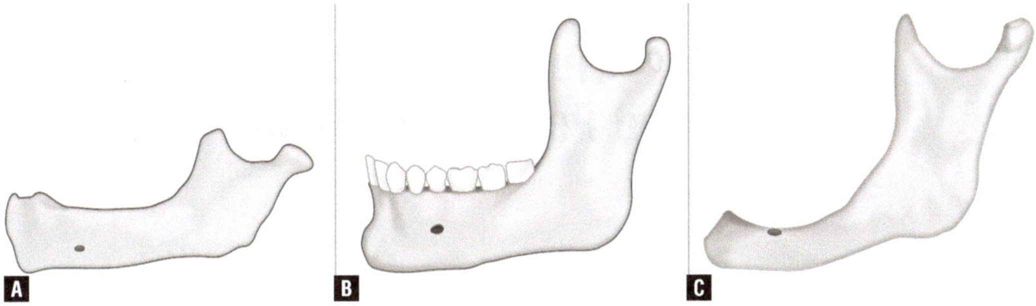

Figs 3.4A to C: Age changes in mandible. (A) Child; (B) Adult; (C) Old

Blood Supply

The external aspect of the mandible is supplied by three main arteries. Inferiorly, the facial artery provides sublingual and submental branches. The lingual artery provides medial branches and the ramus region are supplied by the masseteric and mylohyoid branches of the maxillary artery. The inner aspect of the mandible is supplied mostly by the inferior alveolar branch of the maxillary artery.

Ossification

Mandible is the second bone (next to clavicle) to ossify in the body. Its great part is ossified in membrane. The parts ossifying in cartilage include the incisive part below the incisor teeth, coronoid and condylar processes and upper half of the ramus above the level of mandibular foramen.

Age Changes in the Mandible

- *In infants and children*: Below 5 years of age, the mental foramen is near the lower border and opens below the sockets for the deciduous molars. The mandibular canal runs about 0.5 cm below the occlusal plane due to underdeveloped ramus of mandible, so the needle is inserted below the occlusal plane during inferior alveolar technique (common nerve block for extraction of mandibular teeth). The angle of the mandible is obtuse (140° or more) in children, aged 6 years. Mandibular foramen is usually found at level of occlusal plane, thus needle is inserted at level of occlusal plane (Fig. 3.4A)
- *In adults:* Mental foramen opens in the middle, needle should be placed above the level of occlusion. Angle reduces to 110° or 120° (Fig. 3.4B)
- *In old age*: Both the mental foramen and mandibular canal are close to the alveolar border. The angle becomes obtuse (140°). The human skull is made up of the bones of the cranium and the face (the cranium forms the bony protection for the brain). There are many anatomic landmarks of the skull that the dental assistant should know (Fig. 3.4C).

Human Dentition: Primary and Permanent Teeth

CHAPTER 4

INTRODUCTION

Two different sets of teeth erupt during the course of a human's life, i.e. temporary or primary dentition and the secondary or permanent dentition.

PRIMARY TEETH

This is the first set of teeth in the human beings, which must function until these teeth are replaced by secondary teeth or permanent teeth. Other names are milk teeth, temporary teeth or deciduous teeth because they are shed and replaced by other teeth later in life. These teeth start eruption between 6 months and 8 months of life and are shed by 11–12 years when they are replaced by permanent teeth. They are 20 in number; incisor (8), canines (4), molars (8) as shown in Figure 4.1.

Eruption Sequence

- *Central incisors:* Eruption 7 months, shedding 6–7 years
- *Lateral incisors:* Eruption 8 months, shedding 7–8 years
- *Canines:* Eruption 17 months, shedding 10–12 years
- *First molars:* Eruption 14 months, shedding 10–12 years
- *Second molars:* Eruption 21 months, shedding 10–12 years.

SECONDARY OR PERMANENT TEETH

They begin to erupt at the 6th year and they are meant to function throughout the individual's life. These teeth have no successors except those provided as substitutes artificially. They

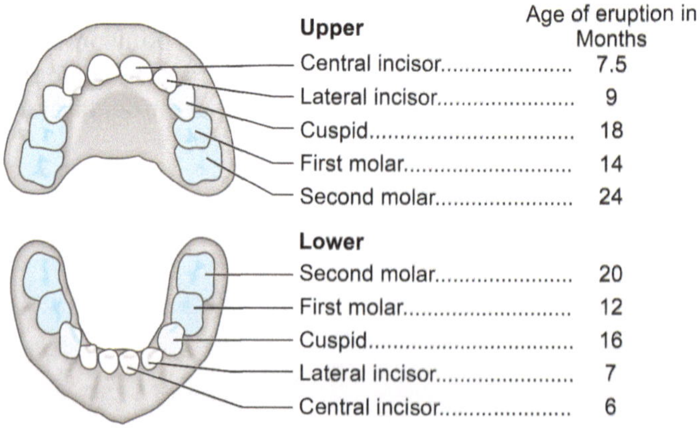

Fig. 4.1: Primary teeth

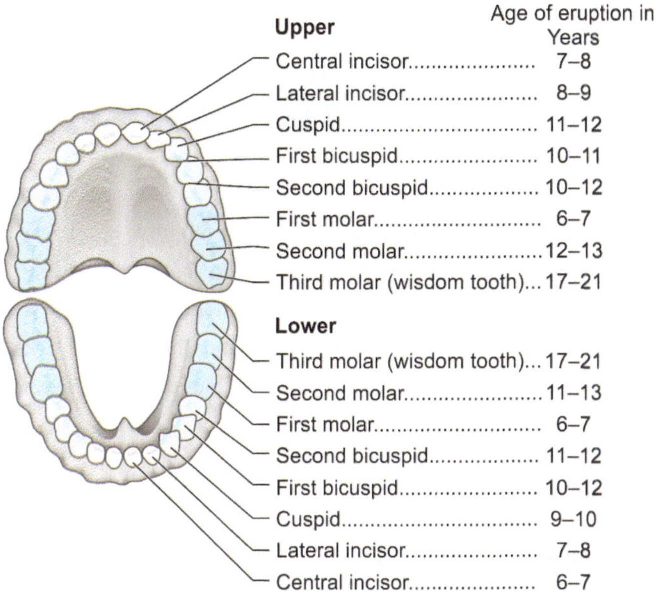

Fig. 4.2: Permanent teeth

are 32 in number; incisors (8), canines (4), premolars (8), and molars (12) as shown in Figure 4.2.

Time of Eruption

- *Central incisors:* 8 years
- *Lateral incisors:* 7-9 years
- *Canines:* 10-12 years
- *First premolars:* 10-12 years
- *Second premolars:* 10-12 years
- *First molars:* 6 years
- *Second molars:* 12 years
- *Third molars:* 17-21 years.

The pattern of tooth eruption and shedding of both deciduous and permanent teeth is depicted in Table 4.1.

TOOTH NUMBERING SYSTEM

The Federation Dentaire Internationale (FDI) two digit tooth numbering system is used in all examinations which is shown in Figures 4.3 and 4.4.

FUNCTIONS OF TEETH

General functions of teeth are mastication, aesthetics, and phonetics.

The word "incisors" is derived from Latin incidere, which means to cut into. They are used for shearing of food and these are forced between the posterior teeth by tongue and cheek muscles. For canines or cuspids, the word cusp refers to the spear-shaped crown of these teeth. They are much thicker because of a strong ridge of enamel on the labial and on the lingual surfaces. This ridge of enamel extends from the tip of the cusp to the cervical line or neck of tooth, and therefore, makes it a strong tooth.

It has also good support in the bone because it has the longest root. It is a corner tooth at the angle of the mouth which helps it to tear the food, e.g. carnivorous animals tear the flesh of their prey and man tears sugarcane.

Bicuspids or premolars mean two cuspids, preceding the molars. They pulverize the food

Table 4.1: Chronology of mineralization and eruption of the human dentition

Tooth	*Initial mineralization*	*Enamel formed at birth*	*Enamel formation completed*	*Root formation completed*	*Eruption*
Deciduous dentition					
Upper/maxillary					
First molar	4 months in utero	Five-sixths	1 ½ months	1 ½ years	7 ½ months
Second incisor	4½ months in utero	Two-thirds	2 ½ months	2 years	9 months
Canine	5 months in utero	One-third	9 months	3 ¼ years	18 months
First molar	5 months in utero	Cusps united	6 months	2 ½ years	14 months
Second molar	6 months in utero	Cusp tips still isolated	11 months	3 years	24 months
Lower/mandibular					
First incisor	4 ½ months in utero	Three-fifths	2 ½ months	1 ½ years	6 months
Second incisor	4 ½ months in utero	Three-fifths	3 months	1 ¾ years	7 months
Canine	5 months in utero	One-third	9 months	3 ¼ years	16 months
First molar	5 months in utero	Cusps united	5 ½ months	2 ¼ years	12 months
Second molar	6 months in utero	Cusp tips still isolated	10 months	3 years	20 months
Permanent dentition					
Upper/maxillary					
First incisor	3–4 months		4–5 years	10 years	7–8 years
Second incisor	10–12 months		4–5 years	11 years	8–9 years
Canine	4–5 months		6–7 years	13–15 years	11–12 years
First premolar	1 ½–1 ¾ years		5–6 years	12–13 years	10–11 years
Second premolar	2–2 ¼ years		6–7 years	12–14 years	10–12 years
First molar	At birth	Sometimes a trace	2 ½–3 years	9–10 years	6–7 years
Second molar	2 ½–3 years		7–8 years	14–16 years	12–13 years
Third molar	7–9 years		12–16 years	18–25 years	17–21 years
Lower/mandibular					
First incisor	3–4 months		4–6 years	9–10 years	6–7 years
Second incisor	3–4 months		4–5 years	10 years	7–8 years
Canine	4–5 months		6–7 years	12–14 years	9–10 years
First premolar	1 ¾–2 years		5–6 years	12–13 years	10–12 years
Second premolar	2 ¼–2 ¾ years		6–7 years	13–14 years	11–12 years
First molar	At birth	Sometimes a trace	2 ½–3 years	9–10 years	6–7 years
Second molar	2 ½–3 years		7–8 years	14–15 years	11–13 years

which has been cut into pieces by incisors and canines.

Molars, this word is derived from Latin "molaris". They are the largest teeth in the mouth because of the size of their crown and because of well-developed two or three roots. Upper molars have three roots and lower two roots. The last molars are the smallest, and least functional.

Maxillary incisors are larger than mandibular teeth. The lateral incisors are more rounded and smaller than the central incisors, which are stronger than their distal neighbors. Lower lateral is a slightly larger than the lower central incisor. The cuspids—maxillary canine is longest tooth in both the arches. It is bigger than mandibular canine. The cingulum or maxillary cuspid is more prominent. Upper 1st premolar has two roots while all other premolars have one root. Lower 1st premolar is smallest of all permanent teeth. Second premolars are more developed for grinding of food. Maxillary 1st molar is largest of all the molars and has three well-developed roots and is the most useful teeth. Third molars are smallest and are called wisdom teeth (Fig. 4.5).

Occlusion

The biting surface of the teeth is called occlusal surfaces of teeth. Occlusion of the teeth means functional relationship of upper and lower teeth when the jaws are closed and teeth meet in contact with each other. Every tooth has two antagonists with the exception of lower central incisors and upper 3rd molars. The study of surface anatomy of the teeth is important in rendering any treatment of the teeth such as dental prophylaxis and dental restoration. The form of the teeth is interrelation to the functions that they are required to perform. The crown of an incisor tooth has an incisal edge and crowns of canines, premolars and molars have cusps. These incisal edges and cusps form the cutting surfaces of tooth crowns.

SURFACE ANATOMY

- Labial surface is the outer surface of the anterior teeth which faces forward towards the lips (Fig. 4.6)
- Buccal surface is the surface of posterior teeth facing the cheeks (Buccinator muscles)
- Lingual surface or inner surfaces of all the teeth in the lower jaw facing the tongue are called lingual surfaces. The corresponding surface of the upper teeth are called palatal surface
- Proximal surface is the area where the mesial surface of one tooth touches the distal surface of another; called also contact area or surface.

Permanent dentition

	Right															Left	
FDI	1.8	1.7	1.6	1.5	1.4	1.3	1.2	1.1	2.1	2.2	2.3	2.4	2.5	2.6	2.7	2.8	**FDI**
Universal	1	2	3	4	5	6	7	8	9	10	11	12	13	14	15	16	Universal
Universal	32	31	30	29	28	27	26	25	24	23	22	21	20	19	18	17	Universal
FDI	4.8	4.7	4.6	4.5	4.4	4.3	4.2	4.1	3.1	3.2	3.3	3.4	3.5	3.6	3.7	3.8	**FDI**

Primary dentition

	Right								Left	
FDI	5.5	5.4	5.3	5.2	5.1	6.1	6.2	6.3	6.4	6.5	**FDI**
Universal	A	B	C	D	E	F	G	H	I	J	Universal
Universal	T	S	R	Q	P	O	N	M	L	K	Universal
FDI	8.5	8.4	8.3	8.2	8.1	7.1	7.2	7.3	7.4	7.5	**FDI**

Fig. 4.3: FDI/Universal tooth numbering system

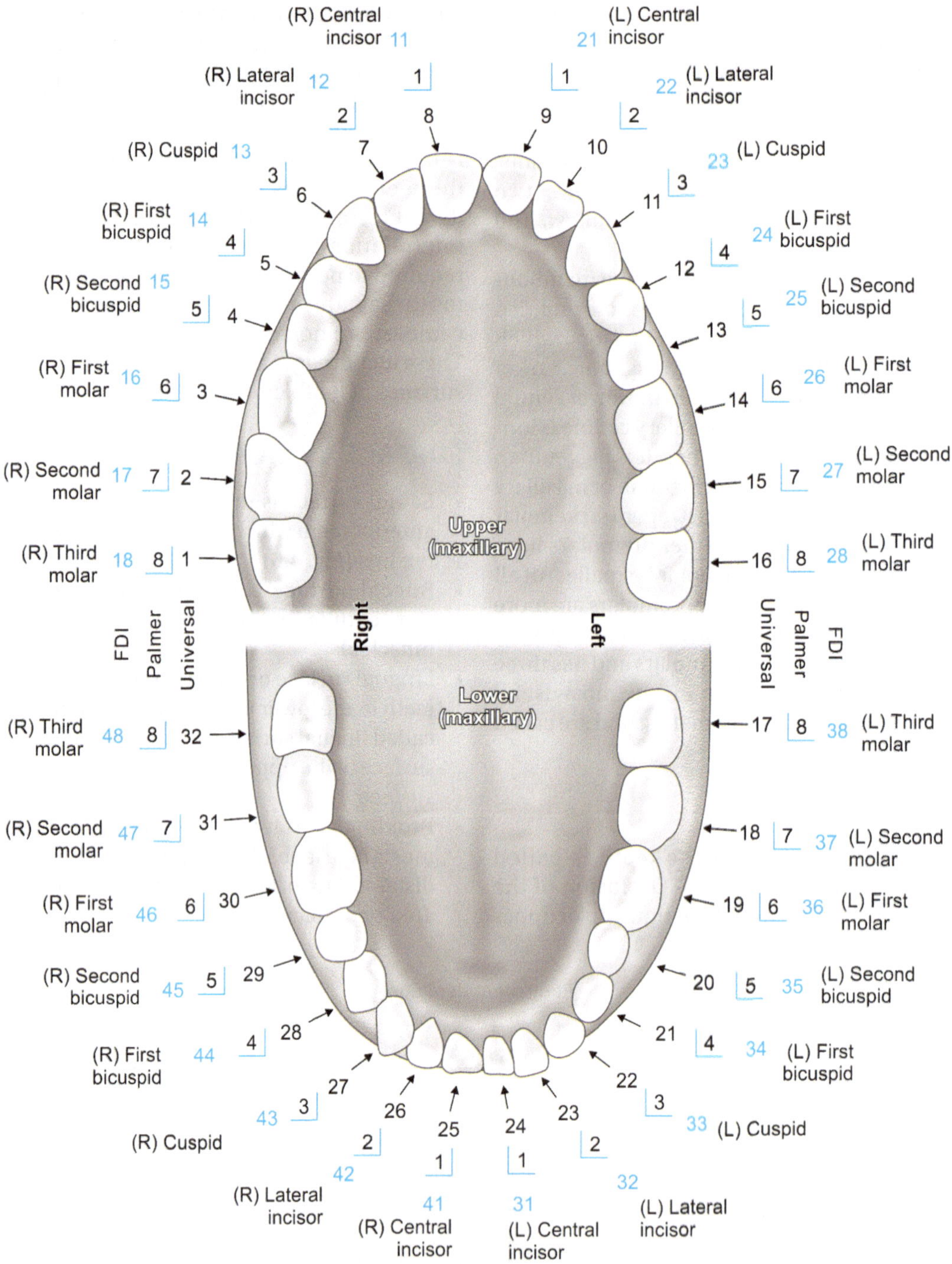

Fig. 4.4: Different types of tooth numbering system

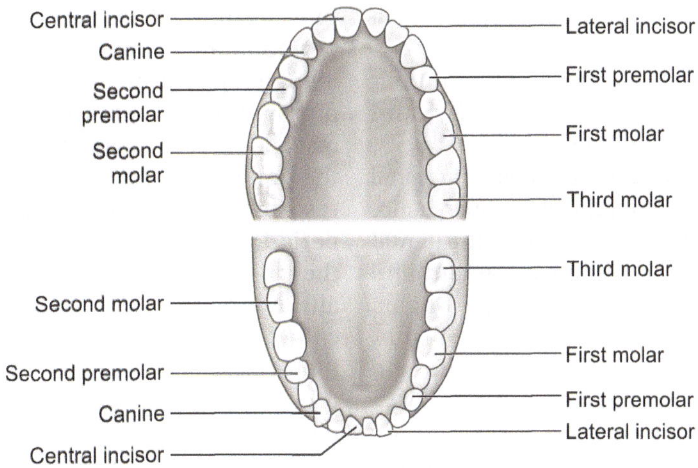

Fig. 4.5: Positioning of maxillary and mandibular teeth in oral cavity

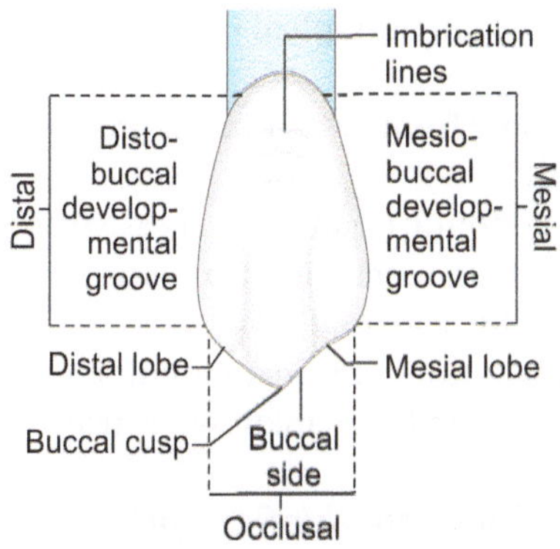

Fig. 4.6: Labial surface of incisor

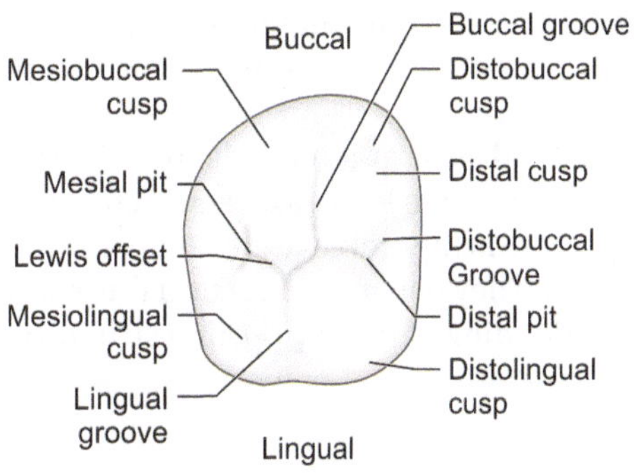

Fig. 4.7: Occlusal surface of molar

- Occlusal surface is the chewing surface of the premolars and molars (Fig. 4.7)
- Line angle is formed by the junction of two surfaces, e.g. mesiolabial line angle of anterior teeth
- Point angle is formed by the junction of three surfaces, e.g. mesiolabioincisal point angle of anterior teeth
- Cusp is a pronounced elevation on the occlusal surface of posterior teeth
- Tubercle is a small elevation on the crown which may not be typical
- Ridge is any linear elevation on the surface of the tooth
- Cingulum is a bulbous convexity near the cervical region of a tooth
- Marginal ridge are ridges at the mesial and distal edges of the occlusal surfaces of posterior teeth
- Fissure is along cleft between cusps or ridges
- A fossa is a rounded depression.

Axial wall is any wall of the pulp chamber which is parallel to the long axis of the tooth.

Maintenance of Tooth Position

The factors which keep the teeth in position are:

- *Occlusal contact:* Two antagonists except lower central incisor and upper 3rd molar
- *Intercuspal relation:* Interlocking of cusps prevent drifting

- *Muscles of face and tongue:* Keep the teeth in natural zone
- *Mesial and distal contacts:* Prevent their movement mesially and distally, and protect gingiva and bone.

Teeth are sustained by their own functional anatomy. Form and function go hand in hand. They help to sustain themselves in the dental arch by assisting in the development and protection of the tissues that support them. The following anatomic features help in this.

- Contours or curves of surfaces of teeth protect food impaction on gums
- Contact and embrasure form provide spillways for dispersion of food during mastication. Normal contact and embrasure form is required for health of tissues
- Mesial and distal edges have elevations of enamel called the marginal ridges. These ridges convey the food in the proper direction.

Occlusal wear gradually decreases crown length of the teeth with edge, and teeth tend to erupt more in the oral cavity to compensate for this loss. They become wider and this results in overloading of the supporting structures.

Resorption of Teeth

Resorption of the roots of the teeth is of two types, which are termed as external resorption and internal resorption.

External Resorption

Physiological resorption occurs in deciduous teeth; there is a gradual resorption of their roots resulting in loss of attachment of their periodontal ligament. The developing permanent successor tooth creates sufficient pressure by its increase in size to produce resorption of the primary tooth root and of the bone surrounding the root. As the root resorbs, the tooth loosens. Eventually, all periodontal ligament attachment is lost and the rootless crown of the primary tooth literally falls off from the jaw and the process is called shedding of teeth. If the permanent tooth does not cause pressure on the primary tooth root, the resorption process may be delayed and continue to function for many years, but quite a few times the primary teeth are lost.

Other causes of external resorption are:

- Low grade periapical chronic inflammation
- Pressure from cysts, tumors and impacted teeth
- Orthodontic treatment excessive pressure
- Traumatic occlusion (excessive pressure of occlusal forces)
- Replantation or transplantation of teeth
- Resorption from unknown causes.

Internal or Idiopathic Resorption

Mouth is the gateway of the body and the teeth are the sentinels to protect it. The periodical visits are required to ensure the oral health. It can be arranged by either carrying out periodical dental inspections by carrying out periodical recalls for dental treatment.

Periodontal Anatomy: Clinical and Histological Characteristics

CHAPTER 5

INTRODUCTION

Knowledge of the anatomy of the periodontal tissues and their associated structures is essential for understanding periodontal diseases. This Chapter describes the clinical and microscopic features of healthy periodontal tissues.

PERIODONTIUM

The tissue that invest and support the teeth including the gingival, alveolar mucosa, cementum, periodontal ligament and alveolar bone is called peridontium (Fig. 5.1).

This means all structures which are around the teeth and provide support to tooth. Periodontium includes two soft tissues and two hard tissues.

Soft tissues of periodontium are:

- Gingiva
- Periodontal ligament.

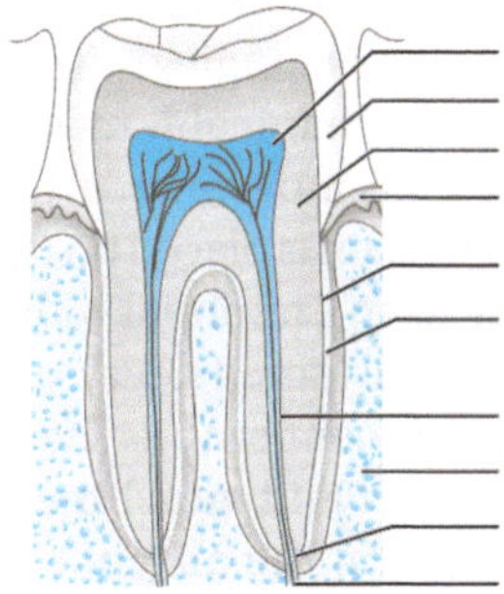

Fig. 5.1: Structure of periodontium

Hard tissues of periodontium are:

- Cementum
- Alveolar bone.

GINGIVA

Gingiva is a kind of masticatory mucosa that envelops the cervical areas of teeth and forms the covering of alveolar process. It is primarily used to prevent an injury to the deeper tissues while permitting a selective interchange with the oral environment. It is composed of underlying connective tissue layer referred as lamina proper and an upper epithelial layer.

Various collagen fibers of the gingival connective tissue provide a rigid structural framework in the gingiva. These fibers are organized into several characteristic and architecturally distinct units that are classified into various groups based on their location, origin, and insertion. They are:

- *Dentogingival fibers*: Inserted into the root surface as Sharpey's fibers and fan out from the root surface adjacent to the junctional epithelium and coronal to the alveolar crest into the gingival tissues
- *Dentoperiosteal fibers:* Inserted into the root surface, run over the alveolar crest and insert into the buccal and lingual periosteum
- *Alveogingival fibers*: Arise from the alveolar crest, traverse coronally, and terminate in the free and attached gingiva

- *Transseptal fibers*: Arise in the cementum, traverse the interdental alveolar crest and reinsert into the cementum of adjacent tooth
- *Circular and semicircular fibers*: Located coronal to the transseptal fibers and run in a circumferential or semicircular manner around the tooth
- *Transgingival fibers*: The fibers traversing from the cementoenamel junction to the free marginal gingiva of the adjacent tooth
- *Intergingival fibers*: These fibers extend along facial and lingual marginal gingiva from tooth to tooth
- *Interpapillary fibers*: Run in a buccolingual direction through the interdental tissue
- *Periosteogingival fibers*: Inserted into the alveolar periosteum and spread out into the attached gingiva
- *Intercircular fibers*: Located both buccal and lingual and run in a mesiodistal manner to join circular fibers of adjacent tooth.

Types

- *Marginal gingiva:* Free or unattached gingiva
- *Attached gingiva:* Firmly attached to underlying tooth and bone
- *Interdental gingiva:* Located between adjacent teeth (Fig. 5.2).

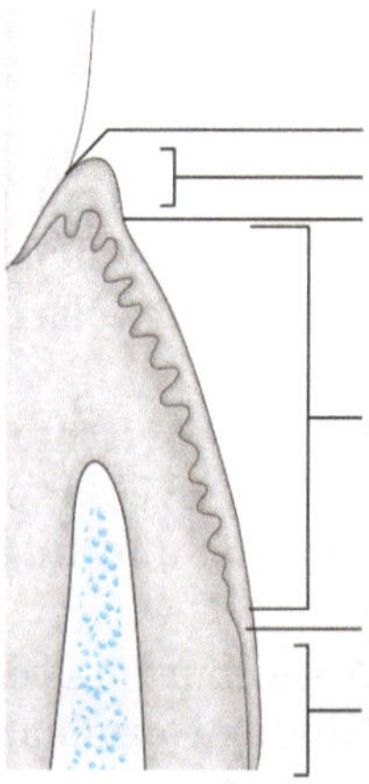

Fig. 5.2: Types of gingiva

Marginal Gingiva

The marginal gingiva is the most coronally positioned portion of the gingiva. It is not attached to the tooth, and it creates the soft tissue wall of the gingival sulcus (the shallow space between the marginal gingival and the tooth). In health, the marginal gingiva is knife-edged in contour, firm in consistency, and smooth in texture. It extends apically to the free gingival groove, the shallow depression in the gingival surface approximately 1 mm wide that corresponds to the most coronal aspect of the gingival attachment to the tooth. In some patients, the free gingival groove is pronounced, while in others it is absent (Figs 5.3A and B).

Attached Gingiva

Just apical to the marginal gingiva and the free gingival groove is the attached gingiva. It is firmly bound to the underlying tooth and alveolar bone. The attached gingiva is tapered in contour, stippled in texture, and firm in consistency. Stippling refers to the irregular surface of the gingiva, which resembles the surface of an orange. The attached gingiva varies in width from one area of the mouth to another and can range from less than 1 mm to 9 mm. The width depends principally on the teeth involved, their buccolingual position in the arch, and the location of frenum or muscle attachments.

In general, the attached gingiva is widest on the incisor teeth, ranging from 3.5 mm to 4.5 mm in the maxilla and 3.3 mm to 3.9 mm in the mandible. It provides gingival tissue that can withstand the mechanical forces of tooth brushing and prevents movement of the marginal gingiva when tension is placed on the alveolar mucosa. In the past, a minimal width of attached gingiva was considered necessary for gingival health, but recent studies have shown that gingival health and attachment levels can be maintained in the absence of attached gingiva. The attached gingiva is bound coronally by the free gingival groove

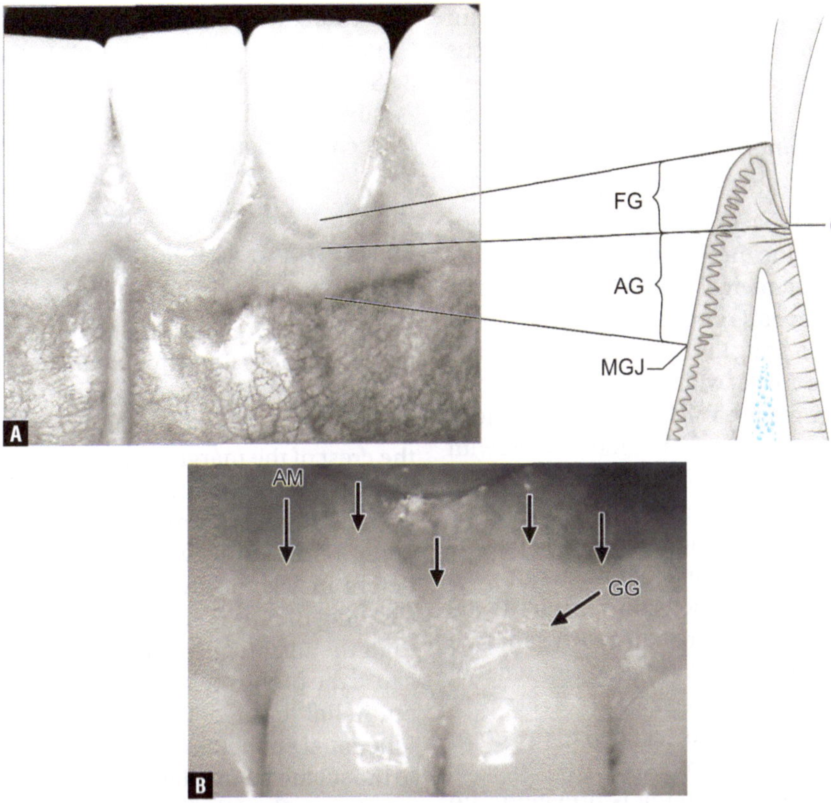

Figs 5.3A and B: (A) Healthy gingival tissue; (B) Tapered contours and pointed interdental gingiva *(For color version of Fig. 5.3B, see Plate 8)*

Abbreviations: GG, gingival groove; AM, alveolar mucosa (stippled texture); MGJ, mucogingival junction; AG, attached gingiva; FG, free gingiva; CEJ, cementoenamel junction.

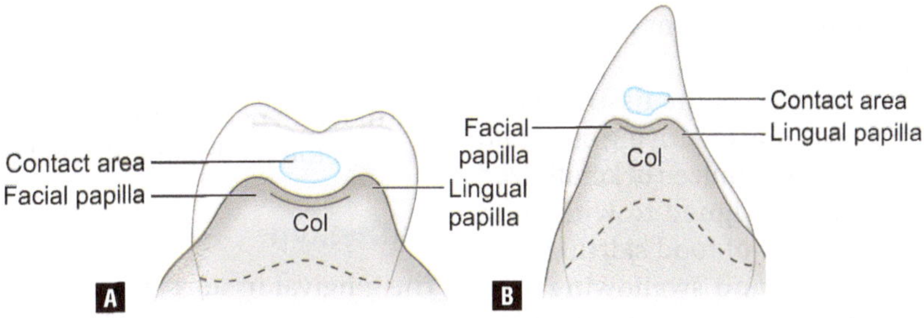

Figs 5.4A and B: Clinical presentation of interdental col. (A) In molar; (B) In central incisor

and apically by the mucogingival junction (Fig. 5.4). The latter marks or demarcate the beginning of the alveolar mucosa, which is loosely attached to the underlying bone, is smooth in surface texture, covered with a thin layer of nonkeratinized epithelium, and generally not as resistant to frictional contact as the attached gingiva.

Keratinized gingiva is covered with keratinized or parakeratinized stratified squamous epithelium. This includes the free or marginal gingiva as well as the attached gingiva and is different from the nonkeratinized epithelium that forms the soft tissue wall of healthy sulcus or pocket.

Interdental Gingiva

The interdental gingiva is located in the interproximal space created by adjacent teeth in contact. In the mesiodistal dimension, the shape of the interdental gingiva, while generally triangular, depends on the proximal contours of the teeth creating the interproximal space. If the contours are flat with broad interproximal contacts, the gingiva will be narrow and short. If the proximal contours are more convex with a small coronally positioned contact area, the interdental gingiva will be broad and high. When teeth overlap, the interdental space is small or absent, resulting in bulbous gingiva. In the buccolingual dimension, the interdental gingiva terminates coronally with separate buccal and lingual peaks of tissue joined by a depression known as the gingival col (Fig. 5.4). If the gingival tissue has receded to the point that it no longer touches the interproximal contact area or if diastema is prevalent, no col will be seen. The col is present only when the gingiva surrounds the gingival surface of the interproximal contact area.

Collectively, all the soft tissues of the mouth are known as the oral mucosa. They are divided into three different types which are as follows:

1. Masticatory mucosa is the tissue that is firmly attached to the underlying bone and covered with parakeratinized or keratinized epithelium. It is designed to withstand the frictional forces of food skirting over it during chewing and swallowing. The gingiva and the tissue covering the hard palate are examples of masticatory mucosa.
2. Lining mucosa is composed of oral tissues that are loosely attached to their underlying structures and covered with nonkeratinized epithelium. The mucosa covering the lips, cheek, floor of the mouth, inferior surface of the tongue, soft palate, uvula, and alveolar mucosa are examples of lining mucosa.
3. Specialized mucosa covers the dorsal surface of the tongue and is adapted to accommodate for the sensation of taste.

Gingival Sulcus, Sulcular and Junctional Epithelium

The gingival sulcus is an area of potential space between a tooth and the surrounding gingival tissue and is lined by sulcular epithelium. Histologically, the sulcus is lined with nonkeratinized sulcular epithelium and extends from the crest of the marginal gingival to the most coronal level of the junctional epithelium. The average depth is 1.8 mm with variation up to 6 mm. The healthy gingival sulcus depth as determined clinically with periodontal probe (probing depth) is slightly deeper (2–3 mm) than the histologically measured depth because the probe often penetrates the delicate epithelial lining of the gingival sulcus. The junctional epithelium, which is located apical to the sulcular epithelium, is approximately 12 mm in length and attaches the gingiva to the tooth. It establishes the histological gingival attachment level and is formed by a uniting of the oral epithelium and the reduced enamel epithelium during tooth eruption.

PARTS OF GINGIVA

The different parts of gingiva are described in detail in the section mentioned below.

Epithelium

The gingival tissues are made up of fibrous connective tissue covered by stratified squamous epithelium. The epithelium that covers the oral surface of the attached and marginal gingiva is either parakeratinized or keratinized, while the sulcular epithelium and the junctional epithelium are nonkeratinized. The sulcular epithelium is thinner, which makes it easier for the products of dental plaque to penetrate into the connective tissue of the gingiva and stimulate inflammation and tissue destruction. The epithelium that covers the alveolar mucosa is thin and nonkeratinized.

Oral Epithelium

The oral epithelium that is keratinized or parakeratinized is composed of four layers of cells (Figs 5.5 and 5.6). The deeper cells are cuboidal in shape (basal cells) and form the stratum basale. The second layer of cells, called the stratum spinosum, is composed of polygonal cells. The next layer is composed of cells that are flattened in shape with prominent basophilic keratohyalin granules in the cytoplasm. This layer is known as the stratum granulosum. The most superficial layer, the stratum corneum, is a cornified layer that may be keratinized (no nuclei), parakeratinized

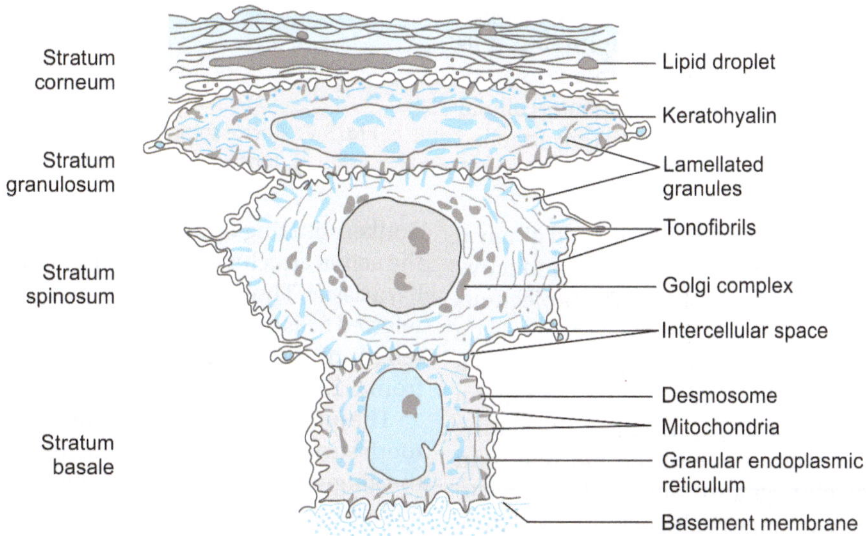

Fig. 5.5: Different types of cells in various layers of oral keratinized epithelium *(For color version, see Plate 8)*

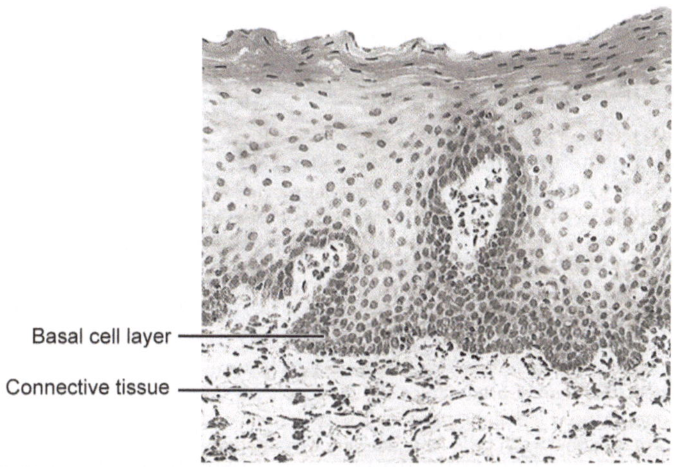

Fig. 5.6: Histological view of oral epithelium and underlying connective tissue *(For color version, see Plate 8)*

(retained nuclei), or both. The epithelial cells are formed as basal cells and gradually change to the characteristics of each of the cell layers as they migrate toward the surface. This process is known as keratinization. The cells are ultimately sloughed from the keratinized surface layer. The cell turnover rate in experimental animals is about 10-12 days for the oral epithelium and 1-6 days for the junctional epithelium. The thickness of gingival epithelium is formed by balance between basal epithelium cell formation and sloughing of older cells at surface. The epithelial cells are joined together by structures known as desmosomes, tight junctions, and intercellular ground substance. The basal cells are attached to the basement membrane by hemidesmosomes.

The junction between keratinized gingival oral epithelium and its underlying connective tissue is usually wavy in shape. The projections of epithelial cells into the connective tissue are known as rete pegs. The intervening projections of connective tissue are known as connective tissue papillae. The alternating pattern of connective tissue papillae and epithelial rete pegs are thought to be related to the stippled (orange peel-like) surface texture of attached gingiva.

Sulcular Epithelium

A balance between new basal cell formation and the sloughing of older cells at the surface maintain the thickness of the gingival epithelium.

The crevicular and the junctional epithelium are not as thick as the oral epithelium and in health, have no rete pegs and are not keratinized. The epithelium in this area is composed principally of the stratum basale and the stratum spinosum (Fig. 5.7).

Junctional Epithelium

The junctional epithelium consists of a collar-like band of stratified squamous nonkeratinizing epithelium, which provides the actual attachment of the epithelium to the hard tissue. Thus, the epithelium is sometimes referred to as the "attachment epithelium". The length of the junctional epithelium ranges from 0.25 mm to 1.35 mm.

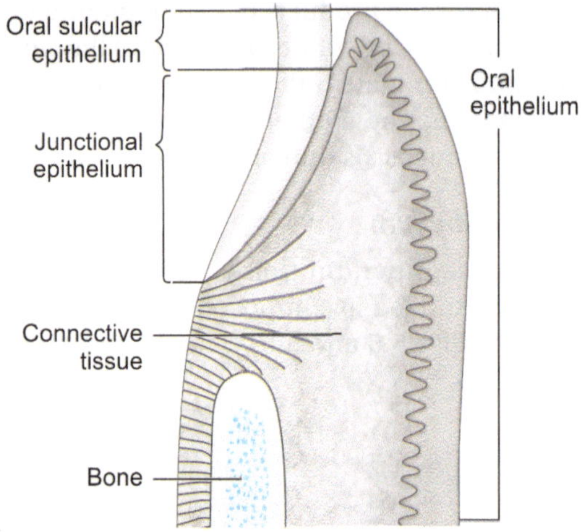

Fig. 5.7: Microscopic view of sulcular and junctional epithelium

The junctional epithelium is attached to the tooth surface or epithelial attachment and to the gingival connective tissue by the internal basal lamina and an external basal lamina, respectively. The attachment of junctional epithelium to the tooth is strengthened by the gingival fibers, which supports the marginal gingiva against the tooth surface. The junctional epithelium and the gingival fibers together form a functional unit known as dentogingival unit (Fig. 5.7).

Connective Tissue

The connective tissue of the gingiva is known as the lamina propria, a highly vascular layer of connective tissue under the basement membrane lining a layer of epithelium. It is divided into two layers:

1. The papillary layer, adjacent to the epithelium
2. The reticular layer, contiguous with the periosteum on the alveolar bone.

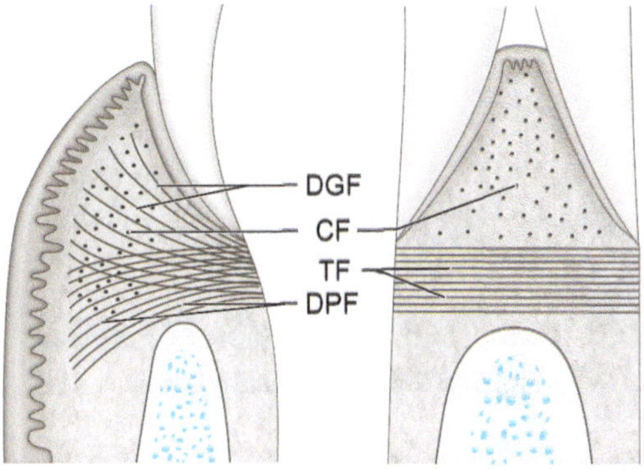

Fig. 5.8: Gingival fibers on the buccal aspect of a tooth
Abbreviations: DGF, dentogingival fibers; TF, transseptal fibers; DPF, dentoperiosteal fibers; CF, circular fibers.

The lamina propria consists primarily of the following:

- Collagen fibers
- Intercellular ground substance
- Cells
- Blood vessels
- Nerves.

The collagen fibers help to hold the marginal gingiva tightly against the tooth and provide a firm junction of the attached gingiva to the underlying tooth, root and alveolar bone. The fibers are grouped into the following types (Fig. 5.8):

- Dentogingival fibers
- Transseptal fibers
- Dentoperiosteal fibers
- Circular fibers.

The dentogingival group runs from the root surface out into the gingiva, the circular group runs circumferentially around the tooth, and the transseptal group runs between the adjacent teeth.

Collagen fibers are strong rope-like cords that bind and hold tissues together in a functioning unit. Their structure consists of three polypeptide chains wound together to form a basic collagen molecule. The molecules aggregate side by side to form collagen filaments, which in turn are accumulated to form the collagen fibril. The collagen fibers found in the gingival fibers are composed of many collagen fibrils held together by proteoglycans. The viscous intercellular ground substance consists principally of mucopolysaccharides and glycoproteins. These substances help to regulate the distribution of water, electrolytes, and metabolites in the tissues.

In contrast to the dense mass of firmly bound collagen fibers found in the gingiva, the connective tissue of the alveolar mucosa is composed of more loosely arranged collagen fibers interspersed with elastic and muscle fibers. They are not firmly attached to the underlying bone, and therefore, this tissue can be moved easily to adapt to the changing shapes and sizes of the muscles during function.

Following are the most prominent cells found in the gingival connective tissue:

- Plasma cells
- Fibroblasts
- Mast cells
- Lymphocytes.

Gingival Crevicular Fluid

The gingival crevicular fluid is continually secreted from the gingival connective tissue into the sulcus through the sulcular epithelial wall. This fluid helps to mechanically clean the sulcus and in addition, possesses antimicrobial properties and antibodies that enhance the resistance of the gingiva to gingivitis. It also contains plasma proteins, which may improve the adhesion of the epithelium to the tooth.

Secretion of the crevicular fluid increases when the tissues are inflamed and when the patient is chewing. It also increases when the patient is pregnant or taking contraceptive medication. This increase is most likely related to the exaggerated inflammatory response to local irritants associated with these hormonal changes. The crevicular fluid is most commonly considered to be inflammatory exudates; however, small amounts are found in clinically healthy gingival sulcus.

CLINICAL DESCRIPTIVE CRITERIA

Gingival Color

The color of healthy gingiva is uniformly coral pink from the attached gingiva through to the crest of the marginal gingiva. However, considerable variation exists depending on the amount of melanin in the tissues, the thickness of the epithelium, the degree of keratinization, and the vascularity of the connective tissue. Dark skinned people often exhibit a dark blue or brown color. Red to bluish red changes are often characteristic of gingival inflammation.

Gingival Contour

The marginal gingiva and attached gingiva are usually tapered in contour, ending coronally in knife-edged margins. The interdental gingiva is generally pointed. However, the contours of the gingiva vary depending upon the shape of the teeth, the buccolingual position of the teeth in the arch, and the size of the interproximal embrasure space. In gingival disease, the contours are often rounded and enlarged because of vascular stagnation and increased formation of collagen fibers.

Gingival Consistency

In health, the gingiva is usually resilient and firm because of the dense collagenous nature of the gingival connective tissue. In gingival disease, the consistency may be soft and boggy, because of vascular stagnation and a decrease in the amount of gingival collagen fibers. In addition, fibrosis can also occur when the amount of collagen formation is very extremely high.

Gingival Texture

The surface texture of the gingiva is described as being stippled like an orange peel or smooth and shiny. The attached gingiva and the central portions of the interdental gingiva are stippled and the marginal gingiva is smooth.

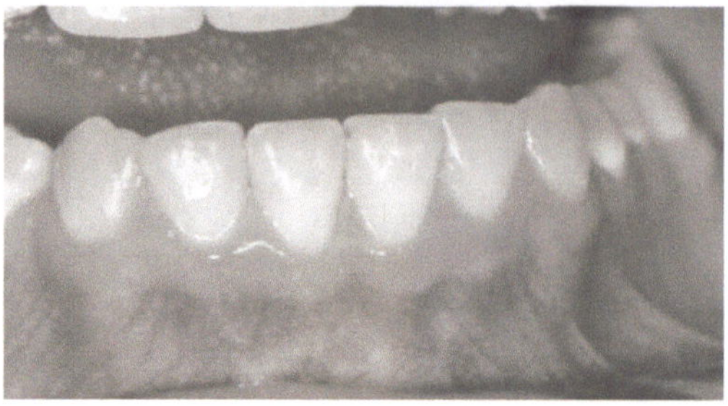

Fig. 5.9: Clinically healthy gingiva

The degree of keratinization and stippling are related and depend on each other (Fig. 5.9).

Gingival Position

The level on the tooth at which the gingiva is attached is known as the gingival position. When teeth first erupt into the oral cavity, the gingival attachments are close to the tips of the crown; however, they gradually shift to cervico enamel junction. During the eruption, aging process, and the periodontal disease and the gingival position (attachment) is found on the root surface. The measurement of gingival level is made with the periodontal probe from the most coronal level of the junctional epithelium to a fixed point on the tooth (most commonly the cementoenamel junction).

PERIODONTAL LIGAMENT

The periodontal ligament, commonly abbreviated as the PDL, is a group of specialized connective tissue fibers that essentially attach a tooth to the alveolar bone within which it sits. It consists primarily of bundles of continuous intermingling collagen fibers arranged into a network running from the tooth to the alveolar bone proper. These fibers are referred to as the principal fibers of the periodontal ligament. In teeth undergoing active eruption, it has been suggested that the fiber bundles consist of three separate sections. One section is located near the cementum, one towards the alveolar bone and one area of splicing known as the intermediate plexus is located midway between the root and the bone. This plexus has not been identified in fully erupted human teeth. The average width of the periodontal ligament of an adult tooth in function is 0.18 mm. However, it has an hourglass shape, being widest in the coronal aspect, slightly narrower near the apex, and narrowest in the middle of the alveolus in the area of rotation. Periodontal ligament fibers have a structural necessity to withstand intensive forces from mastication and to accommodate tooth eruption.

Arrangement of Principal Fibers

The principal fibers are arranged in six groups (Fig. 5.10):

Transseptal Group

- These fibers insert in the cementum of adjacent teeth and extend interproximally over the alveolar crest
- In periodontal disease, these fibers get reconstructed even after destruction of the alveolar bone.

Alveolar Crest Group

- These fibers run obliquely from the cementum below the junctional epithelium to the alveolar crest
- They aid in prevention of the extension of teeth
- In addition, they resist lateral movements of tooth
- Tooth mobility is not remarkably increased by their incision.

Horizontal Group

- This group of fibers runs at right angles to the long axis of the tooth from the cementum to the alveolar bone.

Oblique Group

- These fibers are considered as the largest group in the periodontal ligament which extends from the cementum in a coronal direction obliquely to the bone
- They bear vertical occlusal stress and convert them into tension onto the alveolar bone.

Apical Group

- These fibers radiate from the cementum to the bone at the fundus of the socket
- They are not present on incompletely formed roots.

Interradicular Fibers

- These fibers fan out from the cementum to the teeth on the furcation areas of multirooted teeth.

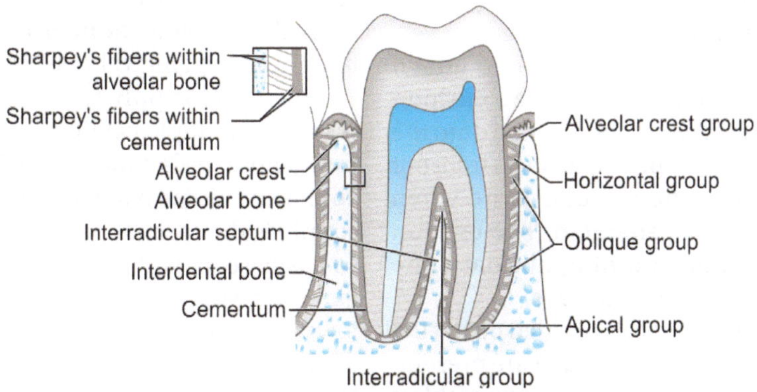

Fig. 5.10: Principal groups of periodontal ligament fibers and their terminal portion *(For color version, see Plate 8)*

The ends of the principal fibers are embedded in cementum on the tooth side and in the alveolar bone proper on the opposite side. The embedded portions of the principal fibers are known as Sharpey's fibers. Surrounding the collagen fibers is a loose type of connective tissue within which cells, blood, lymph vessels and nerves are found.

The blood vessels found in the periodontal ligament are branches from three sources: the apical vessels that supply the teeth, the vessels in the interproximal alveolar bone, and the gingival vessels.

Following are the principal cells found in the periodontal ligament.

- Undifferentiated mesenchymal cells
- Fibroblasts
- Osteoblasts
- Osteoclasts
- Cementoblasts
- Epithelial rests of Malassez.

With the exception of the epithelial rests of Malassez, which are the remnants of the Hertwig root sheath, these cells are involved in the destruction and formation of the tissues of the periodontal ligament, cementum and alveolar bone proper. Small, irregularly shaped calcified structures as cementicles are found in the periodontal ligament.

Following are the functions of the periodontal ligament:

- Mechanical functions
- Formative function
- Nutritive function
- Sensory function.

The mechanical functions are to attach the tooth to the bone and provide a cushion that partially absorbs forces directed onto the teeth. In addition, the principal fibers transmit tension forces to the alveolar bone when occlusal forces are generated. The tension is important in maintaining normal bone position and trabecular patterns.

The formative function is carried out by the many connective tissue cells that are present. Throughout the life of the tooth, cementoblast are continuously forming collagen, and osteoblasts are forming bone. Without an intact periodontal ligament, continuous deposition of cementum and bone is not possible.

The nutritive function is performed by the blood supply of the periodontal ligament when they carry food products to the cells of the area.

The nerves perform the sensory function. Both pain and proprioceptive receptors are present and play an important role in movement of mandible.

The periodontal ligament has also been known as the periodontal membrane. However, since its principal structure and functions resemble those of a ligament more than those of a membrane, the preferred term is periodontal ligament.

Vascular Supply

The blood supply to the periodontium is derived from the following branches of the superior and inferior alveolar arteries.

Supraperiosteal arteries are on the facial, lingual, and palatal surfaces of the alveolar bone.

Interdental arteries are located within the interproximal bone that exit at the crest of the interproximal alveolar processes to supply the gingiva and periodontal ligament.

Periodontal ligament arterioles are the blood vessels found in the periodontal ligament. These branches form from three sources—the apical vessels that supply the teeth, the vessels in the interproximal alveolar bone, and the gingival vessels (Fig. 5.11).

The blood supply to the gingiva is profuse with multiple capillary loops extending throughout the lamina propria and into each connective tissue papilla. This profuse blood supply is the reason for the color variations so easily seen, with the vascular changes of gingivitis. The lymphatic drainage usually follows the blood supply, with the major portion of the lymph drainage from the gingiva going to the submandibular lymph nodes.

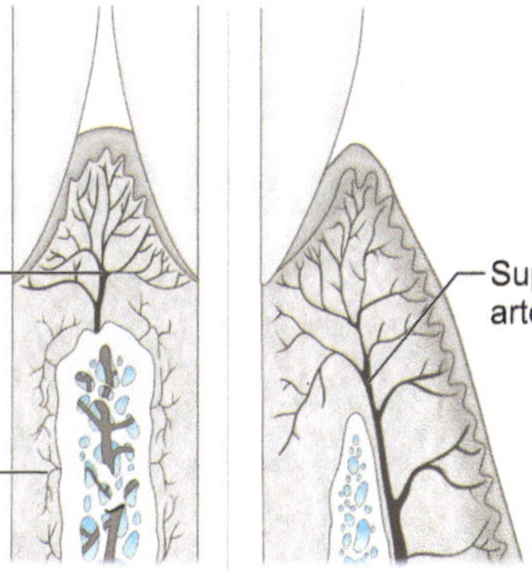

Fig. 5.11: Mesiodistal section of an interproximal area of the periodontium illustrating vascular supply on facial or lingual surface of tooth

Nerve Supply

The innervation of the gingiva is derived from the maxillary and mandibular branches of the trigeminal nerve. Innervation of gums of maxillary arch is derived from the superior alveolar nerves (front, middle and rear branches), infraorbital nerve, and more, the Palatine hill and nasopalatine nerves. Innervation of gums of mandibular arch is derived from mental nerves, nervous tissue, and sublingual branch of the lingual nerve.

ALVEOLAR BONE

The alveolar bone is made up of bony processes that project from the basal portions of the mandible and maxilla. These processes are composed principally of cancellous or spongy bone.

Blood and Nerve Supply of Teeth and Associated Structures

CHAPTER 6

INTRODUCTION

The blood supply of the face, oral cavity and pharynx is extremely abundant. Arterial anastomoses will provide for collateral circulation if vessels are interrupted. The vessels from one side will furnish blood to other through connections in the midline. The veins are more superficial in their location and to form accessory vessels, even plexuses. The blood supply of the face and its various organs is derived from external carotid artery, and the blood eventually finds its way to the internal jugular vein. The veins more or less accompany the arteries and carry the same names.

The nerve concerned with the structures of the face and oral tissues is the peripheral nerve, which is of cranial origin. They are classified as somatic or visceral. The former are concerned with body adjustment to environment which is under the control of the will, whereas the latter have to do with body maintenance. Somatic nerve has both sensory (afferent) and motor (efferent) neurons, and some cranial nerves also have ganglia in which nerve cells are located outside the brain. Oral cavity, teeth, jaws, muscles and face is primarily supplied by two cranial nerves, trigeminal nerve (V) and facial nerve (VII).

EXTERNAL CAROTID ARTERY

External carotid artery is a major source of blood supply to the head and neck. It arises from the common carotid artery where it branches mainly into external and internal carotid artery and supplies blood to the face, jaw and teeth.

Branches of External Carotid Artery

Following are the branches of external carotid artery (Fig. 6.1):

- Superior thyroid
- Lingual
- Facial
- Ascending pharyngeal
- Posterior auricular
- Occipital
- Maxillary
- Superficial temporal.

External carotid artery, just above its division from the common carotid artery, gives off the lingual artery, which supplies the tongue.

Above lingual artery, it give off the facial artery which supplies the soft tissue of the side of the face.

At the level of the lower part of ear, the external carotid divides into maxillary and superficial temporal artery.

Maxillary artery, through various branches, supplies the bones of the jaws, the teeth and their supporting tissue (Fig. 6.2).

Inferior alveolar branch of the maxillary artery supplies mandible and mandibular teeth. It enters the mandible through mandibular foramen.

Posterior superior artery supplies the maxilla and roots of the last maxillary molar teeth, bone and bicuspid teeth.

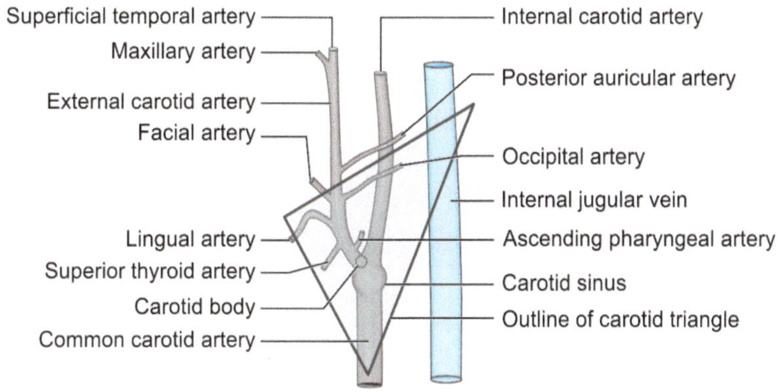

Fig. 6.1: Branches of external carotid artery

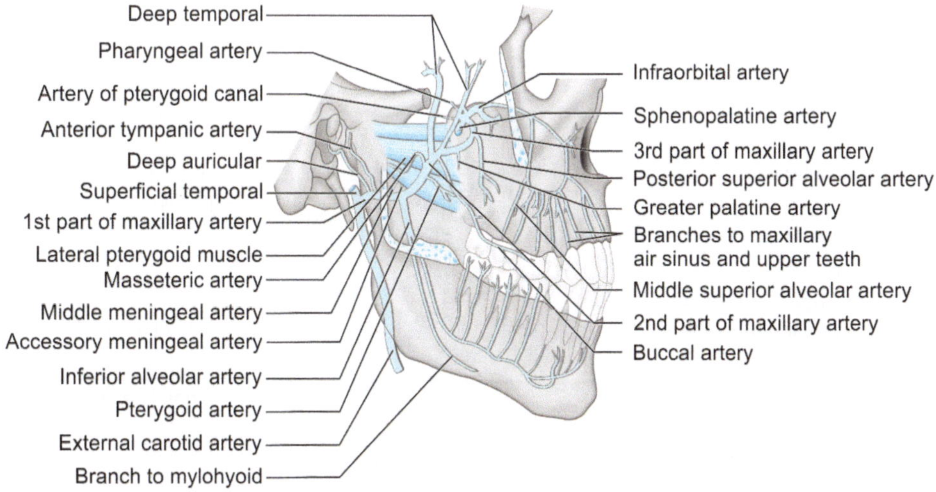

Fig. 6.2: Maxillary artery and its branches

Infraorbital artery supplies incisors and cuspid teeth of the maxilla.

BLOOD SUPPLY OF THE PALATE

Hard palate is supplied by the greater palatine artery, a branch of maxillary artery. It accompanies the greater palatine nerve through greater palatine canal to the roof of the mouth. In the anterior region, it ascends through the incisive canal and anastomoses with sphenopalatine artery in the floor of the nasal cavity.

Soft palate is supplied by the lesser palatine arteries, the branches of maxillary artery. They accompany lesser palatine nerve through lesser palatine foramina and anastomoses with the ascending palatine artery (Fig. 6.3).

NERVE SUPPLY OF THE PALATE

Greater Palatine Nerve

Greater palatine nerve is a branch of maxillary nerve and also carries parasympathetic fibers, emerges from greater palatine foramen and supplies gums, mucous membrane and glands of the hard palate. It communicates in front with the terminal filaments of the nasopalatine nerve.

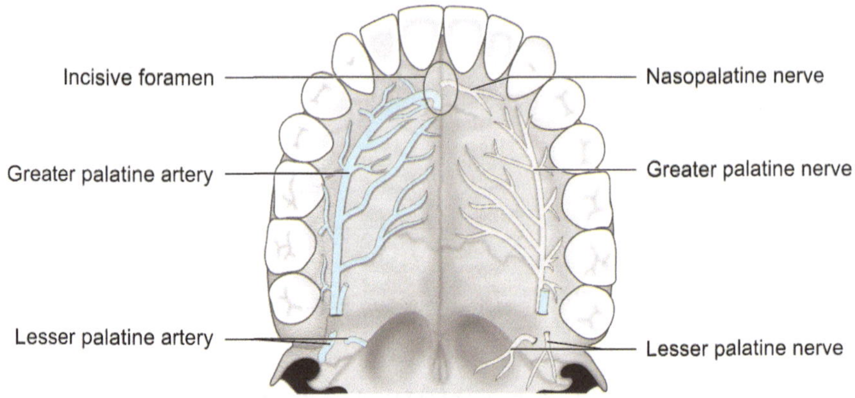

Fig. 6.3: Blood and nerve supply of the palate

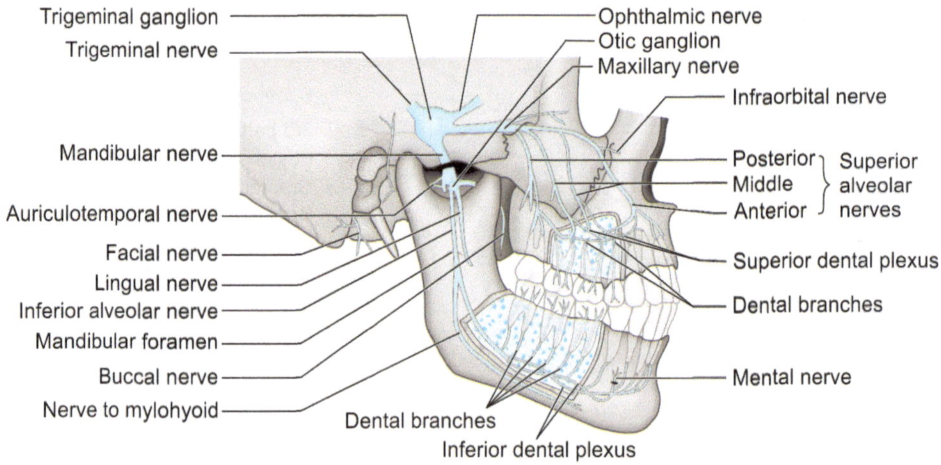

Fig. 6.4: Nerve supply of maxillary teeth

Lesser Palatine Nerve

It is one of the two palatine nerve that descends through the greater palatine canal. It is a branch of the maxillary nerve (V2 cranial nerve). It also has nasal branch that innervate the nasal cavity. It supplies the soft palate, tonsil, and uvula (Fig. 6.3).

NERVE SUPPLY OF THE MAXILLARY TEETH

The maxillary nerve, which in the second division of the trigeminal nerve (V2 cranial nerve), carries sensory fibers to the teeth.

Table 6.1: Nerve supply of the maxillary teeth

Teeth	*Nerve supply*
Anterior teeth (1, 2, 3)	Anterior superior alveolar nerve
Premolars (4, 5) and MB root of 1st molar (6)	Middle superior alveolar nerve
Molars except MB root of 1st molar (6)	Posterior superior alveolar nerve

Abbreviation: MB, Mesiobuccal.

The posterior superior branch of the nerve supplies posterior aspect of the maxillary sinus, maxillary third and second molars, and mucosa around.

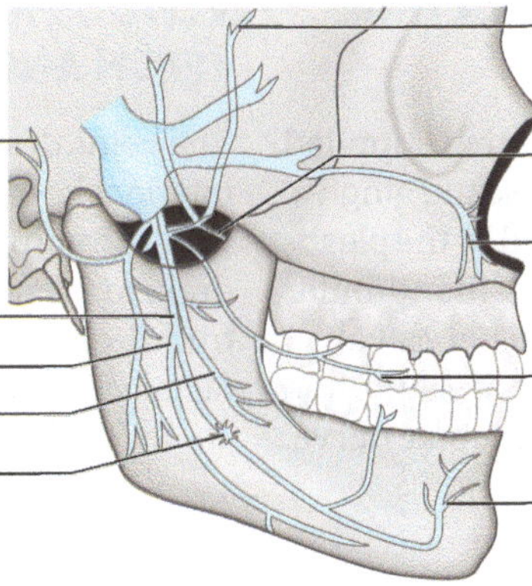

Fig. 6.5: Nerve supply of the mandibular teeth

The middle superior alveolar nerve supplies the medial and lateral aspects of maxillary sinus and the premolars teeth and mesiobuccal root of the first molar, bone and gingiva surrounding it.

The anterior superior alveolar nerve innervates the anterior aspect of the maxillary sinus, incisors and canine teeth as well as bone and mucosa around it (Table 6.1 and Fig. 6.4).

NERVE SUPPLY OF THE MANDIBULAR TEETH

The main nerve supply to the mandibular teeth, the alveolar bone and the periodontal ligament is derived from the inferior alveolar nerve which enters the inferior alveolar canal through the mandibular foramen present on the lingual cortex of the ascending ramus. The nerve travels in the canal through the mandibular foramen present on the lingual cortex of the ascending ramus. At the level of the premolar, the inferior alveolar nerve divides into the incisive nerve and the mental nerve. The incisive nerve continues in the bone and supplies the mandibular anterior teeth and their supporting alveolar bone and periodontal ligament fibers, up to the midline and never crosses over to the other side. The mental nerve makes its exit from the mental foramen situated in the labial mucoperioteum and gingiva of the mandibular anterior teeth, as well as the lining of the lower lip.

The gingiva over the mandibular molars is supplied by the long buccal nerve, which also supplies the mucosa of the cheek up to the level of the corner of the mouth.

The lingual gingival of all the mandibular teeth are supplied by the lingual nerve up to the midline and the lingual nerve also supplies the floor of the mouth and half of the tongue, ipsilaterally (Table 6.2 and Fig. 6.5).

Table 6.2: Nerve supply of the mandibular teeth

Teeth	*Nerve supply*
Anterior teeth (1, 2, 3) and Premolars (4, 5)	• Inferior dental plexus/ mental nerve • Cutaneous coli nerve (branch of cervical plexus C2 and C3) give additional sensory supply for premolars (4, 5) in about 20% of patients
Molars (6, 7, 8)	Long buccal nerve

NERVE SUPPLY TO GINGIVA AND MUCOSA

Lingual gingiva and floor of mouth is supplied by lingual nerve. Mucosa of cheek and gingiva, buccal to molar teeth are supplied by the plexus formed by long buccal branch of mandibular and short buccal branch of facial nerve. Labial gingiva of canine and incisors are supplied by incisive branch of inferior alveolar nerve.

VENOUS RETURN FROM THE TEETH AND THE JAWS

The veins draining the teeth and jaws are the inferior alveolar vein, posterior superior dental vein, infraorbital vein, and palatine vein. They drain to the pterygoid plexus of veins which in turn drains to external jugular vein via deep facial vein.

CHAPTER 7

Cranial Nerves: Trigeminal and Facial Nerve

INTRODUCTION

The 12 pairs of cranial nerves emerge from the brain at various levels (Fig. 7.1). They are numbered according to the order of their emergence. Unlike 31 spinal nerve pairs, which each have a dorsal sensory and a ventral motor root, the cranial nerves may contain afferent (sensory) and/or efferent (motor) fibers. The types of fibers correspond to the function of the nerve. The trigeminal nerve is the major sensory nerve of the face. It has three major divisions: (1) that convey general somatic sensation, touch, pain, and proprioception from the face; (2) mucosa; (3) and supply muscles of mastication. Facial nerve provides innervation to the muscle of facial expression and parasympathetic motor innervations to most of the salivary glands and taste buds of the oral cavity.

TRIGEMINAL NERVE

As it emerges from the lateral surface of the pons, the sensory root is expanded by the presence of many afferent nerve cell bodies into the semilunar ganglion. From the anterior margin; the latter three branches, the ophthalmic, the maxillary, and the mandibular divisions, arise (Fig. 7.2). The motor root accompanies the sensory root and ganglion to join the mandibular nerve near its origin.

Maxillary Division

This passes through the foramen rotundum into the pterygopalatine fossa. Here, it gives off branches to the sphenopalatine ganglion.

The sphenopalatine ganglion is associated with the maxillary nerve, from which it receives its sensory fibers and also with the great superficial petrosal of the facial nerve. It is a small reddish body measuring about 5 mm anteroposteriorly. It lies deep in the pterygomandibular fossa. The vidian nerve supplies parasympathetic and sympathetic fibers.

The branches of the sphenopalatine ganglion contain sensory, vasomotor, and secretory fibers (pharyngeal, palatine, and sphenopalatine).

The pharyngeal branch passes through a bony canal to the mucous membrane of the upper part of the nasopharynx.

The palatine nerves, the major, minor, and medius, pass through the pterygopalatine canal. The major branch emerges through the greater palatine foramen to supply the mucosa and glands of the hard palate. The minor passes through the lesser foramen and enters the soft palate and uvula. They are sensory and not motor nerves. The motor fibers are supplied by the spinal accessory through the vagus branches of the pharyngeal plexus. The medius passes through the lesser foramen also

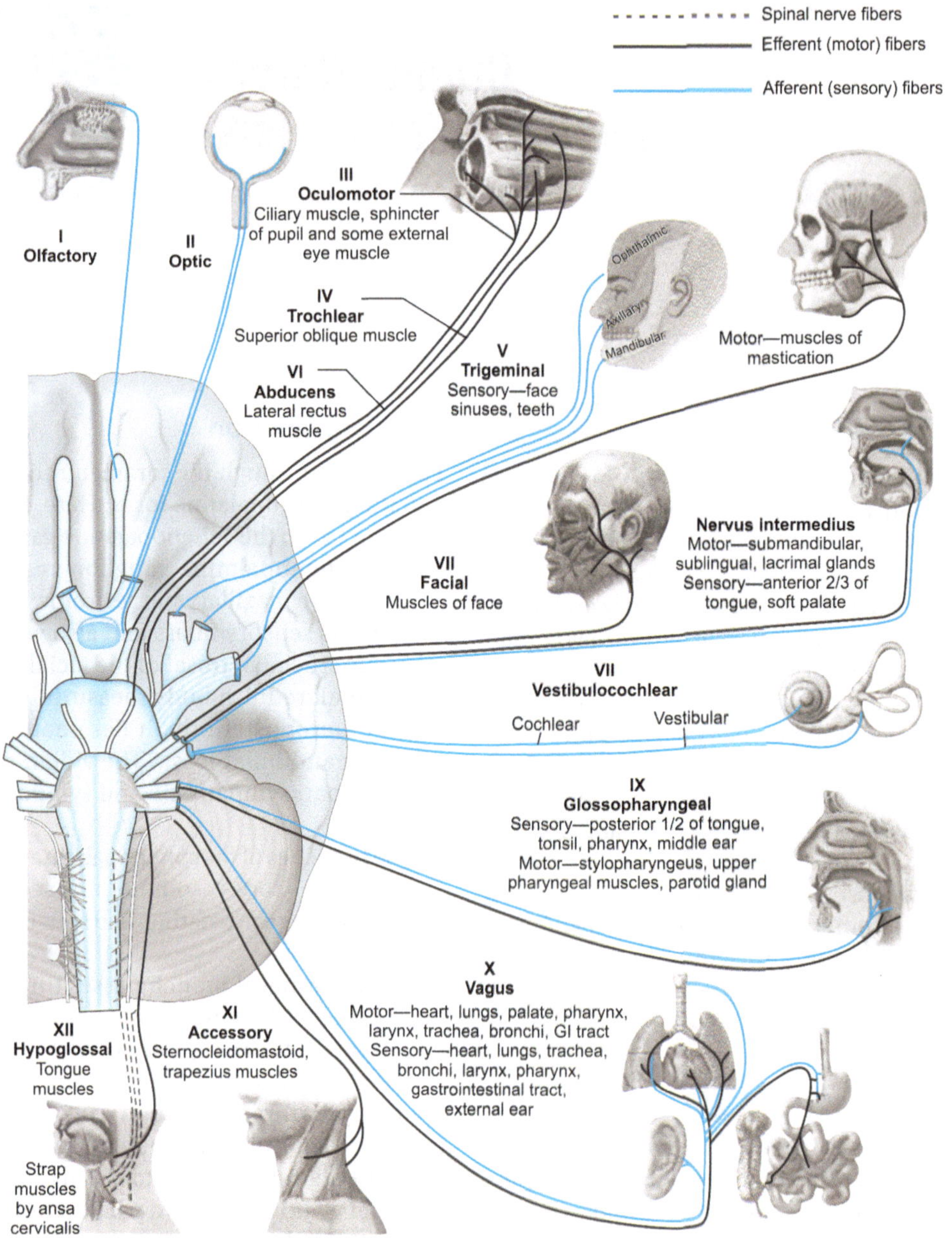

Fig. 7.1: Summary of cranial nerves

and supplies twigs to the tonsil and adjacent part of the soft palate.

A sphenopalatine branch, the largest of the superior nasal branches, which supply the turbinates, nasal septum, and mucosa of the ethmoids, passes through the nasal cavity along the nasal septum and emerges through the incisive foramen to supply the anterior part of the hard palate.

The maxillary division, in addition, gives off the posterior superior alveolar branches, and in the infraorbital canal, where it is called the infraobital, the middle and anterior superior nerve. Upon emerging from the infraorbital

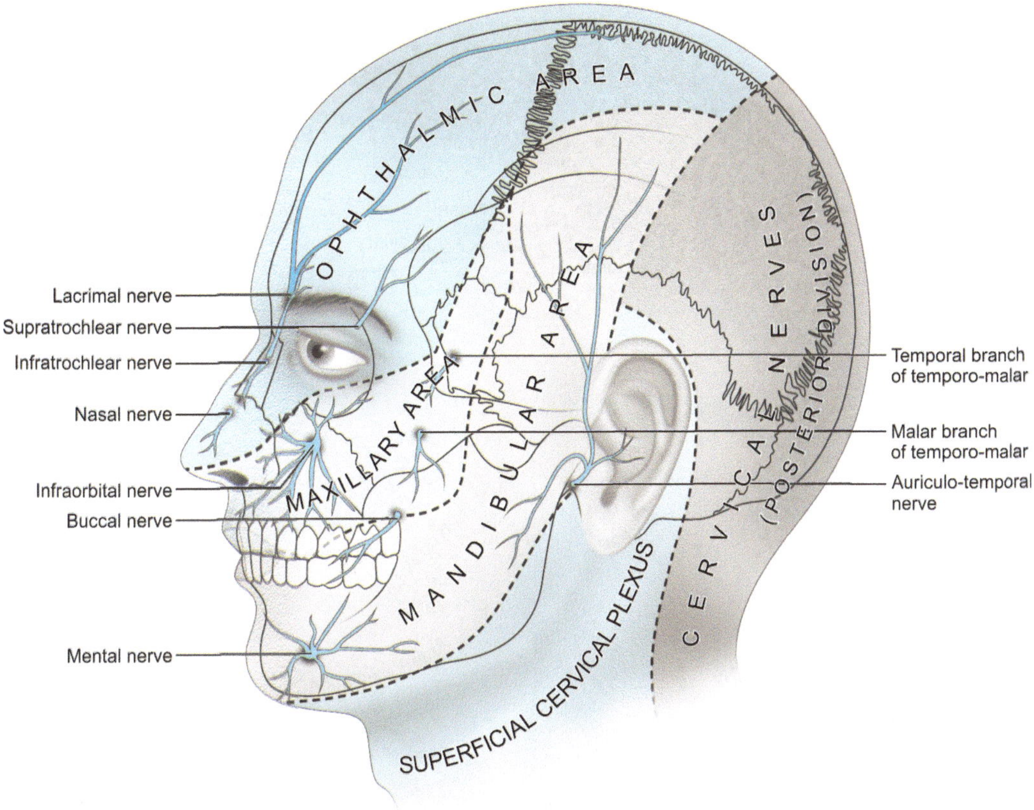

Fig. 7.2: General distribution of trigeminal nerve

foramen, the nerve divides into inferior palpebral, superior labial, and external and internal nasal branches.

The posterior superior alveolar nerves, usually two to three in number, branch off in the pterygopalatine fossa and enter the maxilla above the tuberosity to supply the molar teeth and their investing tissue.

The middle superior alveolar nerve and the anterior superior alveolar nerve with the posterior branches form the superior dental plexus. The middle branch, which descends in a canal, supplies also the mucosa of the maxillary sinus besides the bicuspids. The anterior branch, the largest, descends in the anterior wall of the sinus and supplies the canines and incisors as well as the mucosa of the inferior meatus and anterior part of the nasal cavity. From the plexus, branches are given off to the pulps, periodontal membrane, bone, and covering gingivae. Figure 7.3 illustrates branches of trigeminal nerve.

Mandibular Division

It passes through the foramen ovale into the infratemporal fossa. The following are its motor and sensory branches.

The motor branches are contained in the smaller anterior division and innervate the muscles of mastication, the temporal, masseter, and both pterygoids. The nerve to the internal pterygoids furnishes a visceral motor root to the otic ganglion and small twig to the tensor tympani and tensor palati. The masseteric branch gives off a twig to the mandibular articulation.

The buccinator nerve, which also gives sensory supply to the cheek, passes downward between the two heads of the external

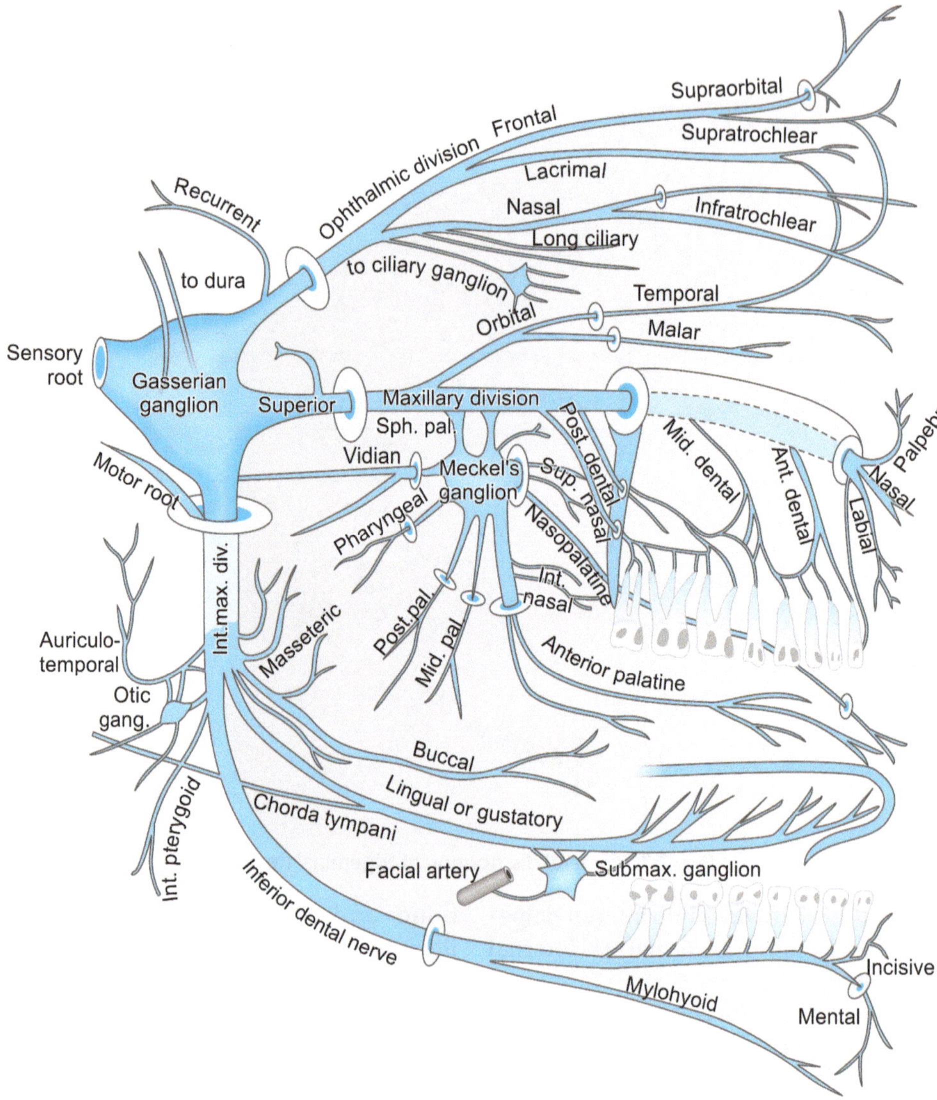

Fig. 7.3: Branches of trigeminal nerve

Abbreviations: Int. max. div., Internal maxillary division; Sph. pal., Sphenopalatine; Post., Posterior; Mid., Middle; Ant., Anterior; Sup., Superior; Inf. nasal-inferior nasal; Mid. pal., Middle palatine; Post. pal., Posterior palatine; Gang. ganglion; Int. pterygoid, Internal pterygoid.

pterygoid muscle. It pierces the sheath of the lower and more tendinous part of the temporal muscle. It passes downward and forward in a lateral direction and breaks into small branches on the external surface of the buccinator muscle. It pierces the muscle and supplies sensation to the mucosa of the cheek as far as the angle of the mouth.

The inferior alveolar nerve descends to the mandibular foramen being, located between the sphenomandibular ligament and the ramus of the mandible. Before entering the foramen, it gives off mylohyoid branch innervating the mylohyoid muscle and the anterior belly of the digastric. It then proceeds through the mandibular canal, supplying the

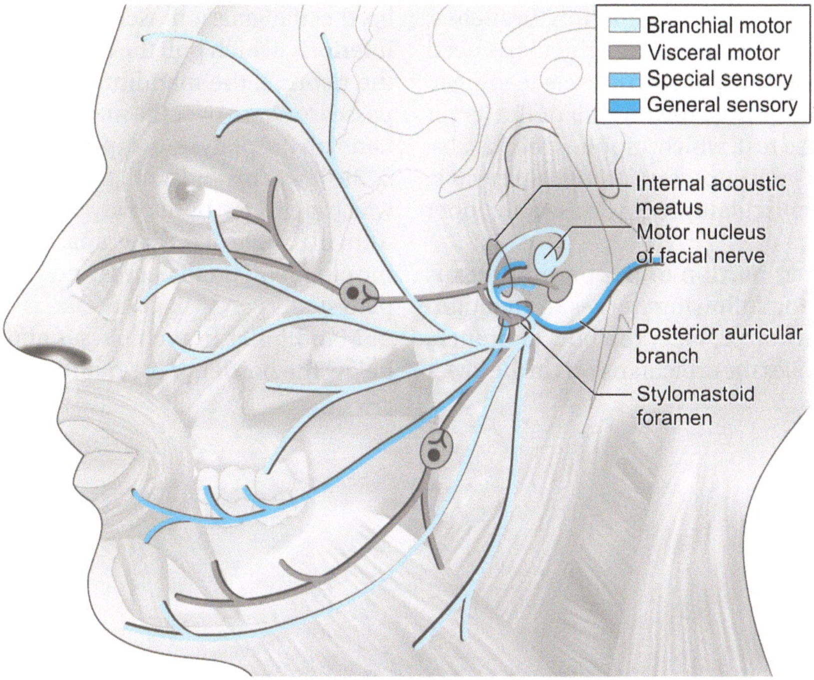

Fig. 7.4: Course of facial nerve

mandibular teeth, including the incisors. It gives off a branch, the mental, which exits through the mental foramen to give sensory supply to the chin and lower lip.

The lingual nerve, after receiving the chorda tympani branch from the facial nerve, runs downward and then forward on the hyoglossus muscle and then passes beneath the submaxillary duct to reach the ventral surface of the tongue. The anterior two-thirds of the tongue is supplied with sensation by the trigeminal nerve.

The mylohyoid nerve leaves the inferior alveolar nerve near the mandibular foramen. It runs forward in the mylohyoid groove and supplies the anterior belly of the digastric and the mylohyoid muscle.

FACIAL NERVE

The facial nerve leaves the cranial cavity by way of the internal acoustic meatus and follows the facial canal to emerge at the stylomastoid foramen, where it gives off branches to the stylohyoid muscle and digastricus (Fig. 7.4). It then runs forward through the substance of the parotid gland. As it is traversing the facial canal, it gives off the greater superficial petrosal nerve which eventually reaches the sphenopalatine ganglion and also the chorda tympani branch which joins the lingual nerve containing special visceral afferent fibers which, as was already stated, take care of the sense of taste of the anterior two-thirds of the tongue. It also gives off fibers which go to the submaxillary ganglion.

In the parotid gland, the nerve divides into branches which leave the anterior border, forming the parotid plexus which varies considerably in different individuals.

The upper portion of the parotid plexus supplies the temporofacial region and consists of the following branches: the temporal branches, which supply the anterior auricularis muscle and the frontalis corrugator supercilii muscle; the zygomatic branches, the temporal part of which supplies the auriculofrontalis and the upper part of the orbicularis oculi muscle, and the remaining branches, which supply the rest of the orbicularis oculi muscle and the zygomatic muscle leading to the orbicularis oris; the buccal, of the larger size than the rest, which supplies the nasalis, quadratus labii superioris, and caninus, i.e. the entire musculature of the nose and upper lip.

The lower portion of the parotid plexus furnishes the following nerves to the mandibular part of the face; the buccal branch, which supplies the orbicularis oris of the lower lip, the triangularis muscle and quadratus labii inferioris, which pull the lower lip down, and the risorius; the mandibular branch, which passes forward over the masseter muscle and beneath the platysma, supplying the muscles of the lower lip and chin; the cervical branch, which is covered by the platysma and descends from the angle of the jaw, anastomosing with the cutaneous colli nerves and supplying the platysma.

Mandibular branch passes about 1–2 cm below the border of the mandible.

Muscles of Mastication

CHAPTER 8

INTRODUCTION

The muscles which are required for mastication (chewing) are known as the muscles of mastication. These muscles help in moving the mandible and not the maxilla as the maxilla is a fixed bone.

Mastication, the initial phase in digestion, is a process by which food gets crushed and ground by teeth. The masticatory process facilitates the surface area of food to permit more effectual breakdown by enzymes.

Muscles of mastication can be divided into two muscles. Which are as follows (Fig. 8.1):

- Primary muscles:
  - Masseter
  - Temporalis
  - Lateral pterygoid
  - Medial pterygoid.
- Accessory muscles:
  - Suprahyoid group of muscles: Muscles which are above the hyoid bone
    - ◊ Digastric
    - ◊ Stylohyoid

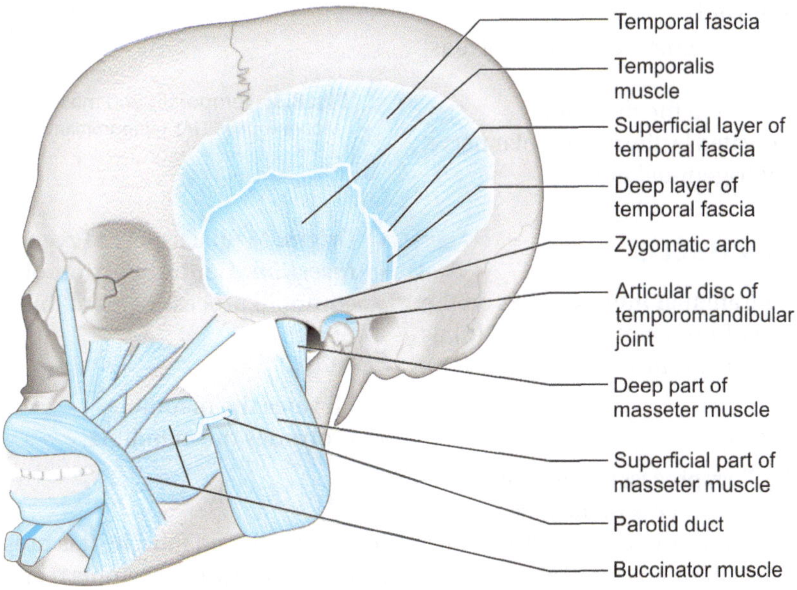

Fig. 8.1: Muscles involved in mastication *(For color version, see Plate 9)*

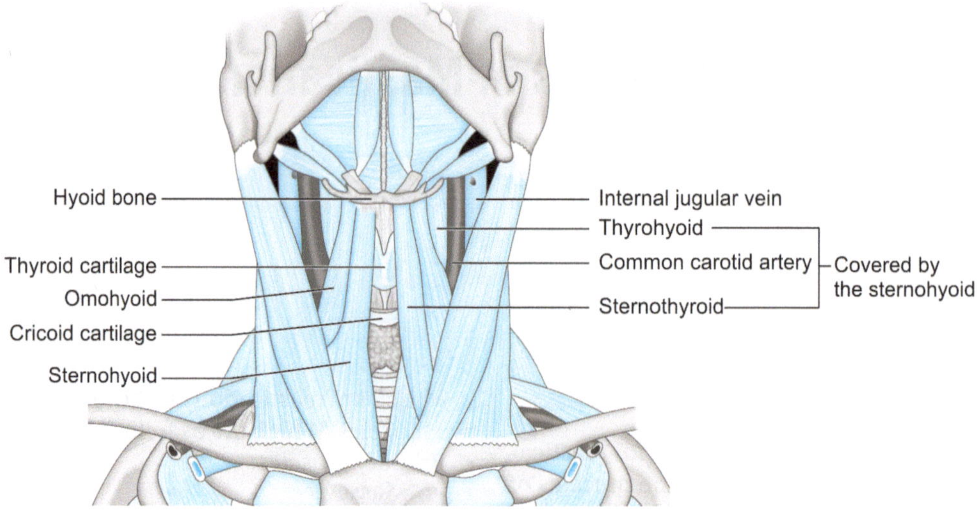

Fig. 8.2: Infrahyoid muscles of mastication

◊ Mylohyoid
◊ Geniohyoid.

- Infrahyoid group of muscles: Muscles which are below the hyoid bone (Fig. 8.2)
  ◊ Sternohyoid
  ◊ Thyrohyoid
  ◊ Omohyoid.

Common characteristic of muscles of mastication are:

- All are inserted to the mandible
- All are innervated by the mandibular nerve, a branch of trigeminal nerve.

MASSETER MUSCLE

It is a flat, quadrangular muscle. It lies on the lateral surface of ramus of mandible. It has two parts; superficial and deep part (Fig. 8.3).

Superficial Part

- *Origin:* Maxillary process of zygomatic bone and zygomatic process of maxilla
- *Insertion:* Angle of the mandible and posterior part of ramus on lateral surface.

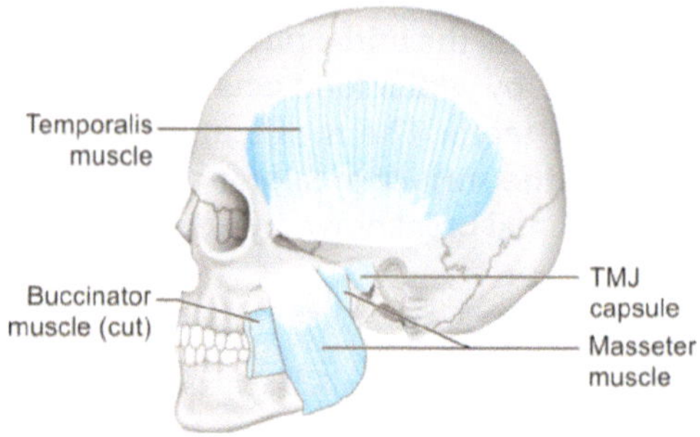

Fig. 8.3: Temporalis and masseter muscles
Abbreviation: TMJ, temporomandibular joint.

Deep Part

- *Origin:* Medial aspect of zygomatic arch
- *Insertion:* Central portion of ramus and coronoid process of mandible.

Functions

- Elevates the mandible
- Protrudes the mandible.

TEMPORALIS MUSCLE

It is a fan-shaped muscle. It is present on the side of the head at the temple region (Fig. 8.3).

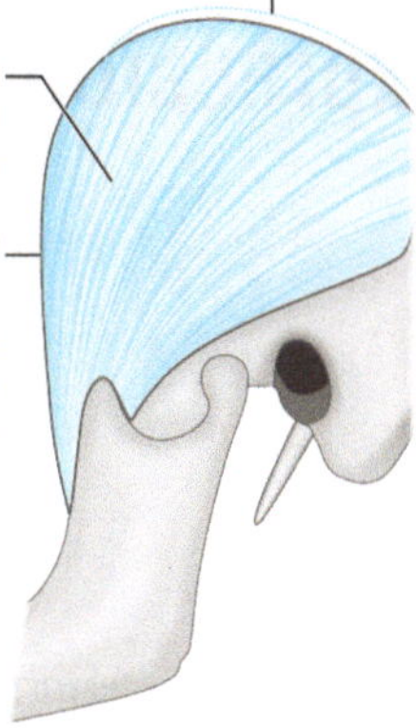

Fig. 8.4: Insertion of temporalis muscle

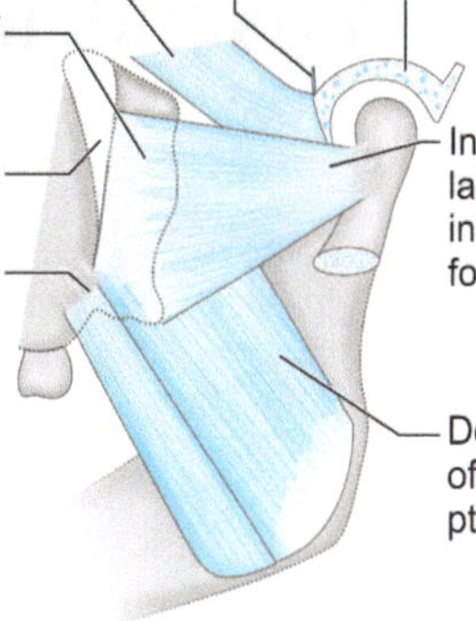

Fig. 8.5: Lateral and medial pterygoid muscles

- *Origin:* From the floor of temporal fossa and from the temporalis fascia.
- *Insertion*:
  - At the apex and deep surface of the coronoid process of mandible
  - Along the anterior border of the ramus (Fig. 8.4).

Function

- Elevates the mandible
- Retracts the mandible.

LATERAL PTERYGOID OR EXTERNAL PTERYGOID MUSCLE

It is a thick and triangular muscle. It has two heads. It is the muscle of mastication that occupies primarily a horizontal position (Fig. 8.5).

- *Origin*:
  - Superior portion—infratemporal surface of greater wing of sphenoid.
- *Inferior portion*:
  - Lateral surface of lateral pterygoid.
- *Insertion*: Fibers are directed backward and laterally to attach to the neck of condyle.

Function

- Depresses the mandible
- Protrudes the mandible
- Side-to-side movement of mandible.

MEDIAL PTERYGOID OR INTERNAL PTERYGOID MUSCLE

It is almost a mirror image of the master muscle. It is rhomboidal and runs practically in the same direction on the inner surface of the ramus of mandible (Fig. 8.5).

- *Origin*:
  - Medial surface of lateral pterygoid plate
  - Posterior surface of the tubercle of palatine bone
  - Tuberosity of maxilla.
- *Insertion*:
  - Medial surface of ramus of the mandible.

Function

- Elevates the mandible
- Protrudes the mandible
- Side to side movements.

Muscles of Facial Expression

CHAPTER 9

INTRODUCTION

The facial muscles, group of about 20 flat skeletal muscles, lies under the facial skin (Fig. 9.1). They originate from the skull or fibrous structures and radiate to the skin through an elastic tendon. However, they are not enclosed by a fascia except the buccinators in contrast to other skeletal muscles.

MUSCLES OF THE MOUTH

- *Orbicularis oris muscle:* Encircles the mouth
- *Buccinator muscle:* Maxilla and mandible (around angle of the mouth). It forms the muscular base of the cheek
- *Levator labii superioris muscle:* Above the infraorbital foramen (upper lip)
- *Depressor labii inferioris muscle:* Mandible underneath the mental foramen (lower lip)
- *Levator labii superioris alaeque nasi muscle:* Medial orbital wall (upper lip and nostrils)
- *Mentalis muscle:* Forms the furrow between chin and lip
- *Risorius muscle (laughing muscle):* Cheek (angle of the mouth)
- *Levator anguli oris muscle:* Underneath the infraorbital foramen (angle of the mouth)
- *Depressor anguli oris muscle:* Lower border of mandible (angle of the mouth)
- *Zygomaticus major and minor muscles:* Zygomatic arch (angle of the mouth).

MUSCLES OF THE NOSE

- *Nasalis muscle:* Maxilla (nasal cartilages)
- *Procerus muscle:* Nasal bridge (skin between eyebrows).

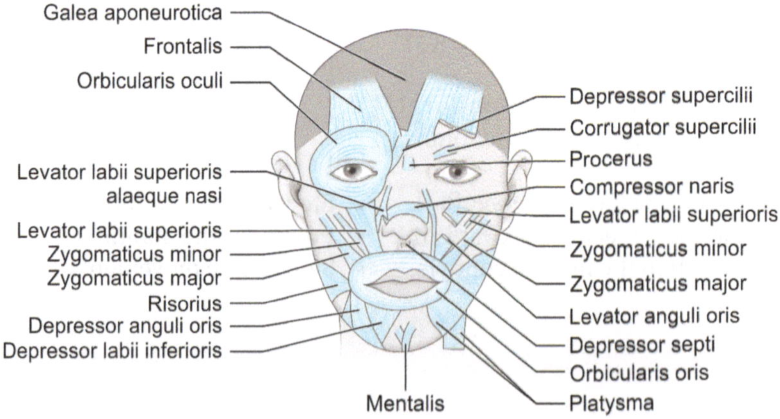

Fig. 9.1: Facial muscles

MUSCLES OF THE EYELID

- *Orbicularis oculi muscle:* Encircles the eye
- *Depressor supercilii muscle:* Medial angle of eye (skin of the eyebrow)
- *Corrugator supercilii muscle:* Above the root of the nose (skin of the eyebrow).

MUSCLES OF THE CRANIUM AND NECK

- *Epicranius muscle:* Forehead, outer surface of the back of the head (occipitofrontalis muscle), above the ear (temporoparietal muscle) fibrous layer on the scalp (galea aponeurotica)
- *Platysma muscle:* Above the mandible (parotid fascia) at the height of the 2nd rib (pectoral fascia).

Biologically, the primary function of the facial muscles is to regulate the facial openings, and the various facial expressions are secondary effects of their contraction (Table 9.1). A few of the common facial expressions and the muscles producing them are given below:

- *Smiling and laughing:* Zygomaticus major
- *Sadness:* Levator labii superioris and levator anguli oris
- *Grief:* Depressor anguli oris
- *Anger:* Dilator naris and depressor septii
- *Frowning:* Corrugator supercilii and procerus
- *Horror, terror and fright:* Platysma
- *Surprise:* Frontalis
- *Doubt:* Mentalis
- *Grinning:* Risorius
- *Contempt:* Zygomaticus minor.

The different action of facial muscles along with their origin and insertion has been depicted in Table 9.2.

FACIAL PARALYSIS

Loss of lower motor neurons causes complete ipsilateral facial paralysis. For example, right of the face paralyzed. Depending on the side of the lesion, additional deficit may be present (decreased lacrimation or salivation, loss of taste sensations). During mastication, food accumulates in the cheek and labial function is impaired.

In loss of upper motor neurons of the facial nerve, only lower part of the face is paralyzed, but the ability to wrinkle the forehead and closer of the eye is intact.

Table 9.1: Functional groups of facial muscles

Opening	*Sphincters*	*Dilators*
Palpebral fissure	Orbicularis oculi	• Levator palpebrae superioris • Occipitofrontalis (frontalis)
Oral fissure	Orbicularis oris	All the muscles around the mouth, except for the orbicularis oris (sphincter), and the mentalis (does not mingle with orbicularis oris)
Nostrils	Compressor naris	• Dilator naris • Depressor septi • Medial slip of levator labii superioris alaeque nasi

Table 9.2: Facial muscles

Muscle	*Origin*	*Insertion*	*Action*
Corrugator supercilii	Medial end of superciliary arch	Skin of mid eyebrow	Vertical wrinkling of forehead: Frowning
• Orbicularis oculi – Orbital part, on and around the orbital margin – Palpebral part, in the lids – Lacrimal part, lateral and deep to lacrimal sac	• Medial part of medial palpebral ligament and adjoining bone • Lateral part of medial palpebral ligament • Lacrimal fascia and lacrimal bone	• Concentric rings return to the point of origin • Lateral palpebral raphe • Upper and lower tarsi	• Closes lids tightly: Winking; protects eye from bright light • Closes lids gently, blinking • Dilates lacrimal sac Directs lac puncta into lacus lacrimalis; supports lower lid
• Orbicularis oris – Intrinsic part, deepest stratum, very thin sheet – Extrinsic part, two strata, formed by converging muscles	• Superior incisivus, from maxilla, inferior incisivus, from mandible • Thickest middle stratum, derived from buccinator, thick superficial stratum, derived from elevators and depressors of lips and angles	• Fibromuscular modiolus at the angle of mouth • Lips and the modiolus	Closes and purses the mouth; numerous extrinsic muscles make it most versatile for various types of grimaces
Buccinator, the muscle of cheek	• Upper fibers, from maxilla, opposite molar teeth • Lower fibers, from mandible, opposite molar teeth • Middle fibers, from pterygomandibular raphe	• Upper fibers, straight to upper lip • Lower fibers, straight to lower lip • Middle fibers decussate before passing to the lips	• Flattens cheek against gums and teeth; inhibits the accumulation of food in the vestibule • Blowing action
Platysma	Upper parts of pectoral and deltoid fasciae. Fibers run upwards and medially	Anterior fibers, to the base of mandible; posterior fibers, to the skin of lower face and lip, and may be continuous with risorius	Releases pressure of skin on the underlying veins; depresses mandible; pulls the angle of mouth downwards as in horror or surprise

CHAPTER 10

Occlusion and Malocclusion

INTRODUCTION

Occlusion is the relationship between the maxillary and mandibular teeth when they approach each other, during chewing or at rest.

Malocclusion is the leading cause of a number of health and dental problems which is defined as the misalignment of teeth and jaws, or more simply a bad bite.

IDEAL OCCLUSION

"Ideal" is a hypothetical concept or a standardized goal. "Normal" implies to the variations around an average mean value.

It is a state of relationship existing when all the teeth are perfectly in the arches of the jaws and they have a normal anatomic relationship to each other. When the teeth are brought into contact, the cusp-fossa relationship is regarded as the most perfect relationship that can be achieved (Figs 10.1A and B).

FUNCTIONAL OCCLUSION

Any tooth contacts made within the functional range, i.e. according to the size of the opposing tooth surfaces. This is an occlusion which is seen during mastication.

BALANCED OCCLUSION

A balanced occlusion is that which is in harmony with temporomandibular joints and the neuromuscular system. It allows an increase in the amount of surface contact in centric closure and offers as much closure contact as possible for horizontal chewing.

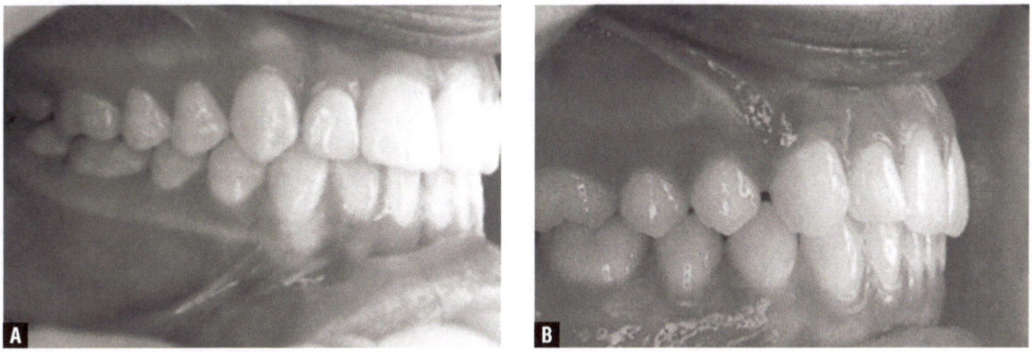

Figs 10.1A and B: (A) Ideal occlusion; (B) Normal occlusion

CENTRIC OCCLUSION

The relation of opposing occlusal surface that provides the maximum planned contact and/or intercuspation. It should exist when the mandible is in centric relation to the maxilla.

CENTRIC RELATION

It is the relationship of the mandible to the maxilla when the condyles are in their most retruded and uppermost position.

CLASSIFICATION OF MALOCCLUSION

Classification of different forms of malocclusion set up by EH Angle, an American orthodontist, is described in Figure 10.2.

The mesiobuccal cusp of the maxillary first molar occludes in the buccal groove of the mandibular first molar.

The mesiolingual cusp of the maxillary first molar occludes in the central fossa of the mandibular first molar.

- *Class I malocclusion:* The molar teeth are in normal occlusion and the mesiobuccal cusp of maxillary first molar fits into the buccal groove of the mandibular first molar
- *Class II malocclusion*: The mandibular molars are one cusp distal to their normal position. The mesiobuccal cusp of the maxillary first molar fits in the interproximal spaces between the mandibular second bicuspid and first molar
  - *Division I:* Labioversion of the maxillary incisors, deep overbite, mouth
  - *Subdivision:* Unilateral distoclusion
  - *Division II:* Retruding or bunched maxillary incisors, deep overbite
  - *Subdivision:* Unilateral distoclusion.
- *Class III malocclusion:* The mandibular molars are one cusp mesial to their position. The mesiobuccal cusp of the maxillary first molar fits into the interproximal space between the first and second mandibular molars
- *Class IV malocclusion:* The teeth are in mesioclusion on one side and distoclusion on the opposite side.

OVERJET AND OVERBITE

Overjet describes the horizontal projection of the maxillary central incisors over the mandibular incisors. Overbite describes the vertical overlapping of the maxillary central incisors over the mandibular incisors.

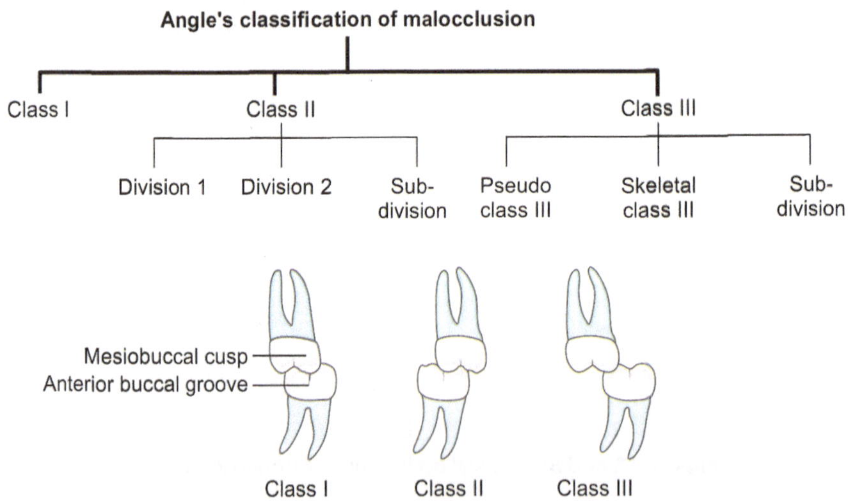

Fig. 10.2: Angle's classification of malocclusion

CHAPTER 11

Alveolar Process

INTRODUCTION

Alveolar process is that part of the jaws which supports and attaches the teeth. It consists of two parts:

1. Alveolar bone proper, which forms the socket wall and gives attachment to periodontal ligament.
2. Supporting bone, consisting of buccal and lingual cortical plates and the cancellous bone in between these plates and the socket walls.

The socket wall is also known as the cribriform plate because of the presence of numerous holes produced by blood vessels. The alveolar process is dependent upon the presence of teeth and is formed after the teeth erupt into the oral cavity. It is reabsorbed after the teeth are lost. The presence of basal bone is independent of the teeth.

CORTICAL PLATE

They are matured lamellated bone. It consists of dense, lamellated haversian system. At the mouth of the tooth sockets, the surface cortical bone is continuous with the alveolar bone proper. The thickness varies in different persons, in different arches and in different areas of the jaws. In general, it is thicker in mandible than in maxilla, thicker posteriorly than anteriorly and thicker lingually than labially. The labial aspects of the plates in maxilla show numerous Volkmann's canals or the entry of vessels and nerves. In mandible, these canals are longer but less frequent.

CANCELLOUS BONE

The cancellous bone lies between the cortical plates and alveolar bone proper. It contains marrow spaces and is continuous with the spongiosa of the body of the jaws. The maxilla has more cancellous bone than mandible. The spongiosa is more on the lingual aspect than on the buccal aspect. It is frequently absent in the anterior region. The amount of cancellous bone increases posteriorly. The spongy bone transmits the masticatory forces from alveolar bone proper to cortical plates. Interradicular and interdental septa consist entirely of spongy bone. These septal transmit blood vessels and the radiolucent lines of these on radiographs are called Hirschfeld's canals.

The spongy bone of alveolus contains fatty marrow. Red marrow may be seen in maxillary tuberosity and mandibular posterior region. The trabeculae tend to be arranged in a horizontal plane near the alveolar bone. They are nearly perpendicular in the interradicular area. By this arrangement, it supports the tooth and resists vertical pressure. The teeth with no antagonists show wider marrow spaces and are almost devoid of any trabeculae. The trabeculae act as buttresses and are referred to as trajectories.

CRIBRIFORM PLATE OR ALVEOLAR BONE PROPER

It is that layer of compact bone which forms the bony wall of the tooth socket. It appears radiopaque in radiograph and is called lamina dura. It is sieve-like because it transmits numerous blood vessels and nerves and is called cribriform plate. It consists of bundle bone and lamellated bone. It gives attachment to Sharpey's fibers. Because of constant mesial and occlusal movement of the teeth, this bone is remodeled constantly. There is resorption on the mesial walls and apposition on the distal walls of the sockets.

BONE

Bone is a connective tissue derived from the multipotential embryonic mesenchymal cell. It consists of the following:

- Cells: Osteoblasts, osteocytes and osteoclasts
- Intercellular substance
  - Collagen fibrils
  - Ground substance calcified.

Types

There are three types of bone tissue:

Mature Bone

They show incremental lines or lamellae and are called lamellated bone. Each lamella is 4–12 μ thick. These lines are parallel to the outer surface. The osteocytes are evenly distributed. It can be compact or spongy. The compact bone is thick and solid. The lamellae are arranged in the form of concentric cylinders surrounding a narrow canal. Each canal is surrounded by 5–20 lamellae. The whole unit is called Haversian system. The central canal is called Haversian canal. Haversian canals of adjacent units are connected with each other by finer canal called Volkmann's canal. Osteocytes through their canaliculi are in communication with the Haversian canals.

Immature Bone

There are more osteocytes than lamellated bone. The cells are arranged haphazardly. The collagen fibrils are not arranged in orderly fashion and are not lamellated. It contains less ground substance and is less calcified. It is always arranged in trabecular pattern.

Bundle Bone

There is less collagen fibrils. Collagen fibers of periodontal ligament known as Sharpey's fibers are seen embedded in it. There is more ground substance and it is more calcified. This type of bone is restricted to alveolar bone proper.

ALVEOLAR PROCESS OF THE MANDIBLE

The mandible is relatively more massive than the maxilla in the posterior region. The outer and the inner plates are strong and they are thin in the anterior region. In the anterior region, the alveolar bone proper fuses with the outer and inner cortical plates and is thin labiolingually. The premolars and first molars are in intimate relationship with the outer alveolar plate. The third molar is in close relationship with the inner alveolar plate. The relationship of the mandibular canals to the roots of the teeth is very important. Molars and premolars are in relation to the mandibular canal. The apices of the third molar are in close relationship to the mandibular canal. In children, the canal is in close contact with the molars. The mental foramen is situated below the first premolar and may be mistaken as a periapical lesion (Fig. 11.1).

ALVEOLAR PROCESS OF THE MAXILLA

The maxillary sinus and the nasal cavity are in contact with upper teeth. The incisors are situated below the nasal cavity. The premolars and molars are generally situated below

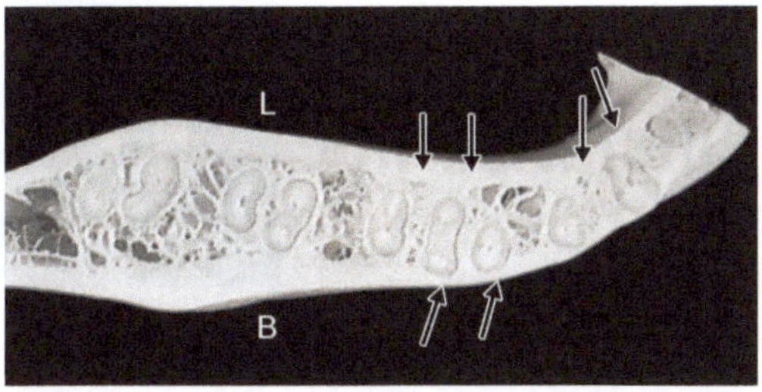

Fig. 11.1: Alveolar process of the mandible (Arrows depict the normal bony surface of the mandible maxilla enclosing the alveolar processes)
Abbreviations: B, buccal; L, lingual

the maxillary sinus. On labial aspect of the anterior teeth, the alveolar bone proper fuses with the external plate to alveolar bone. On the palatal aspect of the anterior teeth, a wedge of spongy bone is seen in between the alveolar bone proper and the inner cortical plate. The relation of the molars with the floor of the maxillary sinus is variable. The apices of the molars and second premolars may lie close to

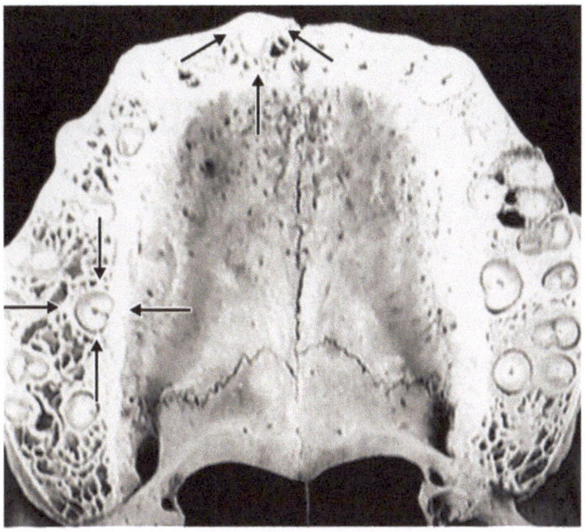

Fig. 11.2: Alveolar process of the maxilla

the floor of the maxillary sinus and may even produce elevation on the floor. On the buccal aspect of the first premolar, the alveolar bone fuses with the outer cortical plate. On the lingual aspect of molars, the alveolar bone proper fuses the inner cortical plate (Fig. 11.2).

CHAPTER 12

Temporomandibular Joint

INTRODUCTION

The temporomandibular joint is a unique joint. It is unique in its anatomy, histology and function. Though, anatomically, there are two joints, a right and a left, yet functionally the joints act as one unit. It is like atlantooccipital joint which is bilateral anatomically but acts as one unit functionally. Therefore, the right and the left joints are really two halves of one joint, the craniomandibular joint (Sicher). Though it is one joint, yet paradoxically there are two compartments—an upper and a lower. No other joint has created so much controversy amongst scientists and investigators regarding its movements during function. The controversy exists because most of the movements are tried on dried skull with no articular cartilage in between. In life, during occlusion, cranial bones and condyle never come in contact, and therefore, the movements in dried skull become unnatural.

STRUCTURE

The temporomandibular joint has the following components:

- Mandibular condyle
- Articular disc
- Synovial cavities
- Mandibular fossa
- Articular capsule.

Mandibular Condyle

It is a semicylindrical structure, the long axis lying at right angle to the ramus. It is convex both anteroposteriorly and mediolaterally. The articular surface is covered by a layer of fibrous tissue consisting of dense collagen and fibroblasts running parallel to articular surface. Lying under this tissue is a plate of hyaline cartilage. Under the cartilage is a layer of calcified cartilage. Under this is a zone of cartilage destruction and under it is the bone. This transition from bone to fibrous tissue is gradual. The growth of condyle occurs in fibrous tissue covering, which is transformed into cartilage and then to bone.

Articular Disc

It is an oval structure attached to the capsule anteriorly, medially and laterally. Its posterior border is thick and is connected with a loose vascular tissue which is attached to the capsule. It consists of dense collagen bundles running in various directions. Elastic fibers are few. The fibroblasts are flat, elongated and has cytoplasmic processes. As age advances, some of these fibroblasts change to cartilage cells. Islands of hyaline cartilage may be seen. Most areas of the disc do not have blood supply except for the posterior part.

Synovial Cavities

The superior and inferior synovial cavities are lined by synovial membrane consisting of thin loose vascular connective tissue thrown into villi. The cavity surface is lined by endothelial cells. They contain clear synovial fluid which lubricates the joint.

Mandibular Fossa

It is concave and situated in the temporal bone. It is covered by dense connective tissue, which is thickest in the anterior part. The deepest layer may be calcified.

Articular Capsule

It consists of dense collagen fibers. It is thick on lateral aspect of the joint and is called the temporomandibular ligament.

ANATOMY

The temporomandibular joint is a bilateral ginglymoarthrodial or sliding hinge joint. The compound synovial joint is formed by mandibular fossa and articular eminence of temporal bone and mandibular condyle with the articular disc interposed in between (Fig. 12.1). The mandible forms joints on both sides of the skull. However, one condyle cannot be moved without moving the other.

The articular disc divides each temporomandibular joint into two compartments.

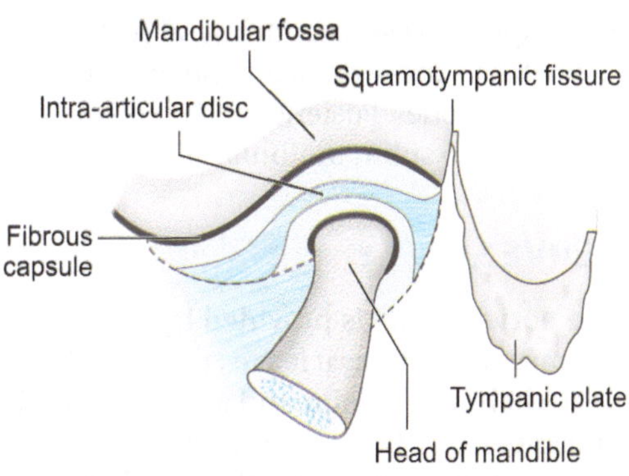

Fig. 12.1: Anatomy of temporomandibular joint

These two compartments are synovial cavities consisting of upper large and lower small synovial cavity. These synovial cavities are filled with the synovial fluid which is produced by the synovial membrane lining the joint capsule.

The condyle of the mandible articulates with temporal bone in the mandibular fossa. The articular surface of the temporal bone has a posterior concave part called as mandible fossa and anterior convex part as articular tubercle or eminence.

The articular eminence has a flat anterior slope and is continuous with infratemporal surface of temporal bone. The portion of temporal bone is connected with spine of sphenoid. The posterior wall is formed by postglenoid process of the temporal bone which lies between mandibular fossa and tympanic bone. The articular fossa is separated from the tympanic bone by the squamotympanic fissure laterally. Medially, this fissure divides into two fissures, an anterior petrosquamosal fissure and a posterior petrotympanic fissure.

The articular fossa is not a functional part of the joint. The fossa comes in contact with only posterior part of articular disc. The condyle rests on the posterior slope of the articular eminence. The fossa is not subjected to any pressure or friction. However, it is the most vulnerable part of the joint during injury. The postglenoid process is not significant functionally. The condyle never braces it in life as is seen to do in dried skull.

Condyle is barrel-shaped measuring 20 mm mediolaterally and 10 mm anteroposteriorly. The perpendicular to ascending ramus of the mandible oriented 10–30° with frontal plane.

The two axis, if extended, form an angle of 150°. If extended medially and posteriorly, the axis would cross at the anterior margin of foramen magnum; this angulation on two sides may be at different axis. The condyle projects to the medial side of the ramus. The sharp border of sigmoid notch leads to lateral tip of condyle and thus three-fourths of condyle lies medial to the ramus and is supported by a triangular buttress.

The capsule surrounds the joint and is loose, funnel-shaped with dense fibrous membrane. It includes articular eminence, the articular disc and the neck of the mandibular condyle.

The temporomandibular ligament is the thickened lateral portion of the capsule, which has two portions, namely, an outer oblique portion and an inner horizontal portion.

The capsule is weak anteriorly and condylar dislocation is not uncommon at this site. The medial aspect of the condyle is strengthened by sphenomandibular ligament. The capsule is attached anteriorly to a muscle, the lateral pterygoid, which pulls the disc forward and downward. Posteriorly, it is attached to the articular fossa, the disc and the condyle.

The intra-articular disc is considered to be the fibrous extension of the capsule which extends between the two articular surfaces of temporomandibular joint. The disc separates the joint into two parts, each with synovial membrane.

The disc also attaches to the condyle medially and laterally by the collateral ligaments. The anterior disc is attached to the joint capsule and the superior head of the lateral pterygoid. The posterior portion attaches to the mandibular fossa and is known as retrodiscal tissue.

Each compartment of the joint cavity has its own synovial membrane, which lines the fibrous capsule and covers the loose retrodiscal pad and is inserted on the neck of the mandible. Therefore, a portion of the neck of the mandible is intracapsular. The synovial membrane is absent over all the four articulating surfaces. The disc is thin at the center. Superior fiber of lateral pterygoid is attached on the articular capsule, the disc and the neck of the condyle. Thus, during the anterior movements of the mandible, the disc also moves forward along with the head on the condyle.

This forward movement of the disc is not due to the pull of the muscle but by virtue of its attachment to both sides of the condyle. The muscle merely stabilizes the disc during mastication.

Anteriorly, the disc blends with the joint capsule and posteriorly, it is attached to the capsule via a highly vascular loose connective tissue known as the retrodiscal pad. When the disc moves anteriorly along with the condyle, the loose connective tissue allows this mobility. The fibrous connective tissue covering the mandibular and temporal surfaces and the central area of the disc is avascular. The avascularity helps in adaptation of the tissue to resist pressure.

The extracapsular ligaments of the joint are:

- The sphenomandibular ligament, extending from the spine of the sphenoid bone to lingual of mandibular foramen. This ligament is a part of remnant of Meckel's cartilage. It supports medial fibers of the capsule.
- The stylomandibular ligament, extending from the styloid process to posterior border of ramus above the angle of the mandible. It separates the submandibular gland from the parotid gland.

BLOOD SUPPLY

- Arterial supply from branches of maxillary artery, branch of external carotid artery
- Veins of the joint drain to superficial temporal veins, pterygoid plexus and maxillary veins
- Lymphatic vessels from lateral surface and anterior surface drain into preauricular and parotid nodes. Posterior and medial surface drain into submandibular nodes.

NERVE SUPPLY

The nerve supply is provided by the auriculotemporal nerve as it leaves the mandibular nerve behind the joint and ascends laterally and superiorly to wrap around the posterior region of the joint. In addition, other nerve innervation is by deep temporal and masseter nerve branches. The articular cartilage and central portion of the disc do not have any nerve supply and blood supply.

DIFFERENT TYPES OF MOVEMENTS

Depression (Opening Movements)

This is a very complicated movement occurring in both upper and the lower of the temporomandibular joints. In the lower compartment, the head of the mandible takes a hinge movement and in the upper compartment the head of the mandible along with the disc takes a gliding movement forwards. In the initial phase, only hinge movement operates and in the later phase, the gliding movement operates. The muscles concerned in this movement are digastric, lateral pterygoid and other suprahyoid muscles. There is combined forward pull of the two lateral pterygoid muscles and backward downward pull of the two anterior bellies of digastric and other suprahyoid muscles. Mandible will rotate around a movable axis which passes through bellies of digastric which further retract the mandible; the pull of suprahyoid muscles will cause a retarded opening movement provided hyoid is stabilized by infrahyoid muscles. Along with contraction of lateral pterygoid, there is relaxation of temporalis, masseter and medial pterygoid muscles (Fig. 12.2).

The movements of mandible are combined results of movements of protrusion, retrusion, depression, elevation and lateral movements. All the muscles that move the mandible are:

- Anterior and posterior belly of digastric
- Geniohyoid
- Muscles of mastication:
  - Lateral pterygoid
  - Medial pterygoid
  - Temporalis
  - Masseter
- Mylohyoid (insignificant, elevates tongue).

All these six pairs of muscles work, as in group. Lateral pterygoid is not the initiator of muscle pull. Some of these muscles act as movers, some act as balancer and some act as holders during any movement. In addition, the muscles of neck and hyoid bone that fixes the head and the hyoid bone, respectively, are also essential. The masseter, medial pterygoid and temporalis are elevator, the lateral pterygoid is the protruser and geniohyoid and digastric are depressors.

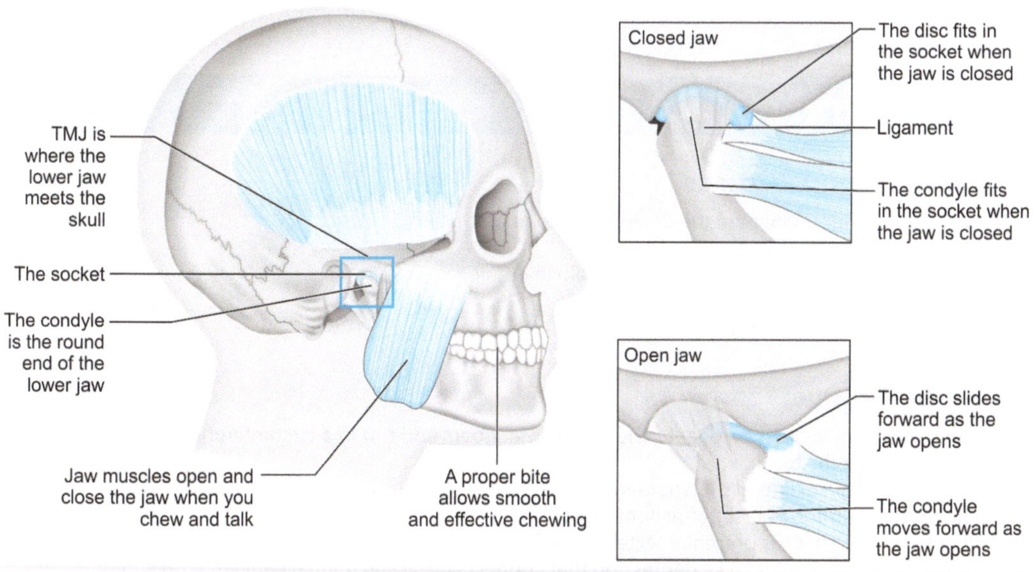

Fig. 12.2: Movement of temporomandibular joint
Abbreviation: TMJ-temporomandibular joint

Elevation (Closing Movements)

This movement is caused by the masseters, two medial pterygoids and two temporal muscles (anterior fibers). During closure with protrusion, the lateral and medial pterygoids contract. The condylar heads remain forward on the articular eminences. During closure with retraction, posterior temporal muscles and masseters contract and the pterygoids relax and the condyles return to glenoid fossa.

Protrusion

The combined pull of the lateral pterygoids moves mandible forward. The posterior horizontal fibers of temporalis relax. The masseters, medial pterygoids and anterior vertical fibers of temporalis remain in tonic contraction and prevent separation of the teeth. The condyles of the mandible with the articular discs move downward and forward by the contraction of lateral pterygoids.

Retrusion

The head of condyle with the articular discs are carried back into the glenoid fossae. The posterior fibers of the temporal muscles of both sides contract along with relaxation of lateral pterygoids. The teeth remain in contact by other muscles.

Lateral Movement

Lateral movements are produced by the combined action of the elevators and retruders on the working side and protruders of the non-working side. The condyle of the side towards which the jaw is moving is carried back into the glenoid fossa by the posterior fibers of the temporalis of that side and held there by the tonic contraction of all the muscles of that side. The other condyle and articular disc is pulled forward and inward by the lateral pterygoids so that the jaw rotates around a vertical axis passing through the fixed condyle.

TEST YOURSELF

Expected Theory Questions

- What is epithelium? What are the different types of epithelium?
- Write a shot note on muscles of tongue.
- What are the various types of gingiva? Explain in detail.
- Elaborate muscles of mastication in detail.
- Write a short note on cranial nerves.

Expected Viva Questions

- Which fibers are located coronal to the transseptal fibers and run in a circumferential or semicircular manner around the tooth?
- What is the origin of lateral pterygoid muscle?
- When is the eruption of first permanent molar occurs?
- What type of cartilage is present in external ear?
- What is the name of valley-like depression that connects facial and lingual papilla?

SECTION

2

General and Dental Physiology and Histology

SECTION OUTLINE

- Development and Growth of Teeth
- Histology of Soft and Hard Dental Tissues
- Salivary Glands
- Saliva
- Blood
- Mastication, Deglutition and Phonation

Development and Growth of Teeth

CHAPTER 13

INTRODUCTION

The tooth germ is formed by an accumulation of cells that eventually forms a tooth. These cells originate from the ectoderm of the first pharyngeal arch and the ectomesenchyme of the neural crest. Tooth germ is composed by three components, namely enamel organ, the dental papilla and the dental sac or follicle.

The enamel organ is made of the outer enamel epithelium, inner enamel epithelium, stellate reticulum and stratum intermedium. These cells give origin to ameloblasts, which forms enamel and, after maturation of enamel, they become part of reduced enamel epithelium. The point where outer and inner enamel epithelium meet is called the cervical loop. The cervical loop cells slowly grow into the deeper tissues giving rise to Hertwig epithelial root sheath, which ultimately gives shape to the root of the tooth. During development of teeth, keratinization and amelogenesis has shown many resemblances between each other. Epithelial cells of tooth germ contain keratin and a recently erupted tooth also shows thin layer of keratin (Nasmyth's membrane or enamel cuticle).

The dental follicle cells differentiate into odontoblasts which form the dentin. Additionally, the crown shape of a tooth is determined by junction between dental papilla and inner enamel epithelium. Mesenchymal cells which are present in dental papilla forms the tooth pulp.

The dental sac or follicle forms three important cell lineages: cementoblasts, osteoblasts, and fibroblasts. Cementoblast lays down the cementum of the tooth. Osteoblasts form alveolar bone around the roots of teeth. Fibroblasts give rise to the periodontal ligament which connects the tooth root to the alveolar bone.

DEVELOPMENT OF TOOTH

Despite the obvious fact that tooth development (as the development of any other organ) is a continual process, it is not only traditional but also didactically necessary to divide the developmental history of a tooth into several "stages". They are named from the shape of the epithelial part of the tooth germ. Since the odontogenic epithelium not only produces enamel but also is indispensable for the initiation of dentin formation, the terms "enamel organ" and "outer and inner enamel epithelium" are best replaced by the terms "dental organ" and "dental epithelium".

The first sign of human tooth development is seen during the sixth week of embryonic life (11 mm embryo). At this stage, the oral epithelium consists of basal layer of high cells and surface layer of flattened cells. The glycogen droplets in their cytoplasm are lost in routine preparations, giving them an empty appearance. The epithelium is separated from the connective tissue by a basement membrane. Certain cells in the basal layer of the oral epithelium begin to proliferate at a more rapid rate than do the adjacent cells. An epithelial thickening arises in the region of the future dental arch and extends along the entire free margin of the jaws. It is the primordium of the ectodermal portion of the teeth that is known as the dental lamina. Mitotic figures are seen not only in the epithelium but also in the adjacent mesoderm.

Dental Lamina

In all teeth except the permanent molars, the dental lamina proliferates at its deep end to give rise to the dental organ of the permanent tooth. While it disintegrates in the region between the dental organ and the oral epithelium, the dental organ is gradually separated from the dental lamina at about the time when the first dentin is formed (Fig. 13.1).

Function of Dental Lamina

The functional activity of the dental lamina and its chronology may be considered in three phases. The first phase is concerned with the initiation of the entire deciduous dentition that occurs during the second month in utero. The second phase deals with the initiation of the successors of the deciduous teeth. It is preceded by the growth of the free end of the dental lamina (successional lamina), lingual to the dental organ of each deciduous tooth, and occurs from about the fifth month in utero for the permanent central incisors to 10 months of age for the second premolar. The third phase is preceded by the extension of the dental lamina distal to the dental organ of the second deciduous molar, which begins in the 140 mm embryo. The permanent molars arise directly from the distal extension of the dental lamina. The time of initiation is about 4 months of fetal life (in the 160 mm embryo) for the first permanent molar, the first year for the second permanent molar, and the fourth to fifth year for the third permanent molar.

It is, thus, evident that the total activity of the dental lamina extends over a period of about 5 years. Any particular portion functions for a much briefer period, since only relatively short time elapses after initiation, before the dental lamina begins to disintegrate at that particular location. However, the dental lamina still is active in the third molar region after it has disappeared elsewhere except for occasional epithelial remnants. The distal proliferation of the dental lamina is responsible for the peculiar location of the germs of

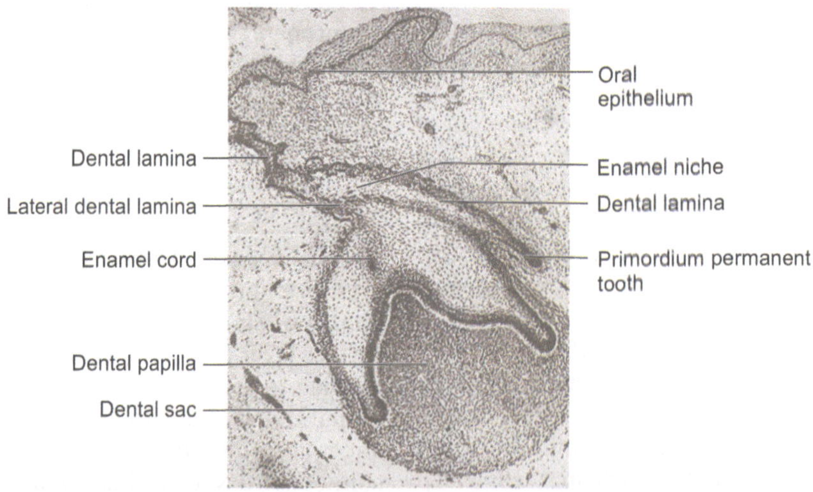

Fig. 13.1: Labiolingual section of tooth bud showing different parts *(For color version, see Plate 9)*

the permanent molars. They develop in the ramus of the mandible and in the tuberosity of the maxilla.

Fate of the Dental Lamina

During the cap stage, the dental lamina maintains a broad connection with the dental organ, but in the bull stage, it begins to break up by mesenchymal invasion, which first penetrates its central portion and divides it into the lateral lamina and the dental lamina proper. The mesenchymal invasion is at first incomplete and does not perforate the dental lamina. The dental lamina proper proliferates only at its deeper margin, which becomes a free end situated lingually to the dental organ and forms the primordium of the permanent tooth. The epithelial connection of the dental organ with the oral epithelium is served by the proliferating mesoderm. Remnants of the dental lamina may persist as epithelial pearls or islands within the jaw as well as in the gingivae.

Vestibular Lamina

Labial and buccal to the dental lamina, another epithelial thickening develops independently and somewhat later. It is the vestibular lamina, also termed lip furrow band. It subsequently follows out and forms the oral vestibule between the alveolar portion of the jaws, and the lips and cheeks.

Dental Papilla

The dental papilla is enclosed in the invaginated portion of the dental organ. The peripheral cells of the mesenchymal dental papilla differentiate into odontoblasts under the organizing influence of the epithelium, before the inner dental epithelium begins to secret enamel. These cells acquire the specific potentiality to produce dentin when they assume a cuboidal and later a columnar form (Fig. 13.1).

Dental Sac

Before formation of dental tissue begins, the dental sac shows a circular arrangement of its fibers and resembles a capsular structure. With the development of the root, the fibers of the dental sac differentiate into the periodontal fibers that become embedded in the cementum and alveolar bone (Fig. 13.1).

Inner Dental Epithelium

The inner dental epithelium consists of a single layer of cells that differentiate prior to amelogenesis into tall columnar cells, the ameloblasts. They are 4–5 microns in diameter and about 40 microns high. In cross section, they assume a hexagonal shape similar to that seen later in transverse sections of the enamel rods. They are the enamel-forming cells. The cells of the inner dental epithelium exert an organizing influence upon the underlying mesenchymal cells, which differentiate into odontoblasts.

Stratum Intermedium

Several layers of squamous, called stratum intermedium, appear between the inner dental epithelium and stellate reticulum. This layer seems to be essential for enamel formation. It is absent in the part of the tooth germ that covers the root portions of the tooth but does not form enamel (Fig. 13.2).

Stellate Reticulum

The stellate reticulum expands further, mainly by increase of the intercellular fluid. The cells are star-shaped, with long processes that anastomoses with those of adjacent cells. Before enamel formation begins, the stellate reticulum shrinks by loss of the intercellular fluid. Its cells then are hardly distinguishable from those of the stratum intermedium. This change begins at the height of the cusp or the incisal edge and progresses cervically.

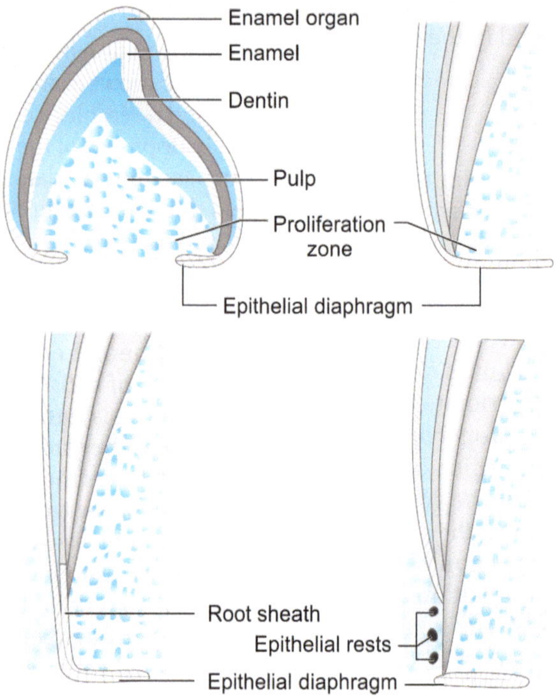

Fig. 13.2: Development of root *(For color version, see Plate 9)*

Outer Dental Epithelium

The cells of the outer dental epithelium flatten to a low cuboidal form. The formerly smooth surface of the outer dental epithelium is laid in folds at the end of the bell stage, preparatory to and during the formation of enamel, thus provides a rich nutritional supply for the intense metabolic activity of the vascular enamel organ; when between the folds the adjacent mesenchyme of the dental sac forms papillae that contains capillary loops (Fig. 13.1).

Tooth Buds (Primordial of Teeth)

Simultaneous with the differentiation of the dental lamina, tooth buds arise from it, in each jaw, round or ovoid swellings at 10 different points, corresponding to the future position of the deciduous teeth, the primordial of the dental organs, and the tooth buds. Thus, the development of the tooth germ is initiated and the cells continue to proliferate faster than the adjacent cells. The dental lamina is shallow, and microscopic section of that shows the tooth buds close to the oral epithelium.

STAGES OF TOOTH DEVELOPMENT

Tooth development occurs into the following stages: The initiation stage, the bud stage, the cap stage, the bell stage, and finally maturation (Table 13.1 and Figs 13.3A and B). The staging

Table 13.1: Stages of tooth growth

Morphologic stages	*Physiologic processes*
Dental lamina	Initiation
Bud stage	
Cap stage (early)	
Cap stage (advanced)	Proliferation
Bell stage (early)	Histodifferentiation
Bell stage (advanced)	Morphodifferentiation
Formation of enamel and dentin matrix	Apposition

of tooth development has been considered in attempt to categorize changes that take place along a continuum; to make the understanding simpler as commonly it is difficult to decide what stage should be assigned to a particular developing tooth. The varying appearance of different histologic sections of the same developing tooth, which can appear to be in different stages, makes this determination further complicated.

Initiation Stage

While development of teeth, one of the initial signs in the formation of a tooth that can be seen microscopically is the distinction between the vestibular lamina and the dental lamina. The developing tooth bud is connected to the epithelial layer of the mouth for a significant time with the help of dental lamina. This is considered as an initiation stage.

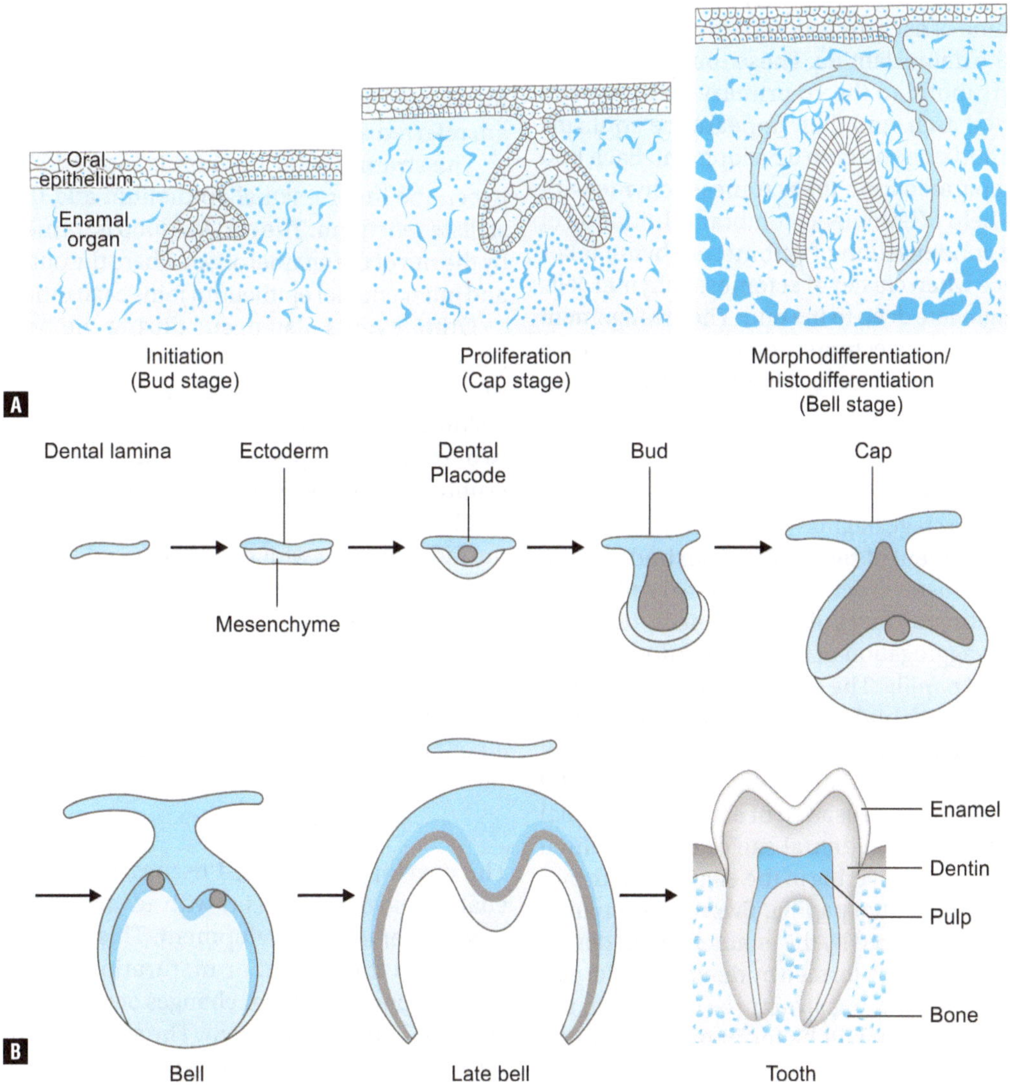

Figs 13.3A and B: Stages in tooth growth *(For color version, see Plate 10)*

Bud Stage

The bud stage can be seen with appearance of a tooth bud without a clear arrangement of cells. Once epithelial cells proliferate into the ectomesenchyme of the jaw, the stage technically begins. Usually, this stage occurs when the fetus is about 8 weeks old. The tooth bud itself is considered as a group of cells at the periphery of the dental lamina.

A bud, 10 round epithelial structures, develops at the distal aspect of the dental lamina of each arch along with the formation of the dental lamina. These round structures correspond to the 10 primary teeth of each dental arch, and their appearance confirms the bud stage of tooth development. Each bud is separated from the ectomesenchyme with the help of basement membrane. Initiation of the condensation of ectomesenchyme takes place when cluster of ectomesenchymal cells congregate deep to the bud. The arrangement of remaining ectomesenchymal cells can be seen as a more or less haphazardly uniform fashion.

Cap Stage

The cap stage begins with the first signs of an arrangement of cells in the tooth bud. Once a small cluster of ectomesenchymal cells cease secreting extracellular substances, it results in an aggregation of these cells known as the dental papilla. The appearance of cap begins as the tooth bud grows around the ectomesenchymal aggregation, which forms enamel organ or (dental) organ covering the dental papilla. A condensation of ectomesenchymal cells called the dental sac or follicle which forms outer covering of the enamel organ and limits the dental papilla. Eventually, enamel will be produced by the enamel organ; dentin and pulp will be formed by dental papilla; and all the supporting structures of a tooth, the periodontium, will be formed by the dental sac or follicle.

Bell Stage

The histodifferentiation and morphodifferentiation in tooth development take place in bell stage. The appearance of dental organ is bell-shaped through this stage, and stellate reticulum cells with their star-shaped appearance forms majority of cells in this stage. The bell stage consists of two stages, the early bell stage and the late bell stage. Cells on the periphery of the enamel organ are composed of four vital layers. Most peripheral cuboidal cells of the dental organ are called as outer enamel epithelium. The innermost columnar cells of the enamel organ close to the enamel papilla are referred as inner enamel epithelium.

The stratum intermedium is located between the inner enamel epithelium and the stellate reticulum. The cervical loop is formed by the rim of the enamel organ where the outer and inner enamel epithelium joins each other.

Other events also occur during the bell stage. Teeth are completely separated from the epithelium of the oral cavity with the disintegration of dental lamina; joining of the two will not take place again until the final eruption of the tooth into the mouth.

The crown of the tooth also takes shape during this stage which is influenced by the shape of the inner enamel epithelium. All teeth undergo this same process throughout the mouth.

Other structures that may be visible in this stage of a developing tooth are enamel knots, enamel cords, and enamel niche (Fig. 13.1).

Advanced Bell Stage

The development of hard tissues, including enamel and dentin, occurs with advancement in stages of tooth development. This stage is named as the crown, or maturation stage. Many important cellular changes occur at this stage of tooth development. The size of tooth bud was increasing in size due to rapid division of cells in prior stages, but rapid dividing known as mitosis ceases during the crown stage at the location where the cusps of the teeth form. The formation of first mineralized hard tissues begins at the location of cusp in teeth. Simultaneously, preameloblasts develop with the change in shape of the cells from cuboidal to columnar.

The cells in dental papilla rapidly increase in size and differentiate into odontoblasts, which are responsible for the formation of dentin.

The organic matrix contains many substances required for the formation of dentin. As predentin formation occurs due to placement of organic matrix by odontoblasts, the cells start traveling gradually towards the center of the dental papilla. Therefore, formation of the dentin begins in the surface closest to the outside of the tooth which then gradually proceeds inward in contrast to the process of formation of enamel.

The cells of the enamel epithelium secrete an organic matrix against the dentin, once dentin formation begins. This matrix instantly mineralizes and forms the initial layer of the tooth's enamel. The newly formed ameloblasts continue the process of enamel formation outside the dentin in response to the formation of dentin, which are cells that always add new material to the outer surface of the developing tooth and enamel formation moves outwards.

CHAPTER 14

Histology of Soft and Hard Dental Tissues

INTRODUCTION

The hard dental tissues include:
- Enamel
- Dentin
- Cementum
- Alveolar bone.

The soft dental tissues include:
- Pulp
- Periodontal ligament
- Gingiva.

ENAMEL

Chemical Composition

• Inorganic substance	95%
• Organic substance	5%
• Water	4.5%.

Inorganic substance: Mainly, calcium hydroxy-apatite crystals. Majority of inorganic elements are calcium and phosphorus. Others are fluorides, silver, aluminum, barium, copper, and magnesium.

Organic substances: Protein in the form of keratin, carbohydrates, lipids, citrates, etc.

Histologically, enamel, the outermost covering of tooth which lies adjacent to the dentin, contains the following (Fig. 14.1):
- Enamel rods
- Rod sheath
- Cementing interrod substances.

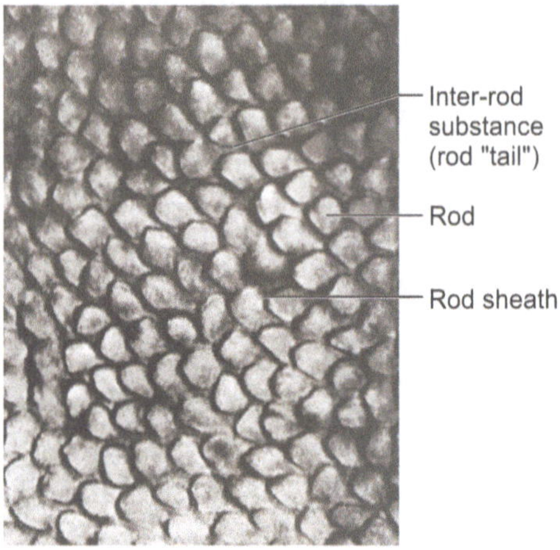

Fig. 14.1: Structure of enamel

Enamel Rods

They arise from dentinoenamel (DE) junction and proceeds uninterruptedly to the external surface of tooth. In general, rods are perpendicular to the DE junction. In cervical region and in the cusps, they are wavy. They appear round or oval in cross section. In permanent teeth, the rods in cervical areas are directed apically and at acute angle with DE junction. In deciduous teeth, rods are oriented perpendicular to DE junction.

Rod Sheath

This is present peripheral to the rods. It is less calcified, contains more organic substance.

Inter-rod Substance

This substance is in between the enamel rods and acts as a cementing substance.

Hunter-Schreger Bands

When a longitudinally ground section of tooth is seen in reflected light, a series of dark and light bands are seen in enamel, known as Hunter-Schreger bands. These are due to differences in degree of mineralization.

Incremental Lines of Retzius

On a ground section of a tooth, when seen under light microscope, concentric brown lines are seen in the enamel that is incremental line of Retzius. They terminate at the enamel surface. These are due to rhythm of mineralization or variations in organic structure. The neonatal line is the line which separates postnatally produced enamel from that produced before birth. It is nothing but an accentuated incremental line.

Enamel Tufts

Unbraided projections seen arising from DE junction into enamel are the enamel tufts, which are like a tuft of grass.

Enamel Spindles

Enamel spindles are short, linear defects found at the DE junction and extend into the enamel, often being more prevalent at the cusp tips.

Dentinoenamel Junction

The dentin at DE junction is pitted; into these pits the rounded projection of enamel are fitted.

Cementoenamel Junction

Cementum may overlap enamel in 65%; meet at edge to edge in 25% and no meeting in 10% (Fig. 14.2).

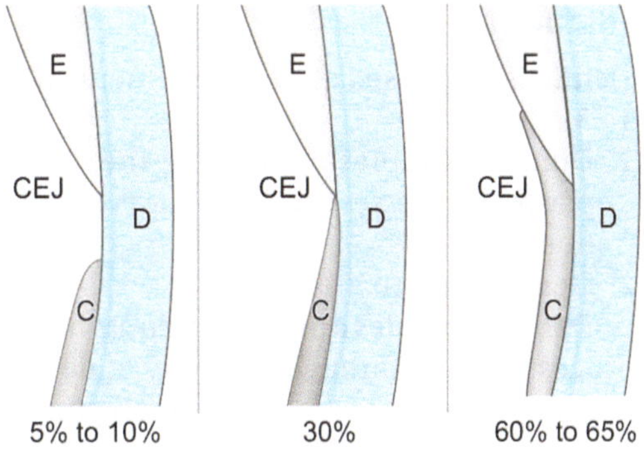

Fig. 14.2: Cementoenamel junction (CEJ)
Abbreviations: E, enamel; D, dentin; C, cementum

Enamel Cuticle

The crown of a newly erupted tooth is covered by a delicate membrane known as enamel cuticle. It gives a protective coating to enamel and a polished surface.

Primary Cuticle

It is formed by ameloblasts, which is a final secretory product.

Secondary Cuticle

It is the cellular layer that has become keratinized.

DENTIN

It forms the largest portion of tooth and gives the basic shape to it.

Chemical Composition

1. Inorganic (70%).
2. Organic (17%).
3. Water (13%).

Majority of inorganic elements are calcium and phosphorus. Organic collagen is 15–17%.

Also found in traces are sodium, potassium, proteins, lipids, magnesium, lead, fluorine.

Histology

Dentin is composed of two constituents (Fig. 14.3):

1. Dentinal tubules containing the protoplasmic processes of odontoblasts (Tomes' fiber).
2. Dentinal matrix.

Dentinal tubules arise from odontoblastic process, extend through the body of dentin, and may extend to enamel as enamel spindles. They contain odontoblast processes which are protoplasmic extensions from odontoblasts. These processes are narrow near to enamel (1 microns in diameter) whereas have 3 to 4 microns diameter near to pulp. They are wider at pulp at end and narrows outwardly. They give lateral branches which anastomoses with the branches of adjacent odontoblastic processes. The dental tubules run as a curved "S" shaped course, starting at perpendicular to the pulp surface. They are straight in the root and under the cusps.

Dentin matrix is calcified collagenous fibrils in the dentin, which is more calcified than adjacent dentin, which is traversed by dentinal tubules. It is divided into:

- *Peritubular dentin:* Immediately around the odontoblastic process, which is more calcified than adjacent dentin
- *Intertubular dentin:* It is present in between the dentinal tubules and is less calcified. This forms the main mass of dentin, containing collagenous material, amorphous organic ground substance, and smaller amount of apatite crystals.

Other forms of dentin are:

- *Mantle dentin:* This is the first formed dentin, which is the most peripheral part of dentin, consisting of Korff's fibers
- *Predentin*: It is the newly formed dentin which is located adjacent to the pulp tissue. It is not mineralized
- *Circumpulpal dentin*: It forms the remaining part of dentin other than mantle dentin. It represents the dentin formed before root completion.

Various histological features of dentin include:

- *Incremental lines of von Ebner* are lines that mark the sites of transition between alternating periods of accelerated and retarded growth
- *Neonatal line* is the hypocalcified band seen in dentin separating the prenatal and postnatal dentin. These are seen only in deciduous teeth and permanent 1st molar
- *Interlobular dentin* is the irregular area of hypocalcified matrix formed due to failure of union of inorganic calcospherite granules.

Dental Junctions

- Dentinoenamel junction
- *Dentino predentin junction*: Interface between calcified and uncalcified dentin

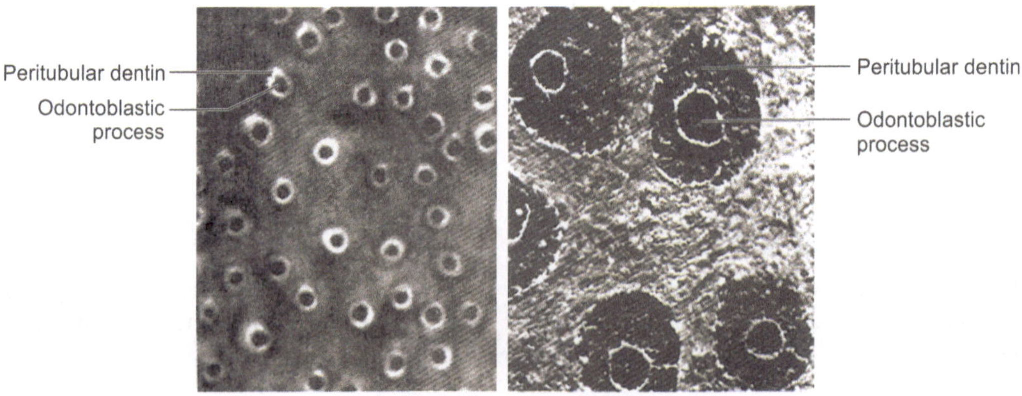

Fig. 14.3: Structure of dentin

- Predentin pulp junction
- Dentinocemental junction.

Types

- *Primary dentin:* Dentin that is formed during the various periods of tooth development to the time when tooth takes its anatomic position in the oral cavity. It represents the dentin which forms before root completion
- *Secondary dentin (regular dentin)* It is seen as a regular, uniform layer around the pulp cavity which forms after root completion
- *Secondary reparative and irregular dentin* It is a localized deposit of dentin on the wall of pulp cavity as a result of erosion, attrition, caries, etc.
- *Sclerotic dentin:* This is formed due to change in structure of primary dentin, as a response to aging, erosion, abrasion. It is commonly seen in roots
- *Dead track:* These are seen as dark lines formed due to groups of dead, degenerated dentinal tubule.

CEMENTUM

Chemical Composition

- Inorganic (45–50%)
  - Hydroxyapatite (Calcium phosphate)
  - Copper, fluorine, iron, lead
  - Potassium, silica, sodium, zinc.
- Organic matter (50–55%)
  - Collagen fiber
  - Interfibrillar substance
    - ◊ Mucopolysaccharides.

There are two types of cementum, acellular cementum (primary) and cellular cementum (secondary) present in teeth (Fig. 14.4).

The acellular layer of cementum is living tissue that does not incorporate cells into its structure and usually forms on the coronal half of the root. Cellular cementum occurs more frequently on the apical half; this is less calcified.

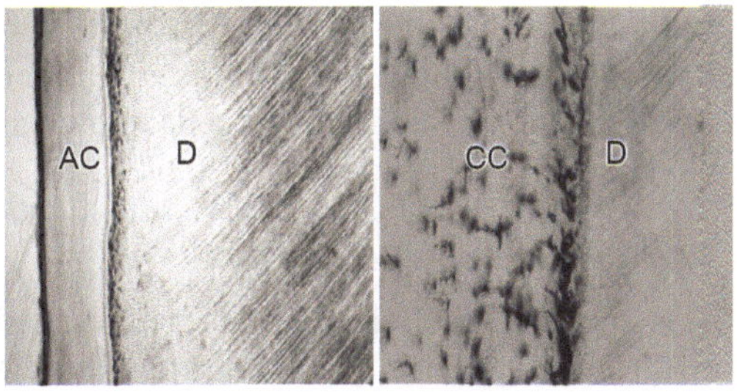

Fig. 14.4: Cellular and acellular cementum
Abbreviations: D, dentin; AC, acellular cementum; CC, cellular cementum

Histology

Cementum covers the dentin of the anatomical root of teeth.

ALVEOLAR BONE

Alveolar bone is the thickened ridge bone that comprises the tooth sockets or alveoli on bones holding teeth. The teeth bearing bones are maxillae and the mandible in humans (Fig. 14.5).

Cells and Intercellular Matrix

Cells are osteocytes, enclosed within lacunae. The processes extend into canaliculi that radiate from lacunae. When there is bone

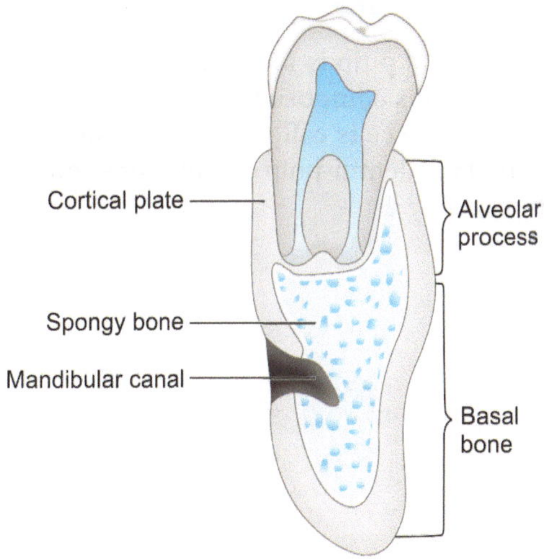

Fig. 14.5: Structure of alveolar bone

resorption, appearance of eroded bone surfaces known as Howships is there. Lacunae are seen with multinucleated cells known as osteoclasts.

Socket Wall

It consists of dense, lamellated bone arranged in Haversian system and bundle bones. Bundle bone lies adjacent to the periodontal ligament containing large number of Sharpey's fibers. The cancellous portion, which is found in interradicular and interdental spaces, contains trabeculae, which encloses irregularly shaped marrow spaces lined with flattened endosteal cells.

Periosteum: This covers the outer surface of the bone, composed of cells that can change into osteoblasts and fibroblasts.

Endosteum: This is the tissue lining the internal bone surface. This is composed of a single layer of osteoprogenitor cells and connective tissue.

Other fibers like elastic and oxytalan fibers are also seen. Interstitial tissues consist of the blood vessels, lymphatics and nerves of periodontal ligament that are contained in spaces between the principal fiber bundles.

DENTAL PULP

The dental pulp is located in the center of teeth and is composed of living connective tissues and cells called odontoblasts. It is a part of the dentin-pulp complex or endodontium.

Cells

- *Fibroblasts and fibers:* Amongst the fibers some are of collagenous in nature. The Korff's fibers originate from among the pulp cells as thin fibers, thickened at the periphery of the pulp to form relatively thick bundles that pass between the odontoblasts
- *Odontoblasts:* They give rise to odontoblastic process. Their body is columnar in shape with an oral nucleus. Each cell extends cytoplasmic process into a tubule in the dentin.

In the crown of the pulp, a cell-free layer can be found just inside the layer of odontoblasts. This layer is known as "zone of Weil" or subodontoblastic layer, which contains a network of nerve fibers, i.e. subodontoblastic plexus.

- *Defense cells:* Histiocytes, undifferentiated mesenchymal cells which are present close to the capillary walls, pericytes
- *Intercellular substance:* They consist of:
  - Ground substance
  - Fibers.

The ground substance is gelatinous and is called the cement substance.

The fibers are of two types:

1. Precollagenous or reticular or Korff's fiber.
2. Collagenous fibers.

Within the ground substance, the blood vessels and lymph vessels are distributed.

CHAPTER 15

Salivary Glands

INTRODUCTION

A gland is a unit of tissue structure and its function involved in the manufacture and discharge of secretion.

CLASSIFICATION OF GLANDS

Glands may be classified in many ways. In using a nomenclature, combination of various classifications is used.

- According to number of cells involved:
  - Unicellular, e.g. goblet cells
  - Multicellular, e.g. salivary gland.
- According to size:
  - Major, e.g. parotid
  - Minor, e.g. mucous glands of cheek.
- According to morphology:
  - Alveolar (acinar)
  - Tubular
  - Tubuloacinar.
- According to branching of the duct:
  - Simple (nonbranching)
  - Compound (branching).
- According to presence of ducts:
  - Exocrine (ducts are present), e.g. salivary gland
  - Endocrine (ductless), e.g. pituitary.
- According to type of secretion:
  - Serous (albuminous), e.g. parotid
  - Mucous, e.g. minor salivary glands of cheek
  - Mixed (seromucous), e.g. submandibular.
- According to damage of secretory cells at discharge:
  - Merocrine (no damage), e.g. salivary gland
  - Apocrine (cells contribute part of their protoplasmic substance to their secretion), e.g. some sweat glands
  - Holocrine (there is extreme damage of the cell, secretion consists of altered cells of the gland itself), e.g. sebaceous gland.

Classification of Salivary Glands

Salivary glands are multicellular, merocrine and exocrine glands. They may be classified according to size, location or type of secretion.

- According to size:
  - *Major (extrinsic):* There are three pairs of major glands—parotid, submandibular and sublingual; flow of saliva is continuous (Fig. 15.1).

    Various characteristics of different major salivary glands have been depicted in Table 15.1
  - *Minor (intrinsic):* Flow of saliva is intermittent, e.g. buccal glands. There are 400–500 minor glands in oral cavity (not seen in gingival and anterior part of hard palate).
- According to location:
  - *Glands whose ducts open in the vestibule:*

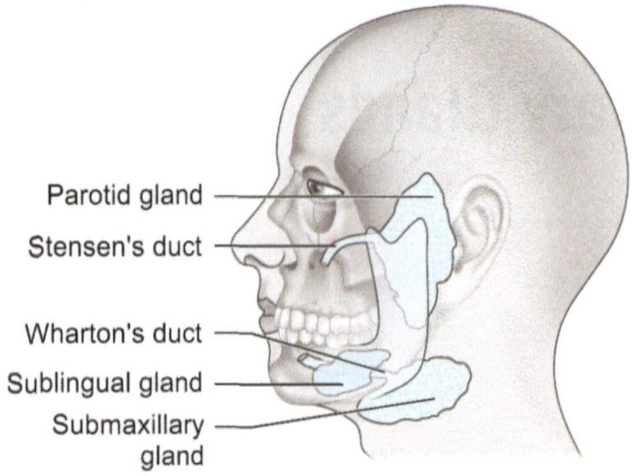

Fig. 15.1: Major salivary glands

◊ Lip: Superior labial and inferior labial
◊ Cheek: Parotid and buccal.
- *Glands whose ducts open in oral cavity proper:*
◊ Floor of mouth
 ▸ Submandibular
 ▸ Sublingual (major)
 ▸ Sublingual (minor)
 ▸ Glossopalatine.
◊ Tongue
 ▸ *Body:* Anterior lingual (of Blandin and Nuhn)
 ▸ *Base:* Posterior lingual
  » Von Ebner (around circumvallate papilla)
  » Tonsil, lingual.
◊ Palate:
 ▸ Palatine.

- According to secretion:
 - *Serous:*
 ◊ Parotid
 ◊ Von Ebner (posterior lingual near vallate papilla).
 - *Mucous:*
 ◊ Palatine
 ◊ Posterior lingual tonsillar
 ◊ Gloss palatine.

Table 15.1: Characteristics features of different types of major salivary glands

Characteristics features	*Parotid*	*Submandibular*	*Sublingual*
Location	In the retromandibular area and extends in front of the external ear	• In the submandibular triangle • Behind and below mylohyoid muscle	In the floor of the mouth at the sublingual fold
Main excretory Duct	• Stenson's duct opens in the vestibule in a papilla • Second molar	Wharton's duct opens on papilla on the floor of the mouth at the side of the lingual frenum	Bartholin's duct opens near the opening of the submandubular gland duct opening
Type	It is a compound, balanced alveolar gland	It is a compound branched alveolotubular gland	It is a compound branched tubuloalveolar gland
Secretion	It is a pure serous gland Through in newborn mucous acini may be seen	It is a mixed, serous elements predominating	It is a mixed gland, mucous elements predominating
Capsule	It is well-capsulated	It is well-capsulated	There is no capsule
Duct system	• Intercalated ducts are long and narrow • Striated ducts are prominent	• Intercalated ducts are short • Striated ducts are longer	• Intercalated ducts are absent • Striated ducts are rare
Caps of serous crescents or demilunes of Giannuzzi	Absent	Frequently seen in mucous alveoli	Occasionally seen on mucous terminal

- *Mixed:*
  - ◊ Submandibular (predominantly serous)
  - ◊ Sublingual (predominantly mucous)
  - ◊ Blandin Nuhn (anterior lingual) predominantly mucous
  - ◊ Buccal (predominantly mucous)
  - ◊ Labial (superior and inferior) predominantly mucous.

STRUCTURAL PATTERN OF THE SALIVARY GLAND

Basically, a salivary gland consists of parenchymatous secretory cells and stromal connective tissue. A capsule may be present. Capsule consists mostly of collagenous tissue with few elastic and reticular fibers.

Trabeculae

Connective tissue strands from capsule traverse the glands and divide them into lobules. These septae carry blood vessels, nerves and excretory ducts. The septal connective tissue consists of mesenchymal cells, fibroblasts, plasma cells, lymphocytes and fat cells. The connective tissue of the septae spreads into the lobules forming stroma for the secretory units.

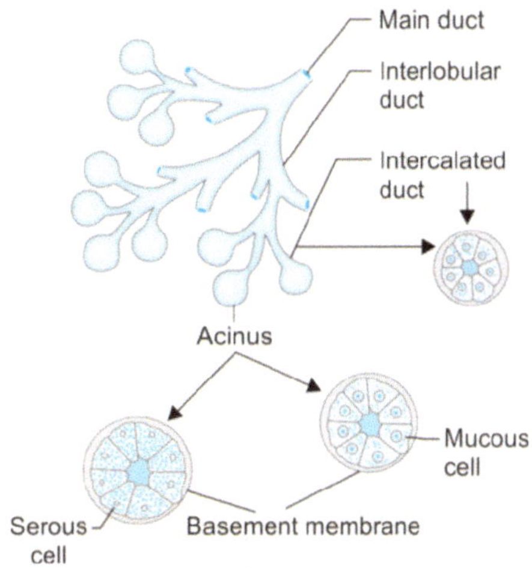

Fig. 15.2: Structure of salivary gland duct system *(For color version, see Plate 10)*

Secretory Cells

The secretory cells are either serous or mucous. They are organized to form acini. The cell morphology varies according to cycle of activity. During the resting phase, there is organization of the cytoplasmic organelles and the nucleus. In the elaborative phase, there is actual synthesis of the secretory product. There is accumulation of the product and the shape of the cell is altered. During the secretory phase, there is actual liberation of the secretory product (Fig. 15.2).

CHAPTER 16

Saliva

INTRODUCTION

Saliva is the fluid released into the oral cavity by salivary glands and is the result of both secretion and excretion.

FUNCTIONS

- Helps formation of bolus by moistening solid food
- Moistens epithelium and teeth and protects them
- Flushes and cleans oral cavity
- Helps in speech by moistening epithelial surface
- Helps digestion via ptyalin and maltose by hydrolyzing starch
- Helps in perception of taste by dispersing and dissolving food
- Excretes body metabolites (electrolytes water and protein)
- Has bacteriolytic action via lysozymes
- Decreases blood clotting time (Oral tissues bleed less than rest of the body)
- Regulation of body temperature—in dogs and cattle.

CHEMICAL COMPOSITION

The composition varies from man to man, from one gland to another, from food to food. In stimulated and resting saliva, average composition is:

- Water 99%
- Solid 0.5%
- Inorganic 0.2%
- Organic 0.3%.

Inorganic constituents are bicarbonates, chlorides and phosphates of calcium, magnesium, potassium and sodium. There are also thiocyanate, bromide, iodide, fluoride, copper, oxygen and carbon dioxide.

Organic constituents are proteins—glycoprotein, intrinsic salivary proteins, serum proteins like albumin and globulin, mucin; enzymes—ptyalin, lysozyme, lipase, phosphates; vitamins—pantothenic acid, riboflavin, nicotinic acid and vitamin K; carbohydrate—galactose, mannose, fructose, glucose; desquamated epithelial cells; and salivary corpuscles (resemble leukocytes, derived from gingival sulcus).

QUANTITY OF SECRETION

The amount of saliva secreted varies from person to person, depending on type of food taken, age, degree of mechanical stimulation, emotional condition, etc. On an average, 1500 mL is secreted per day under normal condition. Salivary flow is continuous. It varies from 3 cc per hour to 110 cc per hour (average 20.6 cc); 25% contributed by parotid, 70% submandibular and 5% sublingual gland. The pH of saliva varies from 5.6 to 7.6 (average is 6.8). The factors that influence pH are the type of diet, time of day, rate of flow, emotional state, etc.

MECHANISM OF SALIVATION

Salivation is controlled exclusively by nervous system. The salivary glands are richly supplied with both sympathetic and parasympathetic nerves. The parasympathetic supply to submandibular and sublingual glands comes via the chorda tympani nerve. These fibers arise in the superior salivatory nucleus in medulla oblongata. The fibers pass through the geniculate ganglion of the facial nerve and descend with this nerve, cross to chorda tympani and proceed along with lingual nerve. It forms synapse with postganglionic fibers from submaxillary ganglion. The postganglionic neurons supply the secretory cells.

The fibers leave the brain stem along with glossopharyngeal nerve (IX), join small superficial petrosal nerve and synapse in the otic ganglion. Postganglionic nerves supply the gland via auriculotemporal nerve. The postganglionic sympathetic supply for all the three glands originates in the superior cervical ganglion. They course along with external carotid artery and its branches. It is believed that there is independent innervation of the serous and mucous cells. Stimulation of parasympathetic fibers produces highly mucous saliva and a sympathetic stimulation produces a serous flow.

Saliva is produced by an active process. It is thought that after an impulse arrives at the neuroglandular junction, a substance is released which alters the permeability of the cells and the cell content is emptied. Most probably, the fibers of different threshold innervate various types of secretory cells. That is why, with increasing stimulation, not only the concentration and volume is augmented, but also the composition is altered.

Unconditional reflex response is evoked by the presence of food in the mouth or movements of the jaws and tongue. The amount and composition of saliva depends on the nature of the stimulation. Palatable food brings a large amount of saliva. Meat produces viscid, mucinous saliva and dry bread produces copious saliva with high ptyalin content. Acids also act as a salivary stimulant. Conditioned reflex response may be provided by smell, sight or even thought of food.

FACTORS AFFECTING SALIVARY FLOW

The secretion of saliva is controlled exclusively by nerves. No hormone has been discovered which controls the rate of flow. It has been estimated that the total volume of saliva amounts to between 1.0 L and 1.5 L a day.

Resting Flow

The resting flow of saliva can be studied some hours after a meal, either by means of Lashley cannula, or by allowing saliva to drain directly into a beaker from the open mouth with the head bent forward to a horizontal position. The average rate has been found to be 26 mL per hour and the range of variation being 3–110 mL per hour.

Psychic Flow

The experiments of Pavlov have proved the existence of conditioned reflexes in the control of the salivary flow. It has been observed that by experience, stimulation primarily connected with food may cause a secretion of saliva in animals. Lashley found that mention of food, even to a hungry individual, had no effect on parotid flow, but the sight of food gave a positive response.

Unconditioned Reflexes

The presence of food in the mouth is a powerful stimulus to salivation, and experiments show that this effect is made up of three main components:

- Taste forms one group of stimuli and there is evidence that different tastes vary in their effectiveness.

- Mechanical stimulation of the oral mucosa by the food
- Masticatory movements which normally follow the taking of food also stimulate human parotid secretion.

Mastication is accompanied by many sensory impulses, such as mechanical irritation of the oral mucosa, pressure on the teeth, and kinesthetic impulses from the masticatory muscle. Salivation is inhibited during muscular exercise and during the application of sensory stimuli to the skin. Mental work increases the secretion rate. The acts of swallowing and yawning are followed by a transient increase in rates of flow from the period and then usually a compensatory pause. Chemical stimuli vary greatly in their effectiveness as salivary stimuli.

Chemical irritation of the lining of the stomach or any other stimulus leading to nausea is also a powerful stimulus to salivation. Since nausea is usually lead to vomiting, the value of saliva in diluting and washing away the irritant is obvious. Animal experiments have shown that the presence of food in the stomach causes a flow of saliva known as the gastrosalivary reflexes. This is difficult to investigate in man. Chronic irritation of the esophagus, resulting from disease, e.g. carcinoma of the esophagus, is often accompanied by excessive salivation.

Saliva is a true secretion due to vital activity of cells of the three pairs of salivary glands and the numerous buccal glands. The passage of various blood elements into the mouth is not well-understood. Its amount and compositions vary in the same individual depending upon various factors. Saliva plays a dual role against the health of an individual. Based upon its constituents, it performs various useful functions in maintaining the oral and general health. On the other hand, it also contributes in giving rise to various pathological conditions in the oral cavity.

SALIVA IN HEALTH

Physical and Mechanical Functions

- *Lubrication:* The mucin and water contents of saliva act as lubricant during mastication, formation of bolus of food and swallowing
- *Taste:* Saliva converts the food materials into solution which is essential for the sensation of taste.

Digestive Function

The only important digestive enzyme present in the saliva is ptyalin or salivary amylase. The amylase contents vary considerably with age, with an average of 25 years, the amount varies between 10 and 15 units of amylase per mL. The enzyme digests cooked starch only. It is the alpha type of amylase, and breaks down the starch molecules simultaneously in many places into large number of dextrin molecules which are then more slowly attacked forming molecules. The action of amylase is inhibited by acids and the optimal pH for its activity is 6.8, therefore the main action of amylase remains in the mouth and in the stomach before secretion of gastric hydrochloric acid.

Antibacterial Function

Mechanical Removal of Bacteria

A large number of microorganisms are present in the saliva which contributes to its antibacterial effect.

Leukotoxin and opsonin: These substances are responsible for the presence of phagocyte activity of leukocytes in saliva. It has been shown that saliva increases capillary permeability and poses chemotactic activity towards leukocytes. The attraction of leukocytes is governed by leukotoxin, polypeptide in the saliva. Opsonin is the substance which is responsible for phagocytes by the leukocytes. It has been seen that in the absence of opsonin, the leukocytes do not show phagocytosis.

Lysozyme: Discovered by Fleming (1922), this enzyme breaks down the polysaccharides; hence, its action is limited only on those bacteria which contain polysaccharides.

Inhibin: Reported by Dold (1934), this substance inhibits the growth of *Lactobacillus* and diphtheria bacilli.

Mutinase: These are the substances in the saliva which render pathogenic organism into nonpathogenic by mutation.

Gamma globulin: The concentration of gamma globulin is more in the gingival sulcus sensitive of the route of entrance for blood elements in the oral cavity. Their action against the bacteria is of two types:

1. Certain gamma globulin known as immunoglobulin possesses antibody properties.
2. The globulin attaches itself to lactobacilli and can both inhibit their growth and cause their lysis.

Bacterial Antagonism

There is evidence that some organisms cannot survive in the mouth in the presence of certain other organisms. The action is based upon their metabolic products. It can be demonstrated that washing of blood agar culture of streptococci colonies produced inhibition effect on the other organisms.

Saliva and Blood Coagulation

When freshly shed blood is diluted with saliva, its clotting time is reduced. Saliva has been found to possess coagulation effects on the blood owing to the presence of factor VII, IX, X plasma thromboplastin antecedent and Hageman factor.

Buffering Power of Saliva

It is the capability of the saliva to resist against the change in pH. Bicarbonate is the strongest buffer in saliva and the phosphate also plays some role, when proteins are chief buffers of plaque. Buffers work by converting highly ionized substance acid or alkali in the more weakly ionized substance. Unstimulated saliva, which has lower bicarbonate content, is a less powerful buffer near naturality.

Water Balance

As shown by Cannoh (1934), the "dry mouth reflex" stimulates the secretion of saliva, which prevents drying of the pharynx and thirst is avoided. But if the body tissues are short of water, the reflex does not occur and the thirst is satisfied by intake of water.

Excretion

Saliva is a route of excretion also, by which certain substances are excreted. It can be effective only for those substances that are either destroyed or rendered insoluble in the gut after swallowing. Mercury and lead are excreted through saliva in poisoning cases but are reabsorbed by the intestine, and cannot be considered as true excretion. On the other hand, excreted glucose in diabetic cases is destroyed in the mouth and excretion of viruses in viral infection also gets destroyed in the gastrointestinal tract, which can be taken as true excretion.

SALIVA IN DISEASE

Dental Calculus

Calculus is believed to be an important factor in causing periodontal disease. Histological studies indicate that all the constituents of calculus are derived from saliva such as mucin, inorganic salts and microorganisms.

Saliva is a saturated solution of calcium phosphate. Some of the insoluble calcium phosphate is present in colloidal form and some is bound to salivary proteins. Various views have been put up regarding the precipitation and formation of calculus. Presence of CO_2 in saliva is important in keeping the calcium in solution form. The loss of CO_2 from saliva resulting in precipitation of calcium salts is the most widely accepted view. Enzyme phosphates release phosphate ions from organic phosphates in saliva, and thus by mass action causing precipitation has also been reported.

Dental Plaque

Dental plaque is a thin, yellowish film found on the surface of teeth which are inaccessible to brushing. Mucin and microorganism from saliva are the main factors responsible for the formation of plaque, which leads to caries and calculus formation. It is firmly held on the tooth surface and cannot be removed by rinsing and stream of water. The microscopic studies show that the plaque consists of closely matted organisms of filamentous type embedded in a matrix of uncertain origin. It also contains various types of bacteria, epithelial cells and food debris.

The factors concerned in the formation of plaque are not well-understood. It is believed that bacteria growing on the tooth surface, by acid production, cause the precipitation of mucin which would entangle bacteria and provide a medium for further growth and repetition of cycle.

Dental Caries

The pH of saliva plays an important role in the incidence of caries. Calcium phosphate is insoluble at neutral pH, but if the saliva becomes acidic of particular pH will be reached at which the solubility of calcium phosphate becomes so high that the concentration of ions in the solution fails to saturate it. Below this critical pH, the inorganic material of the tooth will be dissolved in saliva. This pH is usually between 5.5 and 6.5 resulting in caries.

Role of Salivary Enzymes

The enzyme of saliva is a potential etiologic factor in gingival and periodontal diseases. The enzymes normally contained in saliva are derived from glands, bacteria, tissues and leukocytes. Certain enzymes which increase in saliva during gingivitis and periodontal disease are hyaluronidase, lipase, B-glucuronidase, chondroitin sulfatase, amino acid decarboxylases, catalase, peroxidase and collagenase. Many components of gingival and connective tissues are good substrates for the activity of these enzymes. The acid mucopolysaccharides, hyaluronic acid and chondroitin sulfate in the intercellular substance of the gingival epithelium and connective tissue are destroyed. These enzymes produce a break in the continuity of the oral epithelium. This break in continuity causes invasion of bacteria and their toxins into the tissues giving rise to the pathological conditions.

Blood

CHAPTER 17

INTRODUCTION

Blood is a fluid thicker than water circulating uninterruptedly through the heart, arteries, capillaries and veins of the human body. It carries nutrients and oxygen to body tissues and takes away the waste products to the excretory organs of the body.

Blood is made up of two major components:

- Cellular components: About half of the blood volume is composed of blood cells
  - Erythrocytes, also known as red blood cells, which carry the oxygen to the tissues
  - Leukocytes, also known as white blood cells, which protects the body from infections
  - Platelets are smaller size cells which help in stopping the bleeding from the body. Blood vessels which circulate the blood have very smooth lumen which helps in preventing the blood clotting and maintain the balance of blood-clotting factors.
- Noncellular component or blood fluid is known as plasma, which constitutes the other half of the blood.

COMPOSITION

- *Erythrocytes*: Total number of red blood cells are 4.7 to 6.1 million in male and 4.2 to 5.4 million in female. Red blood cells distribute oxygen and is composed of blood's hemoglobin. Mature red blood cells lack a nucleus and organelles in mammals. Life span of red blood cells is about 120 days in circulation. In addition, these cells together with endothelial vessel cells and other cells are also marked by glycoproteins that define the different blood types. The proportion of blood occupied by red blood cells is known as the hematocrit, and is normally about 45%. The combined surface area of all red blood cells of the human body would be roughly 2000 times as great as the body's exterior surface (Fig. 17.1)

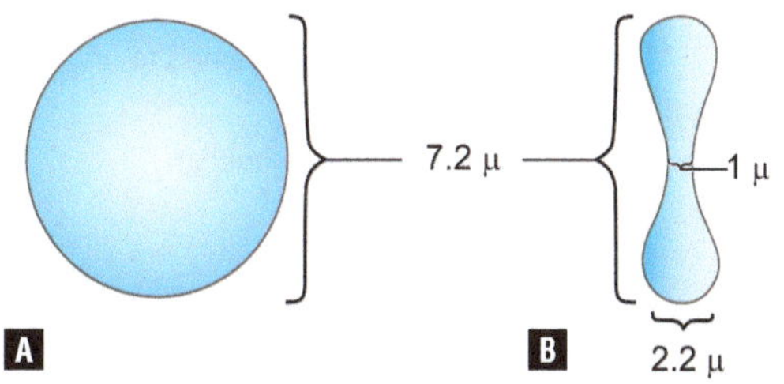

Figs 17.1A and B: Red blood cell (A) Dimension; (B) Surface view

- *Leukocytes:* Total number of white blood cells are 4,000–11,000. They forms an integral part of the body's immune system, destroy and remove old or aberrant cells and cellular debris. In addition, they attack infectious agents or pathogens and foreign substances. The cancer of leukocytes is called leukemia (Fig. 17.2). The various characteristics features of leukocytes are detailed in Box 17.1

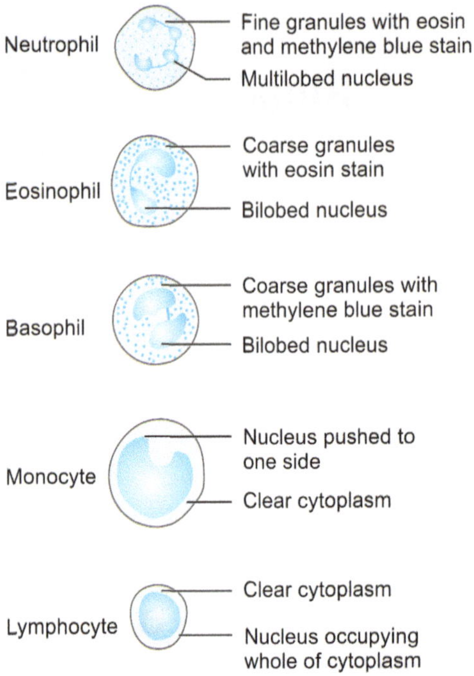

Fig. 17.2: Different types of white blood cells *(For color version, see Plate 10)*

Box 17.1: Various characteristics of leukocytes

- WBCs: 5000–10,000 WBCs/μL blood
- RBCs: Outnumber WBCs about 700:1
- Life span: Typically a few hours to days
- Abnormal WBC counts
  - Leukocytosis: High WBC count in response to infection, exercise, surgery
  - Leukopenia: Low WBC count
- Differential WBC count: Measures percentage of WBCs made up of each of the five types

Abbreviations: WBC, white blood cell; RBC, red blood cell

- *Thrombocytes*: These are 200,000–500,000 in number and are also referred as platelets which take part in blood clotting or coagulation. Fibrin from the coagulation cascade makes a mesh over the platelet plug.

Plasma

About 55% of total volume of blood is plasma. It is a straw-colored, clear liquid. It contains 91–92% water and 8–9% solids. The solids are organic and inorganic substances.

Organic Substances

- Protein: Albumin, globulin, fibrinogen
- Carbohydrates: Glucose
- Fats: Neutral fats, phospholipids and cholesterol
- Amino acid
- Nonprotein nitrogenous substances: Ammonia, creatinine, urea, uric acid, etc.
- External secretions: Hormones
- Enzymes: Amylase, alkaline phosphatase, acid phosphatase, lipase, protease, esterase, etc.
- Antibiotics: Immunoglobulin.

Inorganic Substances

Sodium, calcium, potassium, magnesium, chloride, iron, iodide, copper and phosphates.

Gases Present in Plasma

Oxygen, carbon dioxide.

FUNCTIONS

Blood performs many important functions within the body, including:

- Supplies oxygen which is bound to hemoglobin to tissues
- Supplies nutrients such as glucose, amino acids, and fatty acids (dissolved in the blood or bound to plasma proteins)
- Removal of waste such as carbon dioxide, urea, and lactic acid
- Immunological functions like circulation of white blood cells, and detection of foreign material by antibodies
- Coagulation, the response to a broken blood vessel, the conversion of blood from a liquid to a semisolid gel to stop bleeding
- Messenger functions, including the transport of hormones and the signaling of tissue damage

- Regulation of body pH
- Regulation of core body temperature
- Hydraulic functions.

NORMAL VALUES

The normal values of different blood test has been described in Box 17.2.

The complete blood count (CBC) has been depicted in Box 17.3.

Box 17.2: Normal values of blood tests

- Bleeding time = 1-9 minutes in adults
  1-13 minutes in children
  Longer in female than in male
- Clotting time (or) = 10.5-13.5/14 seconds
  Prothrombin time
- Partial thromboplastin time = 25-35 seconds

Box 17.3: Complete blood count

- WBC: 4,000–10,000/mm^3
- RBC: 4.2–5.9 million/mm^3
- Hemoglobin:
  - Males: 14–18 g/dL
  - Females: 12–16 g/dL
- Hematocrit:
  - Males: 40–50%
  - Females: 37–47%
- MCV: 86–98 μm^3/cell
- MCH: 27–32 μm^3/RBC
- RDW: 11.5–14.5%
- Platelet count: 150,000–400,000/mm^3
- WBC differential:
  - Neutrophils: 40–75%
  - Lymphocytes: 15–45%
  - Monocytes: 1–10%
  - Eosinophils: 1–10%
  - Basophils: 0–2%

Abbreviations: WBC, white blood cell; RBC, red blood cell; MCV, mean corpuscular volume; MCH, mean corpuscular hemoglobin; RDW, red cell distribution width.

Mastication, Deglutition and Phonation

CHAPTER 18

MASTICATION

It is the process of cutting and breaking down the large food particles into small particles and grinding them into a soft bolus.

Significance

It is the first mechanical process to which food is subjected. The following are the significances:

- Breaking down into smaller particles
- Mixing of saliva with food substances thoroughly
- Lubrication and moistening of dry food by saliva so that bolus can be easily swallowed
- Appreciation of the taste of the food
- Increases the surface area of the food for the digestive enzyme to act.

Mechanism

It is mostly a reflex process. It is the result of a highly complex neuromuscular activity. It can be carried out voluntarily also. The center of the mastication is situated in medulla and cerebral cortex. The muscles of mastication are supplied by fifth cranial nerve (Trigeminal nerve).

Teeth, temporomandibular joint and muscles of mastication are responsible for the process of mastication. Tooth contacts occur during most of the chewing strokes. The maximum load on natural teeth during chewing is 500–700 newtons (110–160 lbf). The tongue directs the food between the teeth and exerts a crushing effect by pressing the substance against the hard palate. The cheeks and lips keep the food from escaping between the teeth. Once the bolus formation is ready, it pushes back to oropharynx for deglutition.

DEGLUTITION

The process of swallowing is defined as deglutition. The process of swallowing has been divided into three stages for better understanding:

Stages

Oral Stage

This stage has been considered as an only voluntary stage in the act of swallowing. It consists of bolus formation with mastication of food which can be easily swallowed. Three main muscles involved in the act of chewing are:

- Masseter
- Temporalis
- Pterygoid.

All three muscles are considered as muscle of mastication and they are supplied by the mandibular division of the trigeminal nerve. The tongue plays an important role in this phase which is supplied by the hypoglossal nerve. The buccinator and orbicularis oris is supplied the facial nerve. These muscles play an important role in swallowing, as these muscles contract and inhibit the dropping out of food from the oral cavity by keeping the contents inside the mouth. The paralysis of the buccinator and orbicularis oris is seen in patients with facial palsy and is associated with the drooling of saliva occurring on the side of the mouth.

Pharyngeal Stage

This complex phase aids in passing of the masticated food through the oropharynx to cricopharynx and further into the upper esophagus. This stage is involuntary and passage is allowed due to relaxation of cricopharyngeus muscle while swallowing.

In this phase, nasopharynx gets separated from the oropharynx by the contraction of muscles of soft palate and posterior pharyngeal wall. This, in turn, inhibits nasal regurgitation of masticated food.

In addition to these muscles, laryngeal musculature also constricts to prevent aspiration during this phase. Thus, this stage needs the coordination of many muscle groups including the muscles of the soft palate which is supplied by the 5th, 7th, 9th and 12th cranial nerves.

Moreover, pharyngeal muscles play an important role in propelling the food through the cricopharynx which are supplied by the 9th and 10th cranial nerves. The cricopharyngeus muscle is innervated by the 10th cranial nerve and sympathetic nerves.

Many neurological disorders affect the pharynx and can lead to impairment in swallowing by altering motor and/or sensory functions in the oral and pharyngeal stages.

Esophageal Stage

This is an involuntary stage. It helps in propelling the food bolus down the esophagus. This phase is mainly regulated by the 10th cranial nerve and sympathetic nerves.

This phase primarily involves peristalsis of the esophageal musculature. Peristaltic waves move down the esophagus with waves of positive pressure reaching 50–100 mm Hg while swallowing. There is an initial negative wave caused by elevation of the larynx drawing on the cervical esophagus during the swallowing of liquids and semisolids.

This is followed by an abrupt positive wave which coincides with the entry of the bolus into the esophagus. This wave is referred as primary peristaltic wave.

This wave is further succeeded by a smaller positive wave known as the stripping wave. This wave eradicates the leftover food material from the esophagus.

Further, secondary peristaltic waves begin in the esophagus in response to dilatation of esophagus. Moreover, stage of emotional stress gives rise to tertiary peristaltic waves which are regarded as irregular, nonpropulsive contractions involving the large segments of esophagus. During swallowing in standing position, fluid may be projected from the pharynx to the esophagus gastric junction in approximately 1 second. This process happens well in advance of the peristaltic wave. Thus, it is regarded that this process causes burns due to swallowing of corrosive fluids more at the distal end of esophagus.

The peristaltic wave rate varies in different portions of the esophagus:

- Rapid progression of peristaltic wave in the upper part of esophagus
- Slow progression in the lower third of esophagus.

These differences have been observed due to the variation in the musculature, the musculature is striated in the upper portion of esophagus and smooth at the lower one-third of esophagus.

PHONATION

Phonation or speech is an expression of thought by production of articulate sounds bearing a definite meaning. It is brought about by coordinated activity of different parts of brain, particularly the motor, sensory and psychic areas.

Mechanism

It is through the coordinated activities of central speech and peripheral speech apparatus. The central apparatus consist of higher centers, i.e. cortical and sub cortical centers in brain. Peripheral apparatus includes larynx or sound box, pharynx, mouth, nasal cavities, tongue and lips.

Development

First Stage

In first stage of the development of speech, association of certain words with visuals, tactile, auditory and other sensations occur which is eventually aroused by objects in the external world.

Second Stage

New neuronal circuits are established during the development of speech in this stage.

Nervous Control

Speech is an integrated and well-coordinated motor phenomenon. Therefore, several parts of the central nervous system are involved in this mechanism. In about 95% of human being, the left cerebral hemisphere is functionally predominant in those persons who are right handed.

Disorders

The disorders of speech are as follows:
- Aphasia: Inability to speak words
- Anarthria or dysarthria: Inability or difficulty to articulate remembered words
- Agnosia: Inability to understand the words or inability to recognize a known object.

Test Yourself

Expected Theory Questions

- Explain in detail about various stages of tooth development.
- What is a gland? Please classify.
- Write a note on the histology of dentin.
- What is deglutition? What are the different stages of deglutition?
- Explain the different functions of saliva.

Expected Viva Questions

- What is the average amount of saliva secreted in normal condition?
- What is the percentage of inorganic substance in enamel and dentin?
- What is the normal number of erythrocytes in male?
- When is the first sign of human tooth development seen?
- What are neonatal teeth?

SECTION 3

General and Dental Pharmacology

SECTION OUTLINE

- General and Local Anesthesia
- Antibiotics in Dental Practice
- Hemostatics
- Vasoconstrictors and Vasodilators
- Counterirritant Agents
- Analgesics
- Hypnotics
- Obtundents and Caustics
- Disclosing Agents
- Dentifrices and Mouthwashes
- Local Drug Delivery
- Desensitizing Agents

General and Local Anesthesia

CHAPTER 19

GENERAL ANESTHESIA

General anesthesia (GA) for dental care in children and adult is sometimes necessary in order to provide safe, efficient and effective care. Depending on the patient, it can be administered in an ambulatory or hospitalized case. The safety of the patient and practitioner should be of paramount importance regardless of the method used.

Preoperative Procedure

Although GA can be given in the dental office in presence of a qualified anesthetist and essential equipment, the safest place to administer is the hospital. Parental or guardian written consent must be taken before administering it. Documentation regarding dental treatment needs, unmanageability in dental clinic, and the associated medical problems must be included in the patient's hospital record. With the consulting anesthetist, the dental surgeon should plan the dental procedures in a rigid time schedule.

Anesthetic Procedure

Facilities for artificial ventilation and for the administration of oxygen and aspirating equipment for cleaning mouth, pharynx and trachea should always be available. Nasotracheal intubation is preferred to ensure good access to the oral cavity. The patient's eyes should be covered with damp gauze so as to protect them against dental and material debris. Great care is warranted to inhibit the entrance of blood or any other type of debris into patient's throat. A mouth prop should be used to keep the mouth open. The pharyngopalatine area is sealed off with a strip of moist 3-inch sterile gauze approximately 18 inches long. This throat pack is tightly packed around the tube. This pack prevents the gases to escape and does not allow debris to enter the throat. A rubber dam may be used when carrying restorations for a dry field and better visibility.

The following monitoring equipment are usually available:

- Stethoscope
- Automatic sphygmomanometer
- Electrocardiograph leads
- A temperature monitoring device
- A pulse oximeter and a capnography device.

Indications

- Patients with certain physical, mental or medically compromised patients
- Patients in whom local anesthesia (LA) is ineffective because of acute infection, allergy or anatomic variations
- Extremely uncooperative, fearful, anxious or uncommunicative child.

Contraindications

- Healthy and cooperative patients
- When GA cannot be given on medical grounds.

Agents

Nitrous Oxide

It is a colorless, nonirritating gas with sweet taste. It is also called laughing gas as it produces excitement and delirium. It is used with oxygen and ether and the technique is called "gas-oxygen-ether (GOE) technique". It is the safest of the anesthetic agent with rapid induction, recovery and a better analgesic action in subanesthetic concentration. Nausea, vomiting and irritation are uncommon with nitrous oxide (N_2O).

Ether

Anesthetic ether contains 96–98% diethyl ether. It is highly inflammable, colorless, volatile, and liquid with pungent smell. It is usually used along with oxygen and N_2O. It is also a safest anesthetic agent with excellent analgesia, therefore provides excellent pain relief under light anesthesia. The induction with ether is slow and laryngeal spasm may occur because of pungent smell. Nausea and vomiting appear during recovery and the recovery is slow. Alcoholics are tolerant to ether. It is economical.

Halothane (Fluothane)

It is a heavy colorless liquid with sweet odor supplied in amber colored bottles. It has a fruity odor and readily attacks all metals like stainless steel, brass, copper and rubber elements. A special apparatus is required to achieve precise control of concentration. Halothane (2–3%) in oxygen produces loss of consciousness and the maintenance dosage is 1–2%.

It is noninflammable and does not irritate respiratory passage. Induction of anesthesia is quick and pleasant without laryngospasm. It provides a bloodless field and is preferred for plastic surgery. As it possesses poor analgesic properties, sedative and narcotics may be used for premedication. Halothane is expensive also.

Thiopentone

It is a thiobarbiturate and is used as thiopentone sodium. These are used intravenously to produce anesthesia. The induction is very quick and pleasant with ease in administration. The incidence of vomiting and excitement is less. There is speedy recovery after small doses without postanesthetic complication. Thiopentone sodium 0.5–1 g is used as a freshly prepared and 2.5% solution for intravenous anesthesia. This agent is used for operation of short duration. This anesthesia is contraindicated in presence of hepatic/renal damage in shock, in airway obstruction, in bronchial asthma, and porphyria. When it is used premedication with atropine is a must.

Ethyl Chloride

Ethyl chloride is a nonirritating, highly volatile and inflammable liquid with a boiling point of 12°C. The vapor has a characteristic but not unpleasant odor. It induces GA within two to three minutes. Because of its quick induction property, it is mainly used for induction of GA. When sprayed on the skin, it rapidly evaporates and thus cools the skin thereby producing transient paralysis of cutaneous sensory nerve endings. The LA effect last from a few seconds to a minute and so incision of an abscess can be carried out within this time. If ethyl chloride spray is used as local anesthetic, the skin should be prepared with petrolatum to prevent sloughing. The spray may produce local edema with decreased resistance to infection and delayed wound healing.

Ketamine

It is a new nonbarbiturate general anesthetic agent. It is effective in both intramuscular and intravenous routes. Following a single dose (1–2 mg/kg for IV) it induces a state of dissociative anesthesia characterized by complete analgesia combined with amnesia. Analgesia lasts for about 40 minutes while anesthesia lasts for about 15 minutes only.

The drug increases the blood pressure and can be used in presence of shock.

Other general anesthetic agents are trichloroethylene, methoxyflurane, cyclo-propane, methohexital, etc.

Propofol

Newer group, action not very well understood.

- Duration of action: 5 to 10 minutes
- Dosage: Adults (up to 55 years age) 2.5 mg/kg
- Adverse reactions: Involuntary movements, burning, stinging at site of injection, abdominal cramps.

LOCAL ANESTHESIA

Local anesthesia (LA) is loss of sensation, especially pain in a localized area without loss of consciousness. Loss of sensation in a part of body can be achieved by:

- Refrigeration, i.e. application of ice
- Making tissue anemic
- Use of drugs.

The mode of action of local anesthetics is to block nerve conduction, probably by preventing normal passage of ions through the nerve membrane. All sensation, i.e. pain, temperature, pressure and motor functions are affected by the local anesthetic agent. The type of LA used in dentistry is:

- *Topical or surface anesthesia*: Free nerve endings in accessible areas are rendered incapable of sensation by the application of a suitable local anesthetic drug, i.e. 5% xylocaine jelly. Mucous membrane, abraded skin and the cornea of the eye respond well to topical application of a local anesthetic agent
- *Local infiltration*: The terminal nerve endings in the area of surgery are flooded with the local anesthetic solution making them incapable of transmitting an impulse. The surgery is performed in the area in which the anesthetic solution has been deposited
- *Field block*: The local anesthetic agent is deposited in the proximity of a large terminal nerve trunk. All areas beyond this nerve trunk are anesthetized
- *Nerve block*: The main nerve trunk is blocked by the anesthetic solution and hence the area beyond the blocked region gets anesthetized, e.g. inferior alveolar nerve block.

Indications

- Cavity preparation in painful teeth
- Pulpotomy, pulpectomy and root canal therapy
- Extraction of teeth
- Minor oral surgery
  - Surgical extraction
  - Apicoectomy
  - Gingivectomy, flap procedures
  - Removal of cyst
  - Alveolectomy and alveoloplasty
  - Excision of small growth
  - Biopsy.

Contraindications

- Refusal by patient
- In presence of infection, the LA does not act because of acidic pH
- Allergy to LA
- In children because of lack of cooperation LA may not be used
- In mentally retarded people
- In patients suffering from bleeding disorders like hemophilia, Christmas disease or Von Willebrand's disease.

Method of Induction

- Nerve block—may be obtained either by intraoral or extraoral routes
- Field block and local infiltration
  - Submucosal injection
  - Paraperiosteal injections
  - Intraosseous injections
  - Interseptal injections
  - Intraligamentary injections.

Complications

- *Due to LA solution:*
  - Toxicity
  - Allergy
  - Anaphylaxis
  - Infections
  - Local irritations.
- *Due to needle insertion:*
  - Syncope
  - Pain
  - Needle tract infection
  - Broken needle
  - Hematoma
  - Prolonged anesthesia.

Agents

Lignocaine Hydrochloride

It is the most commonly used drug and is stable and can be stored at room temperature for a long time. It is used as a topical anesthetic agent in concentration of 2–5%. A 2% solution is used together with the small amount of adrenaline (1:80,000). The adrenaline increases the duration of anesthesia by inducing vasoconstriction in the area and thus confining the anesthetic to the site of infection, it has also the advantage of improving visibility by reducing bleeding. This solution is used for nerve block, field block and local infiltration.

The use of adrenaline-containing local anesthetic is contraindicated in patients with ischemic coronary disease, hypertension, taking tricyclic antidepressants or hypotensive drugs such as beta-blocker.

Prilocaine

Prilocaine (3%) with felypressin as a vasoconstrictor can be safely used on patients with coronary disease. It is available in the brand name of Citanest® with Octapressin® as vasoconstrictor.

Equipment

The local anesthetic is provided in a glass, 2 mL cartridge which has thin plastic seal at one end and a rubber bung at the other. When it is placed in syringe, the double-end needle pierces the plastic seal and solution is injected when the plunger at the other end pushes down the rubber bung.

To reduce cross infection, the plastic end of cartridge or needle should not be touched. A pair of fine hemostat should be kept nearby to remove the broken needle while giving anesthesia. Nowadays the aspirating syringe can be used safely to avoid injecting the solution into blood vessels.

In a normal individual, 20 mL is the maximum amount of local anesthetic with a vasoconstrictor which can be safely administrated.

Antibiotics in Dental Practice

CHAPTER 20

INTRODUCTION

Antibiotics are considered as powerful medicines that treat certain infections. They play a vital role in saving the lives of the patients either by stopping bacteria from reproducing or by destroying them. The first antibiotic developed was penicillin.

CLASSIFICATION

According to Chemical Structure

- *Beta-lactum ring:*
  - Penicillins
  - Cephalo-sporins
  - Monobactams
  - Carbapenems.
- *Sulfanilamide:*
  - Sulfadiazine.
- *Diaminopyrimidines:*
  - Trimethoprim.
- *Quinolones:*
  - Nalidixic acid.
- *Tetracyclines:*
  - Oxytetracycline.
- *Nitrobenzenes:*
  - Chloramphenicol.
- *Aminoglycosides:*
  - Streptomycin.
- *Macrolides:*
  - Erythromycin.
- *Polypeptides:*
  - Bacitracin.
- *Nitroimidazoles:*
  - Metronidazole.

According to Mechanism of Action

- *Inhibit cell wall synthesis:*
  - Penicillins
  - Cephalosporins
  - Bacitracin.
- *Inhibit protein synthesis:*
  - Tetracyclines
  - Chloramphenicol
  - Erythromycin.
- *Inhibit DNA gyrase:*
  - Quinolones.
- *Cause leakage from cell membrane:*
  - Bacitracin.
- *Interfere with DNA function:*
  - Metronidazole
  - Rifampicin.
- *Cause misreading of mRNA code:*
  - Aminoglycosides.
- *Interfere with intermediary metabolism:*
  - Sulfonamides.

According to Spectrum of Activity

- *Narrow spectrum:*
  - Penicillin
  - Streptomycin
  - Erythromycin.
- *Broad spectrum:*
  - Tetracyclines
  - Chloramphenicol.

According to Mode of Action

- *Bacteriostatic:*
  - Sulfonamides

- Tetracyclines
- Chloramphenicol
- Erythromycin.
- *Bactericidal:*
  - Penicillins
  - Cephalosporins
  - Aminoglycosides
  - Quinolones.

According to Source

- *Fungi:*
  - Penicillins
  - Cephalosporins.
- *Bacteria:*
  - Bacitracin.
- *Actinomycetes:*
  - Aminoglycosides
  - Tetra-cyclines
  - Chloramphenicol.

PROBLEMS ASSOCIATED WITH ANTIBIOTIC USAGE

- Toxicity—local irritants and systematic toxicity
- Hypersensitivity reactions
- Drug resistance
- Superinfection
- Nutritional deficiencies
- Masking of an infection.

FACTORS FOR ANTIBIOTICS SELECTION

The following factors are required for antibiotics selection:

- *Patient's factors:*
  - Age
  - Renal function
  - Hepatic function.
- *Local factors:*
  - Drug allergy.
- *Impaired host defence:*
  - Pregnancy.
- *Genetic factors.*

Patient's Factors

Age of the Patient

- Age affects the pharmacokinetics of the drug
- Chloramphenicol causes Gray baby syndrome in new born infants
- Sulfonamides causes kernicterus in neonates
- Tetracycline staining is caused due to intake of tetracycline during second and third trimester of pregnancy or in children upto 8 years of age
- Aminoglycosides leads to 8th nerve toxicity in old age.

Renal Function

- *Dose reduction in mild renal failure:*
  - Aminoglycosides
  - Cephalosporins
  - Vancomycin.
- *Dose reduction in moderate to severe renal failure:*
  - Metronidazole
  - Fluoroquinolones.
- *Drugs to be avoided:*
  - Cephalothin
  - Tetracyclines
  - Nalidixic acid.

Hepatic Function

- *Dose reduction in hepatic disorders:*
  - Chloramphenicol
  - Metronidazole.
- *Drugs to be avoided:*
  - Erythromycin
  - Tetracyclines.

Local Factors

Drug Allergy

- History of previous exposure to drug
- *Drugs frequently associated with allergies:*
  - Beta-lactams
  - Sulfonamides
  - Fluoroquinolones.

Impaired Host Defense

Pregnancy

- *Avoid use of antibiotics, if need does exist then, well-tolerated drugs:*
  - Penicillins
  - Cephalosporins
  - Erythromycin.

Genetic Factors

Geneticists have demonstrated that overuse of antibiotics can make non-resistance bacteria resistant because they assume DNA of already resistance bacteria. The mere presence of antibiotics exposes the bacteria to enormous stress, and this stress triggers random behavior.

INDICATIONS FOR ANTIBIOTICS PROPHYLAXIS

- Prosthetic cardiac valve
- Other intravascular prosthesis
- History of infective endocarditis, complex cyanotic heart disease, hypertrophic cardiomyopathy
- Other valvular lesions including mitral valve prolapse and rheumatic valvular disease
- Joint replacement.

Standard Prophylactic Regimen

- Cap amoxicillin 2 g orally 1 hour before
- If nil orally—injection ampicillin 2 g intramuscular (IM) 30 minutes before.

If Allergic

- Clindamycin 600 mg orally or
- Cefadroxil 2 g orally or
- Clarithromycin 500 mg orally 1 hour before.

If Nil Orally

- Injection clindamycin 600 mg IM
- Injection cephazoline 1 g IM 30 minutes before.

ADULT DOSAGE OF COMMONLY USED ANTIBIOTICS IN DENTAL OFFICE

The choice of antibiotic depends on factors which involve the patient and the organism. History of allergy, status of renal and hepatic functions, immune status ability to tolerate drugs by mouth, severity of the disease, and sex are factors related to patient. In case of female patients, additional points such as pregnancy, breastfeeding or use of oral contraceptives should be taken into account.

- Ampicillin 500 mg QID (four times daily/6 hourly)
- Erythromycin 500 mg QID (four times daily/6 hourly)
- Amoxicillin 500 mg TID (three times daily/8 hourly)
- Augmentin 625 mg TID (three times daily/8 hourly)
- Ciprofloxacin 500 mg BD (twice daily/12 hourly)
- Cefadroxil 500 mg TID (three times daily/8 hourly)
- Tinidazole 400 mg BD (twice daily/12 hourly): Alcohol consumption contraindicated
- Metronidazole 400 mg BD (twice daily/12 hourly): Alcohol consumption contraindicated
- Doxycycline 100 mg—two doses stat on first day and then 1 dose once daily on subsequent days)
- Azithromycin 500 mg OD (once daily). It can be administered same as doxycycline.

To be taken 1 hour before meals or 2 hours after meals.

Hemostatics

CHAPTER 21

INTRODUCTION

Hemostatics are the agents which arrest bleeding. When these agents are acting locally then they are called styptics. Bleeding can be from gums, tooth socket, ruptured vein or arteriole, blood vessels of a fractured bone or from adjacent soft tissues. Hemostasis can be achieved by different methods which are as follows:

- *Hemostasis achieved by physical method:*
  - Pressure application
  - Tourniquet
  - Ligation
  - Cold
  - Use of cautery.
- *Hemostasis achieved by using hemostatic agent:*
  - Local acting agents:
    - ◊ Tannic acid/alum/turpentine
    - ◊ Thrombin
    - ◊ Thromboplastin
    - ◊ Fibrin
    - ◊ Gelfoam
    - ◊ Oxidized cellulose
    - ◊ Bone wax
    - ◊ Adrenaline.
  - Systemic acting agents:
    - ◊ Fibrinogen
    - ◊ Antihemophilic globulin
    - ◊ Plasma or blood
    - ◊ Calcium
    - ◊ Vitamin and rutin
    - ◊ Certain snake venoms
    - ◊ Vitamin K
    - ◊ Epsilon-aminocaproic acid (EACA)
    - ◊ Sclerosing agents.

PHYSICAL METHOD

Pressure

Bleeding can be controlled by pressure from swabs and this is undoubtedly the most effective method for almost all intraoral wounds. A dry gauze swab is packed into the wound over the bleeding area and digital pressure is maintained over the swab for a minimum of two and half minutes and pressure should be more than clotting time.

Tourniquet

It reduces the venous drainage thus producing hemostasis.

Ligation

Severed blood vessels may be tied with ligatures. A ligature replaces the haemostat as a permanent method of effective haemostasis. For large pulsatile artery, a transfixation ligature to prevent slipping, is indicated.

Cold

Cold compress produces vasoconstriction thus produces hemostasis.

Use of Cautery

It produces hemostasis by thermal coagulation.

HEMOSTATIC AGENTS

Local acting agents

Tannic Acid

Tannic acid or turpentine applied on gauze packs or cotton wool to stop bleeding. It is dangerous and can cause second degree burns at the angle of the mouth and on the lips if it is applied in a bleeding socket.

Thrombin

Thrombin acts at the end of the clotting cascade, action of agent is unaltered by clotting factors deficiencies or platelets malfunction. It can also be given to patients receiving anti-platelets/anticoagulant therapy. Active topical agents are beneficial in controlling bleeding and provide hemostatics within 10 minutes.

Thrombin therapy is restricted to local application in oozing of blood.

Thromboplastin

It is extracted from brain or lung tissue of freshly killed rabbits. It is used for determination of prothrombin time and as a local hemostatic in surgery.

Fibrin

It is composed of concentrated fibrinogen and thrombin which in combination with blood creates fibrin clot. Higher concentration of both fibrinogen and thrombin at bleeding site causes increased rate of clot formation. Moreover, fibrin sealants control local as well as diffuse bleeding but cannot control vigorous bleeding.

Gelfoam

It is a local hemostatic made of porous pressed form of gelatin sponge which is available as cones, packs, sponges and powder to control ooze from surface wounds. It is moistened with sterile isotonic saline during use which gets absorbed within 4–6 weeks from the operative wound.

Oxidized Cellulose (Oxycel)

It reacts with blood increase in size and forms a gelatinous mass and promotes clot formation. Oxycel is usually absorbed completely within 2–10 days. It interferes with the bone regeneration.

Bone Wax

A purely mechanically acting hemostatic agent is bone wax which consists of bees wax seven parts by weight, olive oil two parts, phenol one part. This substance is racked into bleeding bone ends to control the hemorrhage. It forms wax granules.

Adrenaline

It is used with the help of a gauze or wool pack. Dilution is 1:1,000. It is absorbed from skin or mucous membrane and causes vasoconstriction.

Systemic Acting Agents

Fibrinogen

Fibrinogen, a soluble protein found in the plasma is broken down to fibrin by the enzyme thrombin to form clots. Maximum amount of the fibrinogen in the circulating blood is formed in the liver. The normal level is 200–400 mg/100 mL in plasma. If the concentration is less than 100 mg/100 mL, coagulation gets impaired.

Antihemophilic Globulin

It is a protein which is required for the clotting of normal blood and in patients who are or deficient in hemophilia A. Factor VIII is produced in liver sinusoidal cells and endothelial cells outside of the liver throughout the body.

In active form, this protein gets circulated in the bloodstream and bounds to another molecule called Von Willebrand factor, until an injury that damages blood vessels occurs. This coagulation factor VIII gets activated and separates itself from Von Willebrand factor in case of an injury. The active protein also referred as coagulation factor VIIIa interacts with another coagulation factor called factor IX, which sets off a chain of additional chemical reactions forming a blood clot.

Plasma or Blood

Fresh frozen plasma should only be used to replace single inherited clotting factor deficiencies for which no virus safe fractionated product is available. Currently applies mainly to factor V.

Calcium

Calcium therapy, particularly by parenteral route, is restored to control of bleeding. Except in the presence of calcium deficiency such treatment is not useful.

Vitamin C

Vitamin C can control bleeding only in the presence of scurvy. The oral dose is 50–100 mg of vitamin C, repeated three to four times a day.

Snake Venom

Especially Russell's viper and copperhead snake venoms enhance coagulation by stimulating thrombokinase.

Vitamin K

It is fat soluble vitamin but is not single entity but occurs naturally in the form of at least two distinct substances vitamin K1 and K2. Both are derivatives of naphthoquinone. Vitamin K is essential for the biosynthesis of prothrombin and factors VII, IX and X. Apart from the action on blood coagulation, vitamin K does not possess any other pharmacological actions.

Epsilon-Aminocaproic Acid

Continuous uncontrolled hemorrhage associated with excessive fibrinolytic activity has been considered on indication for EACA therapy. The drug has been used to control hemorrhage in abruptio placentae, postpartum hemorrhage and hemorrhage after some surgical proceedings. Dose is 100 mg/kg, or orally four times a day.

Sclerosing Agents

Sclerosing agents are irritating substances employed to obliterate varicose veins. They have also been employed for fibrosing uncomplicated hemorrhoids.

CHAPTER 22

Vasoconstrictors and Vasodilators

VASOCONSTRICTORS

Drugs which constrict blood vessels are called vasoconstrictors.

Adrenaline

It is sympathetic neurohormonal transmitter of the adrenal medulla. It causes vasoconstriction of the blood vessels when applied locally or given as an intravenous injection. For hemostatic effect, gauze is soaked in adrenaline and applied on mucous membrane or packed into socket. It may be injected subcutaneously and action lasts for 0.5–1 hour. Strong solution produces sloughing and very large amounts may result in dry socket. Intravenous injection increases the rate and the cardiac output of the heart. There is a rise of blood pressure due to vasoconstriction but the vessels of skeletal muscles are dilated. It also produces a thick viscous secretion from salivary glands.

In control of hemorrhage, dose is:

- Topical: 1:1,000–1:20,000 bleeding from arterioles and capillaries
- Use with local anesthetics: 1:800,000–1:200,000
- Intracardiac: 0.2–0.3 mL of 1:1,000
- Ventricular fibrillation: 0.5–1 mg (5–10 mL of 1:10,000 every 5 minutes).

Noradrenaline

A catecholamine secreted from adrenal medulla mainly used for elevating the blood pressure in shock.

Isoprenaline (Isoproterenol)

Isoprenaline is the most powerful synthetic, beta-receptor stimulant drug.

- Dose: 5–20 mg sublingually
- Inhalation: 5 mL of 1:200 solution.

Isoprenaline is sometimes being advocated as a cardiac stimulant in the treatment of bacteremic shock.

Ephedrine

It is alkaloid obtained from plants of genus *Ephedra*. It increases blood pressure both by peripheral vasoconstriction and by increasing the cardiac output. It relaxes the bronchial smooth muscle. It increases the metabolic rate and oxygen consumption.

- Dose: Oral 15–60 mg TID, IM or SC 15–45 mg
- Nasal drops: 1% is used.

It is used for:

- Bronchial asthma
- Nasal decongestion
- Hypotension.

Amphetamine

It increases the systolic and diastolic blood pressure. It does not elevate cardiac output significantly.

- Dose: 5–10 mg given in the morning and at midday.

It is used for:

- Narcolepsy: 30–40 mg/day
- Obesity
- In certain cases of epilepsy.

Metaraminol (Aramine)

It resembles noradrenaline, and it raises blood pressure by vasoconstriction. Rise in blood pressure accompanied by bradycardia. It increases the cardiac output; cardiac metabolism and force of ventricular contraction.

- Dose: IM 2–10 mg, IV 0.5–10 mg.

Methedrine

Action of these drugs is like amphetamine but more prolonged.

- Dose: 5–10 mg
- It is useful for obesity.

Ergot

Powder or crystals are readily soluble in water. It has a vasoconstricting effect on arterioles. Effect lasts for 4–6 hours. It is used in control of uterine bleeding and causes powerful uterine contraction. Accumulative effect results in poisoning, nausea, vomiting, tingling sensation at fingertips and toes and may result in gangrene.

Felypressin (Octapressin)

Synthetic polypeptide resembles vasopressin, the naturally occurring posterior pituitary hormone combined with local anesthetic agent.

- Dose: 0.03/mL (5.4 mg/mL). 3% prilocaine and felypressin—(Citanest)
- Advantage: It can be given to patients with cardiovascular disease.

VASODILATORS

Drugs which reduce systemic vascular resistance.

Amyl Nitrate

When inhaled from broken capsule, it dilates arterioles and causes fall of blood pressure. There is sweating, palpitation, fainting attacks, giddiness, throbbing of head and flushed face.

- It dilates coronary artery and relieves pain of angina
- Dose: 0.5–1 mg sublingually.

Priscol

It is a peripheral vasodilator. It antagonizes the action of adrenaline. It is used in the treatment of Raynaud's disease.

Potassium Thiocyanate

Regulated doses decrease blood pressure. Side effects are nausea, vomiting, diarrhea, and acute poisoning can also occur.

Phentolamine

They produce dilatation of the peripheral blood vessels, particularly the arterioles and capillaries of the skin, increase the mobility of the gut and the secretion of hydrochloric acid. The salivary, lacrimal, respiratory and pancreatic secretions are also augmented.

Prazosin

This drug acts by blocking alpha-receptors. It dilates both arteries and veins, causing reduction in venous return and cardiac output. It is used to treat essential hypertension.

CHAPTER 23

Counterirritant Agents

COUNTERIRRITANTS

This term is applied to a group of irritant drugs which, when applied over skin or mucous membrane produces by sensory stimulation, a local inflammatory reaction of redness with sensations of heat and tingling followed by a moderate degree of local anesthesia from subsequent paralysis of sensory endings. According to intensity of reaction, these drugs are divided into three groups:

1. Rubefacients
2. Vesicants
3. Pustulants.

Rubefacients

Mild irritant acting on the skin or mucous membrane stimulate sensory nerve ending and produce irritation resulting in inflammation, redness, due to increased flow of blood. This increased flow of blood brings more phagocytes to the area so that the bacterial, chemical irritants are combated. The initial stimulation follows fatigue of depression of the nerve so that superficial anesthesia results and local or referred pain is relieved.

The drugs are also capable of producing.

- Acceleration of the heart
- Rise in blood pressure
- Shallow rapid respiration.

Vesicants

These are moderate counterirritant. In the hyperemic area, plasma exudates collect in the stratum corneum and the epidermis is raised to form blisters. Blisters are very painful and undergo resolution after few days.

Pustulants

These are severe irritants and cause rapid painful inflammation and blister formation. Leukocytes are killed by the bacteria and irritants, thus pus is formed in the blisters. The blisters burst and the healing is caused by scar formation.

TYPE OF COUNTERIRRITANTS

Heat

It is applied in the form of hot water bottle on the skin. In oral cavity, it is used as a mouthwash. Application of heat gives relief from dry socket. Hot mouthwashes relieve pain from abscess and ulcers.

Poultice

A kaolin poultice consists of kaolin 52.7% with boric acid, methyl salicylate and thymol made into a paste with glycerin. Action is by heat.

Linseed-Mustard

It has irritant properties. It is added to linseed poultice (2 parts mustard + 28 parts linseed). Mustard leaf can be cut and applied too.

Iodine

Useful mild counterirritant for the oral mucosa and gingival. It is used as 10% solution in glycerin.

Tincture Aconite

Produce tingling sensation, followed by numbness. It is used for deep pocket. 50% of this solution can be used for pain against neuralgias.

Camphor

When rubbed into the skin, it acts as a counterirritant to relieve neuralgia.

Menthol

It is used as 15% in cones, ointments and 20% in liniments along with clove oil.

Turpentine Oil

It is a very powerful counterirritant.

CHAPTER 24

Analgesics

INTRODUCTION

Analgesics are drugs which relieve pain without producing unconsciousness. As the treatment of pain is one of the prime functions of dental practitioner, it is important that he should not only be familiar with the various technical procedures, but that he should also be conversant with the types of classes of drugs necessary to relieve or control this symptom in his patients. Analgesics may act centrally (selective depressant effect on the central nervous system) or may act peripherally due to a direct effect on pain receptors.

It can be classified as:

- Opioid analgesics
- Nonsteroidal anti-inflammatory drugs (NSAIDs).

OPIOIDS

- *Properties:*
  - More potent
  - Useful in severe visceral pain
  - High abuse potential
  - Euphoric feeling after intake
  - Can cause respiratory depression
  - Drugs include morphine, pethidine, pentazocine.

Morphine

- Dosage:
  - Adult: 10–50 mg 4 hourly (Severe pain)
  - Child: 5–10 mg.

Pethidine

- Dosage:
  - 25–100 mg subcutaneous (SC)/intramuscular (IM) or
  - 25–50 mg intravenous (IV) 3 hourly.

Pentazocine

- Dosage:
  - Adult: 25–100 mg QID
  - Child: 25 mg QID.

Newer Opioids

Tramadol

- Excellent analgesic
- Reduces respiratory depression
- No dependence
- Postoperative pain relief
- Dosage:
  - Adults—100 mg SC/IM/IV
  - Child—11.5 mg/kg.

NONSTEROIDAL ANTI-INFLAMMATORY DRUGS

- Properties:
  - Commonly used
  - Cannot be used for severe pain
  - Safer analgesics
  - Anti-inflammatory
  - Antipyretic.

- Non steroidal anti inflammatory drugs (NSAIDs) further classified as:
  - Nonselective cyclooxygenase-2 (COX-2) inhibitors
  - Selective COX-2 inhibitors.

Nonselective COX-2 Inhibitors

It includes aspirin, paracetamol, piroxicam, ibuprofen, diclofenac, indomethacin.

Aspirin

- Relief is provided when pain is of aching type, as in headache, temporomandibular joint (TMJ) dysfunction and dry socket
- Adverse reactions:
  - Gastrointestinal disturbances may lead to gastrointestinal bleeding
  - Prevents platelet aggregation. Therefore, cannot be given in bleeding disorders
    - ◊ Dose: 300 mg 8 hourly
    - ◊ Aspirin, phenacetin: 250 mg, codeine phosphate: 8 mg.

Paracetamol

- This mild analgesic is the principal metabolite formed in the liver from phenacetin and acetanilide
- It is used in patients who are sensitized to aspirin, have history of peptic ulcer or suffer from hemophilia or other bleeding disorders
- Dose: 500 mg 8 hourly.

Ibuprofen

- This is a mild analgesic commonly used in dentistry. It has minimal side effects. It has got excellent anti-inflammatory properties generally used in soft tissue inflammation and postextraction
- Dose: 200-400 mg orally every 4–6 hours.

Indomethacin

- It has moderate analgesic properties along with anti-inflammatory property. It causes severe gastric irritation and bone marrow depression
- Dose: 50 mg two to three times a day.

Piroxicam

- Dose: 20–40 mg OD.

Diclofenac

- It has potent anti-inflammatory, analgesic and antipyretic
- Available as sodium and potassium salts
- Dose:
  - Adult: 50 mg BID
  - Child: 13 mg/kg/day.

Selective COX-2 Inhibitors

Nimesulide

- Potent anti-inflammatory
- Inhibits histamine release
- Dose:
  - Adult: 100 mg BID
  - Child: 5 mg/kg/day in divided doses.

Meloxicam

- New NSAID of oxicam group
- Selective action on COX-2
- Dose: 7.5–15 mg OD.

Celecoxib

- Antirheumatic drug
- Dose: 200 mg daily.

Newer Nonsteroidal Anti-inflammatory Drugs

Ketoprofen

- Propionic acid derivative
- Dose: 50 mg BD/TID, 300 mg in severe cases.

Ketorolac

- Belongs to NSAID
- More potent analgesic
- Dosage: 10–20 mg initially followed by 10 mg 6 hourly.

Hypnotics

CHAPTER 25

INTRODUCTION

A drug, such as a barbiturate or antianxiety agent depresses the activity of the central nervous system (CNS) and is used to relieve anxiety and induce sleep. A hypnotic drug is one which produces sleep resembling natural sleep. A sedative, on the other hand, is drug used to calm and relieve anxiety. These drugs are dose-dependent—lower dose having calming effect and larger dose producing sleep.

CLASSIFICATION

- Urea derivatives
  - Diureides: Barbiturates
  - Related ureides: Glutethimide, methyprylon.
- Benzodiazepines
- Alcohols: Chloral hydrate
- Aldehydes: Paraldehyde
- Acetylated carbilols: Ethinamate
- Miscellaneous: Meprobamate, methaqualone, antihistamine and scopolamine
- Inorganic ions: Bromide.

Drugs like morphine and pethidine, besides its analgesic property, also possess hypnotic property. Hence, they are grouped as anodyne hypnotic. It must be emphasized, that they should not be used as hypnotics in the absence of severe pain.

Barbiturates

It is a derivative of barbituric acid and in the past the most commonly employed hypnotics. It is colorless, odorless, crystalline solids with a bitter taste and is sparingly soluble in water. They dissolve rapidly in the organic solvents like chloroform and ether. Conventionally, the barbiturates are divided according to their duration of action as:

1. Long-acting (8 hours or more), e.g. phenobarbitone.
2. Intermediate acting (4–8 hours), e.g. amylobarbitone, butobarbitone, pentobarbitone.
3. Short-acting (less than 4 hours), e.g. secobarbitone, hexobarbitone.
4. Ultrashort-acting [intravenous (IV)], e.g. thiopentone, methohexitone.

Pharmacological Action

Barbiturates cause reversible depression of the activity of all excitable tissue, the CNS being exquisitely sensitive. However, hypnotic drugs produce very little effects on cardiac, smooth or skeletal muscles.

- *Central nervous system*: Barbiturates can achieve various depth of depression of CNS
  - *Sedation and hypnosis*: The long- and intermediate-acting barbiturates are used for this purpose. Thus, phenobarbitone given in the dose of 15 mg three to four times daily

- *Anesthetic effect*: The short-acting thiobarbiturates administered IV produce basal or general anesthesia dose—thiopentone sodium, i.e. 0.5–1.0 g powder. It is used as a freshly prepared 2.5% solution for IV anesthesia, as basal or for induction
- *Anticonvulsant effect*: All the barbiturates administered anesthetic doses are capable of inhibiting or abolishing drug-induced convulsions
- *Analgesic effect*: Barbiturates cannot reduce pain without producing a loss of consciousness
- *Spinal cord*: Reflexes of spinal cord are depressed by barbiturates
- *Eyes*: Hypnotic doses have no effect on the eyes but moderate increase in the dose elicit nystagmus.

- *Cardiovascular system (CVS)*: Therapeutic doses may cause slight fall in blood pressure and decrease in heart rate
- *Gastrointestinal tract (GIT)*: Sedative doses of barbiturate have no effect on GIT. Toxic doses of barbiturate retard peristalsis
- *Kidney*: Intravenous barbiturates results in reduction in urinary output
- *Liver*: No significant effect.

Absorption Rate and Excretion

Barbiturates and their salts are readily absorbed orally and intramuscularly. They are weak acids and the maximum absorption occurs from the stomach where the barbiturates exist in an unionized form.

Therapeutic Uses

- As sedative and hypnotic
- As anticonvulsant
- Preanesthetic medication
- General anesthetics
- As antipsychotic drugs.

Adverse Reaction

- *Intolerance:* Urticaria, angioneurotic edema, etc.
- Prolonged therapy may produce megaloblastic anemia
- May depress fetal respiration
- *Drug interaction*: Barbiturates when combined with other CNS depression drugs such as alcohol, benzodiazepine may cause severe depression
- *Drug dependence*: Repeated administration of barbiturates causes drug dependence. Manifestation of chronic barbiturate intoxications is thick slurred speech, ataxia, impaired superficial and deep reflexes, hypotonia, nystagmus and difficulty in accommodation
- *Acute barbiturate poisoning*: Results from ingestion of an overdose either accidentally or with suicidal intent. It is characterized by depression of the CNS particularly the respiration and peripheral circulatory collapse.

Benzodiazepines

These are mainly used in anxiety states and neurosis. Benzodiazepines usually exhibit the similar pharmacological properties such as anxiolytic, sedative, hypnotic, skeletal muscle, relaxant, amnesic and anticonvulsant.

All benzodiazepines have a hypnotic action. Diazepam (5–10 mg), flurazepam (15–30 mg) and nitrazepam (5–10 mg) have proved highly effective hypnotics. These drugs cause sedation, hypnosis, decreased anxiety, muscle relaxation and some of them also possess anticonvulsant activity. The benzodiazepines are adequately absorbed when given orally.

Alcohol

It is a colorless, volatile, flammable, water miscible liquid with pungent and ether-like odor.

It possesses burning taste with intoxicating principle of fermented liquors. Moreover, it is produced by yeast fermentation of certain carbohydrates, grains, molasses, starch, or sugar.

Along with the popular of ethanol as a sedative, it also provides the sense of happiness at low doses. This attributes to the fact that low doses of ethanol sedate the parts of the brain involved with tension and anxiety which in turn makes the person consuming it, achieves a sense of joy. However, its higher doses demoralize brain centers involved in vital functions such as pain sensation, coordination and balance. It is often used in medicine as an antidote to treat the effects of some other kinds of drugs.

Chloral Hydrate

It is a white crystalline substance, readily soluble in water.

- Doses:
  - As a mixture 0.5-2.0 g
  - Children syrup 125 mg/year to maximum 375 mg
  - Infants syrup 50-75 mg/dose.

Paraldehyde

It is colorless, transparent and inflammable liquid with a characteristic odor. Paraldehyde is given by rectal or intramuscular route to produce hypnosis.

- Dose:
  - Injection 5-10 mL intramuscularly
  - Injection 15-30 mg rectally.

Ethinamate

It has been used for the short-term treatment of insomnia; however, it generally has been replaced by other sedative-hypnotic agents.

Miscellaneous

Meprobamate is used to treat anxiety disorders for short-term relief of the symptoms of anxiety. Meprobamate is in a class of medications called tranquilizers. It works by slowing activity in the brain to allow for relaxation.

Methaqualone is a depressant that affects the central nervous system. Although completely unrelated, it is said that this drugs effects are similar to those of barbiturates.

Antihistamines are popular as nonprescription (over-the-counter) sleep remedies (e.g. diphenhydramine, doxylamine) in which case their sedative side effect is used as the principal effect.

Scopolamine is used to prevent nausea and vomiting caused by motion sickness or from anesthesia given during surgery. Scopolamine is also used to treat certain stomach or intestinal problems, muscle spasms, and Parkinson-like conditions.

Inorganic Ions

Potassium bromide (KBr) is a salt, widely used as an anticonvulsant and a sedative in the late 19th and early 20th centuries. Its action is due to the bromide ion. Potassium bromide is used as a veterinary drug, as an antiepileptic medication for dogs.

Obtundents and Caustics

CHAPTER 26

OBTUNDENTS

Obtundents are drugs used to dull or abolish the sensation or sensitiveness of dentin to allow its painless excavation.

Their action is by:

- Paralyzing the nerve fibril, e.g. local anodynes
- Precipitating proteins and killing nerve tissue, e.g. caustics.

A good obtundent should act painlessly, penetrate dentin rapidly, but not too deeply as it may cause inflammation or necrosis of pulp and that it should not stain enamel or dentin.

Types

Phenol

It is a protoplasmic poison. It causes tingling and then numbness. It acts rapidly but does not penetrate deeply, because it is not soluble in saline or albuminous fluids. It does not stain healthy dentin but darkness infected dentin. 80% phenol is used, and is vaporized with hot air syringe to promote penetration. It is neutralized with alcohol, glycerin or all.

Creosote

It acts as an anodyne on exposed pulp. At first irritates and paralyzes sensory nerve endings causing numbness and analgesia. Penetration is deeper than phenol. It is vaporized with hot air syringe.

Clove Oil

It paralyzes nerve fibrils. It penetrates slowly so requires to be sealed into the cavity for few days. It stains dentin yellow. It is a common ingredient of antiseptic pastes or temporary filling for sensitive dentin.

Camphor, Thymol, Menthol

These volatile oils act like clove oil. Spirit of camphor, alcoholic solution of menthol dried with hot air syringe are good obtundents. Thymol crystals are sealed in cavities. Thymol (2 parts), phenol (2 parts), camphor (1 part) applied to treat sensitive dentin.

Dentalone

It is a saturated solution of chlorbutol. It is a mixture of oil of cloves, cassia and wintergreen. It is nontoxic, obtundent for exposed pulp and sensitive dentin.

Alcohol

It dehydrates and precipitates proteins and is used in 70–95% strength, in a dry cavity. It is painless, does not stain and is nontoxic to the pulp.

Zinc Chloride

It is an astringent caustic. It precipitates proteins. On application, there is brief acute pain and then desensitization. It does not penetrate deeply, does not stain and is a safe drug. It's 5–10% solution is used.

Silver Nitrate

It is a safe caustic, is less painful than zinc chloride. It acts rapidly and is precipitated as phosphate or chloride. It does not penetrate deeply. It stains dentin black and used as 10% solution.

Paraformaldehyde

From this drug, formal-dehyde is liberated which precipitates proteins. Obtundent action is slow and painless. It does not stain. It penetrates deeply.

Paraformaldehyde Plus Zinc Oxide

Made into a paste with clove oil can be sealed into cavities for 6–7 days.

Arsenic Trioxide

It is toxic on living cells. It penetrates deeply and rapidly. In deep cavities, it is not to be used due to chances of necrosis. It is very painful and toxic.

Liquor Soda Ethylate

About 18% solution of sodium ethylate in 95% alcohol. It turns brown on standing and must be freshly prepared. In presence of water, it decomposes into alcohol and sodium hydroxide. It causes slight pain, rapid obtundent effect and does not penetrate deeply nor stains.

CAUSTICS

Caustics are drugs that cause necrosis or tissue death and dissolution of tissues.

- Acids:
  - Nitric
  - Trichloroacetic
  - Lactic and chromic.
- Alkalis:
  - Sodium and potassium hydroxide.
- Metallic salts:
  - Silver nitrate
  - Zinc sulfate and chloride
  - Copper sulfate.
- Protoplasmic poisons:
  - Phenol and arsenic trioxide.

Types

Nitric Acid

It is useful caustic. It acts superficially as it does not dissolve the protein precipitates. It is painful, stains yellow and erodes enamel and dentin. 10% solution is used to devitalize pulp. It is neutralized with sodium bicarbonate.

Trichloroacetic Acid

It is an antiseptic and rapid caustic. It is less painful and more suitable for mucous membranes. 50% solution cauterizes gums, polyp, etc. 5–20% solution is used on aphthous ulcers, Vincent's infection, gingival pockets. Dilute solutions remove tobacco stains.

Lactic Acid

It is very useful caustic for oral use due to low toxicity. It can be applied in cases of leukoplakia and aphthous ulcers. It is used for removing diphtheroid membrane.

Chromic Acid

About 10–20% solution is used on acute ulcerative gingivitis and cancrum oris. It is an antiseptic, caustic, oxidizing and antibacterial agent.

All acids are toxic to cells and have following properties:

- Withdraw water
- Neutralize alkalinity
- Precipitate proteins and dissolve acid albumins.

All alkalis are caustic and have following properties:

- Withdraw water from cells
- Form alkaline albumins with proteins and soaps with fats

- They are less painful and deep penetrating. They gelatinize tissues.

Sodium and Potassium Hydroxide

These are unsuitable for dental treatment. (syringe with water to neutralize and prevent deep penetration).

Metallic Salts

They are caustic due to toxic metallic ions. They precipitate proteins. They do not penetrate deeply and so have to be applied repeatedly. They are painful.

Silver nitrate 10%, zinc sulfate, zinc chloride 10% solutions are used on aphthous ulcers, and for desensitizing dentin.

Copper sulfate is a very painful caustic.

Phenol

It precipitates proteins. It penetrates deeply.

Arsenic Trioxide

It is a protoplasmic poison and causes necrosis of tissue cells, nerve fibrils, lymph and blood vessels. It is toxic and causes acute pain.

Disclosing Agents

CHAPTER 27

INTRODUCTION

A disclosing agent is a selective dye in solution, tablet, or lozenge form used to visualize and identify dental biofilm or dental plaque on the surfaces of the teeth and restorative materials. A disclosing agent is used for the identification of bacterial plaque, which might otherwise be invisible to the naked eye (Figs 27.1A and B).

An individual is usually not aware of the quantity or the location of dental plaque present in their mouth. Dental plaque is commonly transparent, colorless and not easily visible, thereby warranting the need of plaque disclosing compositions to identify areas of the mouth rich in plaque.

DISCLOSING SOLUTION

Basic fuchsin: 6 g
Ethyl alcohol: 100 mL
Add two drops water in a dappen dish
Potassium iodide: 1.6 g
Iodine crystal: 1.6 g
Water: 13.4 mL
Glycerin: 30 mL.

Disclosing solutions are applied to teeth surface with cotton swab diluted in water. They produce heavy staining of plaque and soft tissues.

It is an acceptable method for plaque control. If no stains are detected that means the personal oral hygiene of an individual is at its optimal health state.

WAFERS

Disclosing wafers are crushed between teeth and swished around the mouth for 30 seconds without swallowing (Fig. 27.2).

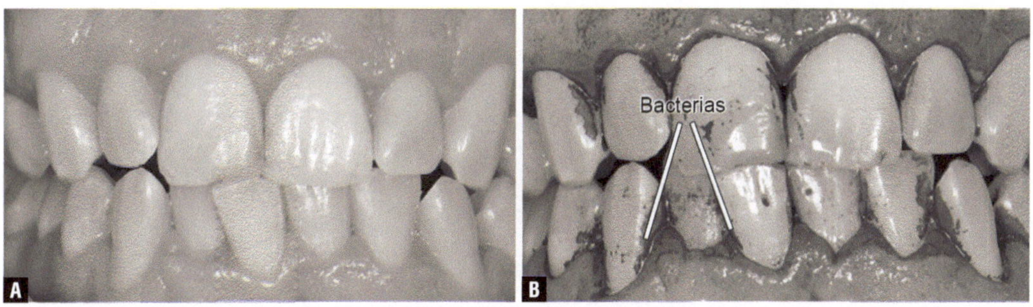

Figs 27.1A and B: (A) Bacteria invisible to naked eye; (B) Bacteria visible after applications of disclosing agent *(For color version, see Plate 11)*

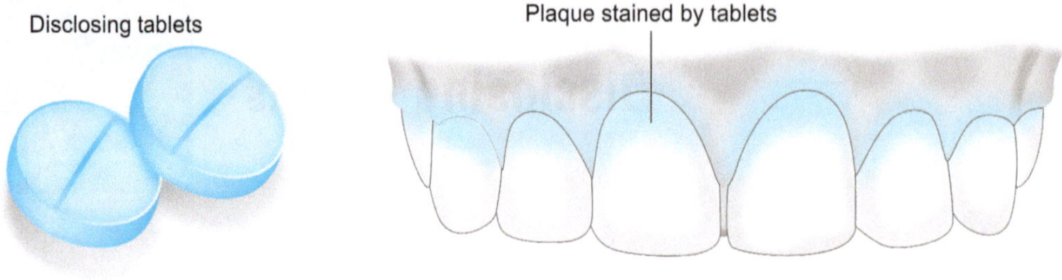

Fig. 27.2: Use of wafers as disclosing agents

Composition

- Erythrosine: 15 mg
- Sodium chloride: 0.747%
- Sodium sucaryl: 0.747%
- Calcium stearate: 0.995%
- Soluble saccharin: 0.186%
- White oil: 0.124%
- Flavoring agent: 2.239%
- Sorbitol: 7 g.

Dentifrices and Mouthwashes

CHAPTER 28

DENTIFRICES

Tooth powders or toothpastes are mechanical aids to cleansing and polishing of teeth with brush. They consist of the following ingredients:

- An abrasive
- Detergent or cleansing agent
- An antiseptic and fluorides
- Flavoring agent
- Coloring agent
- Sweetening agent
- Humectant
- Thickening agent.

Abrasive

These are fine powders which help mechanically the action of a toothbrush. To remove gritty particles, it is passed through 60 mesh powder sieve. Dibasic calcium phosphate has least abrasive action. Calcium carbonate and chalk are used.

Abrasive agents commonly used are:

- Calcium carbonate—a white fine antacid powder
- Chalk—a white amorphous, antacid powder
- Calcium phosphate—a white amorphous powder.

Other agents are:

- Milk of magnesia, kaolin, aluminum oxide, silicon oxide
- Precipitated chalk is frequently combined with magnesium carbonate or oxide or magnesium hydroxide in proportion 1:4.
- Stannic oxide 5–10% may be added if a very high polish is required. pH of saliva is 6.6 but varies. Slight acidity of dentifrice stimulates flow of saliva; on the other hand, alkaline dentifrice neutralizes acids of formation, and also dissolves mucin
- Sodium benzoate 5% dissolves calcium in a kaolin base.

Detergent or Cleansing Agent

These act as:

1. Lowering surface tension, e.g. soap.
2. Dissolving proteins, e.g. soluble alkalis.
3. Evolving oxygen, e.g. peroxides.

The most commonly used is hard soap. Hard soap acts as emollient and cleansing agent by dissolving fatty material and mucin plaques. (It lowers surface tension and loosens debris adherent to teeth and is added from 5% to 25% in the pastes). It acts as a lubricant and foams on teeth. Others used are sodium lauryl sulfate and sodium lauroyl sarcosinate.

Sodium ricinoleate is a valuable soap for treating gingival infections. Soluble alkalis—potassium hydroxide, sodium bicarbonate dissolves protein debris. Sodium, calcium, magnesium perborates and magnesium peroxide liberate oxygen and help to detach debris and exfoliated epithelium. These also act as deodorants.

Antiseptic

These are included in dentifrices but their value in bacterial growth restriction is limited.

- Phenol, thymol, menthol: 0.25–1%
- Eugenol: 1%
- Clove oil, cinnamon: 1–3%
- Potassium chlorate: 2–3%
- Boric acid: 2–5%
- Camphor, borax: 5–10%.

Fluorides

Fluoride tooth paste helps prevent tooth decay and strengthen the tooth enamel by remineralization of the enamel surface. It also helps in minor tooth repair after decalcification. Fluoride in tooth paste is good for people who are at a high-risk for tooth decay and cavity formation.

Flavoring Agent

Mostly these are volatile oils, e.g. thymol, clove, wintergreen, cinnamon, rose. These also act as antiseptics.

Sweetening Agent

Lactose up to 10% is used. It does not ferment. Saccharin sodium is best. It is 200 times sweeter than sugar and does not ferment and 0.1% is added.

Coloring Agents

These are added to toothpastes, which contain toxic antiseptics. Patients are attracted to pleasing colors. Chlorophyll green is in demand at present. Liquor Carmini 2% is also used.

- Methylene blue: 0.001% blue
- Magenta: 0.5%.

Humectants

It binds all ingredients together and keeps dentifrice moist, e.g. glycerin and sorbitol.

Thickening Agents

These are carboxymethyl cellulose, alginate and amylase.

TOOTHPASTES

Tooth powders are converted into pastes by use of syrup, honey, glycerin. Tragacanth (0.1–0.2%) may be added to improve consistency. 1% liquid paraffin may be added so that it can be removed from a tube with ease.

Formula

Composition of a toothpaste is provided in Table 28.1.

For desensitizing and anticariogenic action, sodium fluoride, stannous fluoride, sodium monofluorophosphate have been added. Sensodyne toothpaste contains 10% strontium chloride. Emoform, having 10% formaldehyde acts on hypersensitive dentin. Colgate total, a newly marketed dentifrice contains triclosan, fluoride and Gantrez for added protection.

DEODORANTS

These eliminate halitosis and leave behind freshness and tingling sensation.

- Chlorophyll—deodorant, bacteriostatic
- Oxidizing agent—peroxide in some form

Table 28.1: Composition of a toothpaste

Ingredient	*Percent by weight*
Calcium pyrophosphate	40.00
Sorbitol (70% aqueous solution)	20.40
Glycerine	10.20
Sodium coconut monoglyceride sulfonate	0.82
Sodium lauryl sulfate	0.80
Sodium carboxymethyl cellulose	1.00
Magnesium aluminum silicate	0.40
Stannous fluoride	0.40
Flavor (spearmint)	0.90
Color	0.05
Sweetener (potassium salt of 6-methyloxathiazinone dioxide)	0.05
Water and minors	balance

- Hexachlorophene: It is a coal tar derived antiseptic and deodorant.

MOUTHWASHES

It is used as an aid to physiotherapy. Simple rinsing of the mouth with plain water will remove mechanically any detachable or soluble debris. It removes bacteria and their products by its irrigation power. The mechanical action is increased if used with compressed air and carbon dioxide sprays. Various chemicals have been now incorporated based on rational to make them:

- Anticaries
- Anticalculus
- Desensitizing
- Preventive and therapeutic.

According to mode of action, they can be considered as the following:

- Oxidizing
- Acid and alkalis
- Coal tar agents
- Desensitizing
- Physical agent
- Therapeutic for diseases.

Oxidizing

This action is due to nascent oxygen and effervescence. The mechanical action helps in cleaning deposits. The antiseptic action may be effected by free radicals and bleaching agents are also added. Drugs added are hydrogen peroxide 1 to 3% or 3% of 20 vol potassium permanganate as 1 in 5,000 to 1 in 10,000. These produce stains. Potassium chlorate 2% may also be used. Perborate was marketed as Amosan.

Acids and Alkalis

This makes a soothing and bland mouthwash. It withdraws water from bacteria. Detergent action neutralizes acids of fermentation. Sodium bicarbonate is used 2% strength. Chelating agents have a capacity to remove calcium salts from mineral structure. Thus, it prevents incorporation of calcium in the soft enamel matrix. 5–10% solution in water is used. It has a good smell and a cooling effect.

Astringents

Astringents act by precipitating the proteins on the surface to produce a protective layer against bacterial invasion. Alum, tannic acid 5 g in one fluid ounce is useful for tender swollen gums and helps heal ulcerations. Other drugs are zinc chloride, zinc acetate, acetic and citric acids.

Coal Tar Derivatives

Phenol has a caustic or corrosive action. In small concentrations, it is an anodyne antiseptic useful for aphthous ulcer and dry sockets.

Physical Agents

It acts by mechanical rinsing action and high osmotic pressure. Normal saline is used as a cleaning mouthwash. Hypertonic saline has cleansing and protein solvent action used after prophylaxis and gingivitis.

Anesthetic Mouthwash

This produces and acts as surface anesthetic. It is useful in painful oral ulcers and acute necrotizing ulcerative gingivitis (ANUG). It must be used 30 minutes prior to meals or must be used in between meals. These are anodyne mouthwashes.

Proprietary group (Amosan) "Sodium perborate monohydrate" (BNA O3.)

This yields 65% more O_2 than sodium perborate. Cases show better healing, when one spoonful is used in 100 mL of water.

Ascoxal

It has been tried and compared with hydrogen peroxide in management of ANUG. It reduces the viscosity of saliva. It is demucopolysaccharide with antimicrobial effect. There is marked inhibiting of calculus formation. It is pleasant in taste. Available in tablet and contains vitamin C 100 mg. Sodium bicarbonate 75 mg, copper sulfate as a catalyst only in traces.

Bocasin

One tablet is put in a glass of water. It is effective in ANUG which shows 75% improvement in 48 hours. It is buffered with sodium bitartrate.

Dettolin

It contains chloroxylenol 1.02% w/v, menthol 0.12% w/v and absolute alcohol 60.8% w/v.

Listerine

It is essential oil mouthwashes which coagulate organic matter. It reduces secretion of saliva and washes away the mucin. It acts as a deodorant and removes halitosis.

Chlorhexidine

Chlorhexidine (CHX) is a diguanidohexane with pronounced antiseptic properties. 10 mL of 2% or 15 mL of 1.20% aqueous solution of CHX mouthwash done twice inhibits development of dental plaque. Its side effect is brown staining of teeth, tongue and resin restorations.

Antiseptics used in mouth rinses:

- Triclosan
  - Broadspectrum of activity
  - Effective against Gram-positive and Gram-negative bacteria
  - Antiplaque efficacy
  - Used in combination with zinc citrate.
- Metal ions
  - Stannous fluoride (reduce acid formation in plaque)
  - Antigingivitis effect
  - Reduce halitosis by eliminating volatile sulfur-containing compounds (SCC).

MEDICATED DENTIFRICES

Antiplaque and Antigingivitis Dentifrices

- Chlorhexidine (1%)
- Triclosan (in combination with zinc citrate).

Anticalculus Dentifrices

- 2% zinc chloride
- 1.25–5% pyrophosphate salts
- Triclosan (0.2%).

Anticaries Dentifrice

These contain fluorides in form of:

- Sodium fluoride
- Sodium monofluorophosphate
- Stannous fluoride
- Potassium fluoride
- Aluminum fluoride.

Maximum permissible concentration of fluoride:

- Adults: 1,500 ppm
- Child (<7 years): 250 ppm.

Local Drug Delivery

CHAPTER 29

INTRODUCTION

Local drug delivery (LDD) is the evolved method of delivering the medication within the gum around the teeth. Its advantage include a controlled method of delivering the drug with a standard dose over an extended period of time.

Accumulation of bacteria on hard oral surface is considered the primary cause of gingivitis and periodontitis. Traditionally mechanical/surgical treatments have been the foundation of periodontal treatment along with antimicrobials. Antimicrobial agents can be used for the treatment of periodontal pocket through systemic and local route of delivery. It has been observed that local route of drug delivery can achieve 100-fold higher concentrations of an antimicrobial agent at subgingival sites in contrast to a systemic drug regimen. This decreases the total patient dose by over 400-fold which in turn reduces the potential problems with the use of systemic route of drug administration and development of drug-resistant microbial populations at nonoral body sites. These are well-tolerated in medically compromised patients for whom surgery is not an option.

Controlled delivery systems are designed in such a way that they release drug slowly for more prolonged drug availability and sustained drug action into periodontal pocket. However, drug is released without any mechanism to retain therapeutic levels for prolonged period of time. Therefore, this form of drug delivery is beneficial as it penetrates into the base of periodontal pocket and is maintained for an adequate time for the antimicrobial effect to occur.

Criteria for an Agent to be Effective

- Should inhibit/kill the microorganism
- Reach the site
- Attain adequate concentration
- Stay long enough
- Should not be harmful.

LOCAL DRUG DELIVERY SYSTEMS

Presently, five local delivery systems are available:

1. Tetracycline fibers (Actisite, periodontal AB Plus).
2. Metronidazole gel (Elyzol).
3. Chlorhexidine chip (Periochip).
4. Doxycycline gel (Atridox).
5. Minocycline microspheres (Arestin and periocline).

Tetracycline Fiber (Actisite)

- Placement of tetracycline, loaded ethylene vinyl acetate fibers into periodontal pockets establishes a drug concentration of approximately 0.06%
- It consists of a polymer, ethylene vinyl acetate, 25% saturated with tetracycline HCl

- Length is 2.3 mm, 0.5 mm diameter and contains 12.7 mg of tetracycline HCl
- The fiber releases tetracycline for 14 days.

Metronidazole Gel (Elyzol)

- It contains 25% metronidazole
- It is in fluid form and is injected with a syringe
- It is effective even in lower concentrations and especially against anaerobic bacteria.

Chlorhexidine Chip (Periochip)

Periochip is a biodegradable chip containing 2.5 mg of chlorhexidine gluconate which has been shown to be a beneficial and well-tolerated adjunctive therapy. It reduces depth of pocket in patients with adult periodontitis with a pocket depth (PD) greater than or equal to 5 mm, when used with scaling and root planing (SRP). Periochip (chlorhexidine gluconate) 2.5 mg releases chlorhexidine in vitro in a biophasic manner, initially releasing approximately 40% of the chlorhexidine within the first 24 hours and then releasing the remaining chlorhexidine in an almost linear fashion for 7–10 days.

Doxycycline (Atridox)

- Doxycycline polymer (liquid polymer and powdered doxycycline polymer) needs to be mixed on the chairside before application
- Delivers 10% of doxycycline hyclate into the pocket.

Minocycline (Arestin and Periocline)

- Periocline contains 2% minocycline hydrochloride
- Applied with syringe
- Also available as injectable microspheres (Arestin).

INDICATIONS OF LOCAL DRUG DELIVERY SYSTEMS

- Maintenance patient
- Medically compromised patient unfit for surgery
- Recurrent pockets
- Nonresponding pockets
- Failing implant
- Prior to regenerative treatment
- Periodontal abscess.

ADVANTAGES OF LOCAL DRUG DELIVERY SYSTEMS

- Easy to use
- Achieve high concentration at site
- Does not depend on patient compliance
- Resistance incidence reduced
- Fewer side effects.

DISADVANTAGES OF LOCAL DRUG DELIVERY SYSTEMS

- Expensive
- Do not kill organisms in nontreated sites
- Time consuming if more number of pockets.

Desensitizing Agents

CHAPTER 30

INTRODUCTION

Dental hypersensitivity is characterized by short, sharp pain arising from exposed dentin in response to stimuli such as thermal, evaporative, tactile, osmotic, or chemical and which cannot be ascribed to any other form of dental defect or pathology. Large number of population suffers from symptoms of dentin exposure at some time during their life time.

ROOT SENSITIVITY

Root sensitivity commonly occurs in the cervical area of the root, where cementum is extremely thin. This cementum may get removed during scaling and root planing which in turn leads to hypersensitivity.

Odontoblastic process or hydrodynamic mechanism aids in transmission of stimuli from the surface of dentin to the nerve endings located in dental pulp or in pulpal region of dentin.

Clinical Features

The main symptoms of sensitivity of root include pain induced by cold or hot temperature, more frequently by cold, citrus fruits or sweet, or by contact with a toothbrush or dental instrument.

Plaque control is an important role in reducing or eliminating hypersensitivity. The patient should be informed about the possibility of root hypersensitivity before undergoing any therapy.

The following factors related to hypersensitivity are as follows:

- Hypersensitivity occurs due to exposure of dentin which is inevitable, if calculus and plaque are embedded in the surface of the root
- It slowly disappears over few weeks
- Plaque control is primarily important for the reduction of hypersensitivity
- Action of desensitizing agent takes few weeks to occur.

Agents Used for Desensitization by Patients

The most frequently products used by the patients to relieve pain from hypersensitivity are desensitizing dentifrices, particularly toothpaste containing potassium salts, (potassium nitrate, potassium citrate, and potassium chloride).

The potassium ion has depolarizing effect on electrical nerve conduction causing nerve fibers to be less excitable to the stimuli which thus reduces the patient's sensation. Others agents such as Colgate toothpaste contains 8.0% arginine and 1,450 ppm fluoride in a calcium carbonate base. Sensodyne toothpaste contains 2% potassium ion as 5% potassium nitrate and 1,450 ppm fluoride in a silica base.

Agents Used for Desensitization in Dental Office

Several agents have been used in the form of varnishes, bonding agents, restorations that also reduce caries activity.

Patients should be advised not to rinse, eat or drink for 1 hour after application as some agents like chlorhexidine reduce the ability of fluoride to bind with calcium on root.

Recently to improve the longevity of treatment neodymium-doped yttrium aluminium garnet (Nd:YAG) lasers have been used, but laser treatment is expensive and has potential to cause pulp damage.

Following desensitizing agents are also being used by dental professionals world over:

- Cavity varnishes
- Anti-inflammatory agents
- Treatment that partially obturates dentinal tubules
  - Burnishing of dentin
  - Silver nitrate
  - Zinc chloride
  - Formalin.
- Calcium compounds: Calcium hydroxide
- Fluoride compounds
  - Sodium fluoride
  - Stannous fluoride.
- Iontophoresis
- Strontium chloride
- Restorative resins
- Dentin bonding agents.

Test Yourself

Expected Theory Questions

- Write a short note on various agents used in general anesthesia.
- What are antibiotics? Classify them.
- Explain in detail about local anesthesia along with indications and contraindications.
- Elaborate counterirritant agents in detail.

Expected Viva Questions

- What is the other name for nitrous oxide?
- What is the suitable local anesthetic drug used for topical or surface anesthesia?
- Name some locally acting hemostatic agents.
- What are the characteristics of acute barbiturate poisoning?
- What are the agents used by patient to reduce hypersensitivity?

SECTION 4

Pathology and Microbiology: General and Dental

SECTION OUTLINE

- Inflammation
- Degeneration
- Oral Immunology
- Anomalies of the Teeth
- Fluorosis of the Teeth
- Attrition, Abrasion and Erosion
- Oral Manifestation of Systemic Disease
- Bacteriology and Virology of Oral Cavity
- White Lesions of Oral Cavity
- Oral Cancer
- Dental Caries
- Infection Control Protocol in Dental Practice
- Sterilization and Disinfection
- Biomedical Waste Management

Inflammation

CHAPTER 31

INTRODUCTION

Acute inflammation is the fundamental reaction of the body to injury. Many different agents may cause injury, but they all produce the same basic response. Long ago in the first century AD, Celsus described the cardinal signs of inflammation as rubor, tumor, calor and dolor, which anyone who has suffered from a boil will recognize as redness, swelling, heat and pain. A century later, Galen added function laesa, or loss of function, the fifth cardinal sign.

Causes of Acute Inflammation

There are many and varied causes of injury and, therefore, acute inflammation may be classified as follows:

- *Physical agents:* These include mechanical trauma, heat, extreme cold, ionizing radiation and electricity
- *Chemical agents:* A wide range of chemicals may cause injury to the tissues including all strong acids and alkalis
- *Microorganisms:* Acute inflammation is frequently a feature of infection of the tissues by microorganisms
- *Antigens:* The immune response is discussed in detail in Chapter 33 Oral immunology
- *Interruption of blood supply:* If cells are cut off from their supply of oxygen and nutrition, they die. This is referred to as necrosis and it causes acute inflammation in the surrounding tissue.

Stages of Acute Inflammation

Vascular Response

Following injury, the arterioles in the affected area at first constrict, causing a blanching of the area for a short time, and then dilate. The vasodilatation allows more blood to enter the area (i.e. hyperemia, making it red and hot). This vascular response can easily be demonstrated by running the fingernail firmly across an area of skin. At first, a white line will appear and a red line will gradually replace this.

Emigration of the White Blood Cells

The rate of flow of blood through the affected tissues becomes much slower and eventually stops. The neutrophil polymorph nuclear leukocytes, instead of passing by rapidly, come to lie close to the endothelial cells and gradually work their way through into the tissues, the endothelial gap closing behind them. Neutrophil leukocytes are both mobile and phagocytic, allowing them to scavenge around on the tissues, picking up any minute foreign particles such as bacteria or cell debris. The neutrophils are the first line of defense and they are gradually replaced by the larger monocytes, termed macrophages, in the tissues; these clear up the debris from the whole area. The emigration of the white blood cells is often referred to as the cellular exudates.

Fluid Exudates

While the cells are passing into the tissues, fluid is also exuding from the blood vessels into the tissues, as a result of three changes:

1. The blood pressure within the capillaries is increased by the vasodilatation of the arterioles.
2. The capillary walls become more permeable.
3. The osmotic pressure in the tissue is increased by the breakdown of large protein molecules into numerous smaller osmotically active fragments.

Fate of Acute Inflammation

The changes, which follow acute inflammation, depend on two factors; removal of the cause and damaged amount of tissue.

If the cause is removed, the sequelae will depend on the amount of tissue damage.

- *Resolution:* When little damage has occurred, the area is cleared by the phagocytic action of the macrophages. The causative agent, cell debris, necrotic leukocytes and fibrin are all removed in this way. The excess fluid is drained by the lymphatics and the tissue returns to normal. This is termed as resolution
- Suppuration: When much tissue damage has been produced by the causative agent, return to normal is not possible. In this case, pus is formed and the lesion is called an abscess. Pus consists of dead leukocytes, fibrin, microorganisms, tissue debris and exuded fluid. It tends to track in the route of least resistance and eventually discharges through the body surface. Dental abscesses very often track through the alveolar bone to discharge through the attached gingival, but they may also discharge onto the face or through the periodontal ligament. Once the abscess has discharged and drained, it will heal up if the cause has been removed.

If the cause remains, the inflammatory response will continue alongside the tissue's attempts at repair. This produces a lower grade of inflammation called chronic inflammation.

CHRONIC INFLAMMATION

Clinically, the features of chronic inflammation are not as pronounced as those of acute inflammation. For example, it will be seen that in chronic gingivitis the gingivae are not as red as in acute gingivitis, and chronic gingivitis is normally fairly painless, while acute gingivitis can be exceedingly painful.

Causes of Chronic Inflammation

It has already been mentioned that chronic inflammation occurs when the causative agent persists, i.e. it is not easily removed from the tissues. In this respect, insoluble particles like silica and asbestos are well-suited to causing it. Also, microorganisms which are inadequately eliminated by the body defences cause a prolonged chronic inflammatory response, which may be classified as being either specific or nonspecific.

- Specific—caused by single identifiable organism (e.g. tuberculosis and syphilis)
- Nonspecific—caused by a number of different microorganisms (e.g. chronic gingivitis).

Fate of Chronic Inflammation

In chronic inflammation, the inflammatory process, already described, continues alongside the tissue's attempts at repair. Repair of tissues is achieved by the formation of granulation tissue, which is therefore a prominent feature of many chronic inflammatory lesions.

Granulation Tissue

When a tissue has been damaged, the defect is filled by fluid exudates and a fibrin clot is formed. Endothelial cells from the adjacent blood vessels begin to form side shoots which grow into the fibrin clot, eventually forming new blood vessels. Fibroblasts are also present, laying down collagen and thus forming scar tissue. It is common, in chronic periodontal disease, to find defects in the alveolar bone filled with granulation tissue.

In some chronic inflammatory lesions, the repair process seems to be excessive, resulting in hyperplasia. The reason for this is not known, but chronic gingivitis may often produce gingival hyperplasia.

Degeneration

CHAPTER 32

INTRODUCTION

The cells after injury undergo degenerative changes and become dead. The most common pattern of cell death recognized is necrosis, called by progressive degenerative action of the enzymes on the lethally injured cells. There are two steps that occur when a cell dies:

1. Protein inside the cell breaks down.
2. The body releases enzymes that digest these cells.

Degeneration initiates inflammatory response in the surrounding tissue. This attracts leukocytes and nearby phagocytes at the site and these cells start eating and eliminating the dead cells by phagocytosis. Nevertheless, microbial infection produces toxic substances released by leukocytes which in turn have the potential to cause collateral damage to surrounding tissues. Such collateral damage in excessive rate would impede the healing process. Therefore, necrosis left untreated results in a pile-up of decomposing dead tissue and cell debris at or near the site of the cell death, e.g. gangrene.

ETIOLOGY OF NECROSIS

There are two broad pathways suggested for progression of necrosis in an organism.

Initially, the pathway involves oncosis which signifies swelling of the cells. The cell consequently proceeds to blebbing, which is followed by pyknosis, in which nuclear shrinkage transpires. Furthermore, the nucleus is dissolved into the cytoplasm, which is known as karyolysis.

The second pathway out of the two pathways includes secondary form of necrosis which happens after apoptosis and budding. Cellular changes involved in this form of apoptosis are referred as karyorrhexis, where the nucleus breaks into fragments.

TYPES OF NECROSIS

Coagulative Necrosis

In this type, there is increasing intracellular acidosis which denatures structural proteins. The process of coagulative necrosis is characteristic of hypoxic death of cells in all tissues like kidney and heart, except the brain. Coagulative necrosis is typified by the formation of a gelatinous substance in dead tissues in which the architecture of the tissue remains maintained. It can be observed by light microscopy. The process takes place due to the denaturation of protein which further causes albumin to transform into a firm and opaque state. This type of necrosis is usually seen in hypoxic or low-oxygen environments such as infarction and is most frequently seen in cases of severe ischemia. It occurs chiefly in tissues like kidney, heart and adrenal glands.

Liquefactive Necrosis

Liquefactive necrosis, also known as colliquative necrosis, it is caused by the digestion of dead cells to form a viscous liquid mass. This type of necrosis is typical of bacterial or sometimes fungal infections due to their potential to start an inflammatory response. The necrotic liquid mass is commonly creamy yellow due to the presence of dead leukocytes, referred as pus. This type of necrosis is usually seen in hypoxic infarcts in the brain because the brain constitutes little connective tissue but its digestive enzymes and lipids are in higher amount, and cells hence can be easily digested by their own enzymes.

Gangrenous Necrosis

It is regarded as a type of coagulative necrosis which is similar to mummified tissue. It is generally found in cases of ischemia of lower limb and the gastrointestinal tract. If superimposed infection of dead tissues occurs, then liquefactive necrosis may happen, which is referred as wet gangrene.

Caseous Necrosis

It is an amalgamation of coagulative and liquefactive necrosis. It is a hallmark of mycobacteria infection (e.g. tuberculosis), some fungi and foreign substances which elicits chronic granulomatous response.

Fat Necrosis

It is a special form of necrosis of fat tissue caused due to the action of activated lipases on fatty tissues. It can be seen in cases of pancreatitis; calcium, magnesium or sodium may bind to these lesions to produce a chalky-white substance.

Fibrinoid Necrosis

It is a specialized necrosis often caused by immune-mediated vascular damage. It is found in walls of arteries described as "immune complexes" deposited within arterial walls together with fibrin.

CELLULAR CHANGES

It consists of the nucleus changes and characteristics of this change are determined by the manner in which its DNA breaks down:

- *Karyolysis:* The chromatin of the nucleus fades due to the loss of the DNA by degradation
- *Pyknosis:* The nucleus shrinks and the chromatin condenses
- *Karyorrhexis:* The shrunken nucleus fragments to complete dispersal.

Plasma alterations such as cell blebbing and the loss of microvilli are also seen in necrosis. Plasma membranes appear discontinuous when visualized with an electron microscope.

Oral Immunology

CHAPTER 33

INTRODUCTION

Immunity is the response of the body to microorganisms and foreign materials.

TYPES

Immunity may be innate, i.e. inborn, or acquired, i.e. developed after birth.

Innate

Humans are immune to many diseases which affect other animals. For example, humans are not affected by the disease of rabbits, myxomatosis, and conversely, the more virulent human diseases, such as syphilis, affect few other animals. This innate immunity is a feature of the species to which humans or other animals belong and does not depend upon any defense mechanism being set up after birth.

Acquired

Acquired immunity is developed during life and may be either active, resulting from antibodies formed by the body, or passive resulting from antibodies donated from another animal. It may also be either naturally or artificially acquired.

- *Active natural immunity:* It follows a natural infection. In some cases, such as chickenpox and measles, it lasts for life and in others, like influenza and the common cold, the period of immunity is much less
- *Active artificial immunity:* It is acquired by vaccination, which is a simulated infection. Although the vaccine injected is either killed or harmless, the immunity produced is effective against the natural infection. The body's response with both types of active immunity is usually termed as the immune response
- *Passive natural immunity:* It is found in newborn babies. Antibodies from the mother's serum cross the placenta and enter the fetal circulation, conferring a degree of immunity for the first 36 months of life
- *Passive artificial immunity:* It involves the injection of antibodies into the blood stream of an individual who has come in contact with an infection to which he or she has no immunity. In the past, the injected antibodies were usually obtained from animals, often horses, but modern techniques of genetic engineering may soon permit the production of antibodies in the laboratory.

IMMUNE RESPONSE

The acquired immune system is able to recognize and react specifically to foreign material (usually called an antigen), but does not normally react to the body's own component. Antigens are substances which have a large molecular size, usually proteins, and defense actions. Bacteria entering the tissues, for example, may be killed, but if toxins are produced, these will require to be neutralized. Thus, different responses will occur depending upon the type of antigen.

Two main types of immunological defense reactions can be triggered by antigens entering the body—the humoral and the cell-mediated. Both responses are usually involved simultaneously but it is simpler to consider them separately.

Humoral Immunity

In this type of reaction, the antigen is attacked by specific proteins released from immune cells. The immunoglobulins are types of serum globulins called gammaglobulins, and each one is specific to the antigen which triggered its formation.

The antigen is phagocytosed by macrophages which process the antigen and instruct a lymphocyte (the B lymphocyte in this case). The B lymphocyte, once stimulated by the antigen, changes into a plasma cell and produces immunoglobulins which react with the antigen. This type of response is referred to as humoral because the immunoglobulins can be released some distance from the site of infection and are carried in the blood to the area.

Cell-mediated Immunity

In this response, the T lymphocyte is activated to produce local factors—the lymphokines. The T cell is attracted to the site of the antigen and interacts directly to destroy it. The lymphokines have a whole range of effects, one of which is damage to cell membranes. Although this may destroy foreign microbes, the potential also exists for damaging the body's own cells. The lymphokines also initiate and increase the body's inflammatory responses. A factor which activates osteoclasts to resorb bone, osteoclast activating factor, has been identified and is thought to be formed by activated lymphocytes.

Components

It can be seen that the immune response consists of certain cell, proteins and tissues which function together to provide protection from foreign material entering the body. The commonest sources of danger are the millions of organism, both commensal and pathogenic, which exist in our environment, but a splinter of wood embedded in the skin will provoke the same defences.

Cells

The lymphocyte is the most important cell in the immune response. There are two types of lymphocytes—the B cell, which arises initially in the collections of lymphoid glands (bursa) surrounding the gut, and the T cell, which arises from the thymus. The origins of these cells are not really of significance to the dental hygienist, but they explain the choice of the letters B and T. Once produced, the B- and T lymphocytes colonize the lymphoid tissue scattered throughout the body and produce clones of cells with similar defensive abilities.

Other cells are also important. Neutrophil polymorphs act to phagocytose the antigens and damaged tissues. Large macrophages found throughout the body also phagocytose antigens, process them and instruct the B and T cells, so initiating the immune response. The mast cell is also important. These are found attached to the walls of small blood vessels, and in certain immunological reactions, they release histamines and other similar substances, which cause many of the vascular changes seen in hay fever and other allergic conditions.

The proteins involved in immune reactions are very complex and only an outline of their functions will be discussed.

Complement is a series of proteins and enzymes present in the blood, which is activated by the combination of immunoglobulins and antigens. Its main function is to assist in the destruction of organisms or to promote their phagocytosis. In addition, complement factors trigger the inflammatory response.

Immunoglobulins (antibodies) are produced by plasma cells and released into the bloodstream. Their functions range from helping polymorphs to phagocytose bacteria, to neutralizing toxins. Once the body has been stimulated to produce immunoglobulins, long-lived memory cells remain in the circulation, which can be triggered to initiate the production of large amounts of plasma cells and hence immunoglobulins, should antigen be encountered again. This is why, once we suffer with some diseases, we obtain lifelong immunity (but not, regrettably, to caries or periodontal disease).

The immunoglobulins are given alphabetical letters—G, M, A and E—to distinguish them. Immunoglobulin G is the commonest antibody in serum and can cross the placenta and protect the fetus and baby in the early months of life. Immunoglobulin M is a very large protein which is mainly in body secretions such as saliva, milk and tears. It defends mucosal surfaces, such as in the oral cavity, from bacterial invasion. Immunoglobulin E is found in serum and on the surface of mast cells. It is responsible for many of the features of allergic reactions. Immunoglobulin A (IgA, also referred as SIgA) is an antibody that plays an important role in immune function in the mucous membranes. More IgA is produced in the mucosal linings in contrast to all other types of antibody combined.

The lymphokines are produced by activated T cells when simulated by contact. They perform various functions, including attracting other lymphocytes, attracting and activating macrophages and damaging bacterial cell walls. However, they also cause local damage and this is believed to be one of the sources of tissue damage in periodontal disease.

The tissues of the immune system produce the various cells. The main ones are the bone marrow and the lymph nodes scattered throughout the body.

PATHOGENICITY OF ORGANISMS

As stated at the beginning of this Chapter, microorganism may be divided into pathogenic and commensal types. Pathogenic microorganisms are capable of producing agents called toxins, which are harmful to the tissues. These are of two types: exotoxins and endotoxins.

Exotoxins are given off by the organism and circulate freely throughout the body. They are extremely potent, causing a great deal of damage in small quantities. A typical feature of diseases caused by exotoxins is that the microorganisms remain localized in one area which exotoxins cause widespread damage, as happens in diphtheria and tetanus.

Endotoxins are produced within the organism and are only released when it dies and breaks up. They are less potent than exotoxins and, if they produce generalized symptoms, it is because of the invasiveness of the organism. In other words, the microorganisms themselves disperse throughout the body. Tuberculosis and syphilis are examples of such diseases.

Endotoxins may also be produced as a result of the breakdown of the cells of necrotic commensal organisms. Commensal organisms do not produce potent toxins but are capable of producing low-grade damage as in, for example, periodontal disease. The commensal organisms colonizing the tooth surface irritate the gingival and provoke the inflammatory and immune responses in a number of ways. The main methods are by the presence of enzymes, endotoxins and other antigens in the plaque bacteria.

Enzymes help to damage the crevicular epithelium and make it more permeable to the infiltration of other microbial byproducts such as endotoxins. They are also proteins and as such are antigenic and therefore provoke the immune response. The endotoxins are produced when cell wall components are released from plaque organism after they are lysed. These infiltrate through the junctional epithelium and are very potent initiators of both the inflammatory and immune responses. The organism, their enzymes and endotoxins are, therefore, all be seen to be powerful inducers of the immune response, of both cell-mediated and humoral type.

Role of Immune Response in Periodontal Disease

Initially, the immune response appears to play a protective role, preventing plaque microorganism from penetrating the gingival tissues.

However, whilst being a defensive mechanism for the whole body, the immune response is capable of being locally harmful. This is illustrated by the intense local reaction which may result from injecting certain antigens subcutaneously. This reaction may prevent spread of the antigen, but is locally damaging.

With continued, low-grade, long-term stimulation of the humoral and cell-mediated responses, plaque products will initiate and cause the progression of periodontal disease, with the body's own mechanism being responsible for most of the breakdown of the periodontal tissues.

ABNORMALITIES OF THE IMMUNE RESPONSE

Hypersensitivity

Hypersensitivity is the technical term for allergy and can be defined as an immune reaction which produces tissue damage in the host. The immunological reactions which result in tissue damage are identical with those which destroy microorganism. As already noted, the immune response, whilst being a defensive mechanism, can under certain circumstances cause tissue damage.

Hypersensitivity does not imply an exaggerated immune response, but merely a response which happens to cause tissue damage to the host.

Examples of hypersensitivity are asthma, hay fever and allergic reactions to certain drugs, including penicillin. In relation to drugs, the hypersensitivity reaction to the first exposure to the drug may produce relatively mild symptoms, such as nausea, pyrexia or skin rashes. However, the secondary exposure to the same drug is likely to have a much more severe systemic effect, known as anaphylaxis. Such a reaction can, of course, even result in death.

Autoimmunity

Autoimmunity means the production of an immune response to the host's own tissues. There is a failure of the immune system to recognize "self" proteins. This is usually due to these proteins becoming slightly altered by relatively simple compounds or elements being attached to them. An example of this is the contact dermatitis which occasionally results from substances such as iodine coming in contact with the skin. The same effect can result from antigens coming in contact with tissue cells and attaching themselves to the cell membrane. There is, as a result, an immune reaction against the intact tissue cell, which has the antigen as an integral part of it.

It is this type of reaction which causes rheumatic fever. An exotoxin secreted by bacteria lodged in the throat circulates in the blood and becomes attached to the synovial membrane of joints and valves of the heart. The resulting immune response causes an inflammatory reaction in these tissues. Autoimmunity is also associated with certain relatively uncommon oral conditions, such as pemphigus.

CHAPTER 34

Anomalies of the Teeth

INTRODUCTION

Anomaly is derived from "anomalia", a Greek word meaning developmental disturbance. Teeth are of importance for aesthetics, speech, mastication and development of occlusion. These anomalies have effect on functions of teeth.

Hypoplasia has an effect on aesthetics and causes psychological inferiority complex. Position, size and number of teeth have adverse effect on quality of speech. It has effect on mastication especially anodontia. Premature loss or retention of primary teeth results in malocclusion. Social stigma, e.g. Hutchinson's teeth has powerful effects.

CAUSES

- Hereditary
- Systemic disease
- Intake of drugs, e.g. tonic containing metallic and antibiotics
- Excessive fluoride content or water
- Trauma
- X-ray radiation
- Infections
- Nutritional deficiencies.

Anomalies will occur if these factors come into play during formation of enamel, dentin and cementum.

CLASSIFICATION

Anomalies can be categorized under the following headings namely; size, number, form, structure, and eruption.

Size

- *Microdontia:* The teeth are smaller in size than normal teeth. The disturbance may be localized in areas of permanent lateral incisors or third molars. The lateral incisors may be peg or cone shaped. Rarely, the condition may be generalized (Fig. 34.1)
- *Macrodontia:* Teeth are larger in size. The disturbance may be localized or generalized. Roots are abnormally long. This is rarely seen.

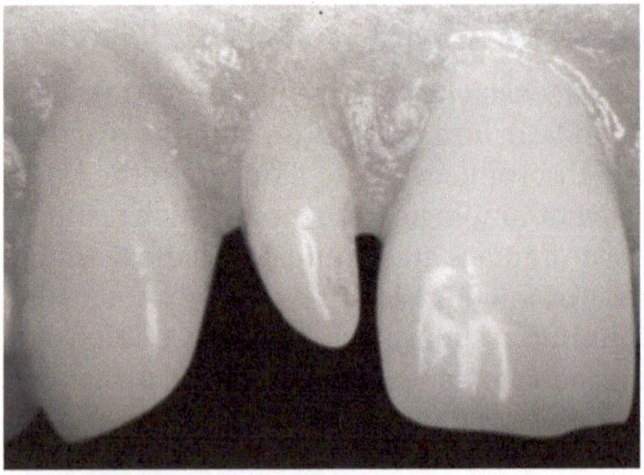

Fig. 34.1: Peg-shaped lateral incisor

Form

- *Dilaceration*: This refers to a bend in the root or crown of a forming tooth. Due to trauma, crown or root may form at an angle and this presents problem at the time of extraction (Fig. 34.2)
- *Fusion*: Fusion of two teeth results from union of two normally formed teeth from separate tooth germs. This fusion may be partial or complete
- *Concrescence*: Fusion in this case occurs after root formation has been completed. The roots are united by cementum
- *Gemination*: This can occur in temporary as well as permanent dentitions. In this, two teeth are produced from single bud. The result is a tooth with two crowns, common pulp chamber and single root
- *Dens in dente*: This odontoma is thought to arise from invagination of developing crown before calcification. It varies in extent from an exaggerated lingual pit to the appearance or a complete tooth within a tooth
- *Taurodontism*: It is a condition in which the pulp chamber is elongated and extends deeply into the region of the roots. As a result, the floor of the pulp and furcation of the tooth move apically down the root (Figs 34.3A and B).

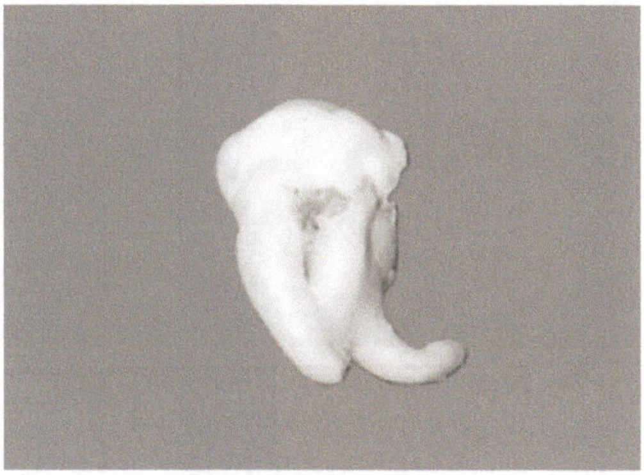

Fig. 34.2: Dilaceration

Number

- *Anodontia*: There may be complete absence of both dentitions in one or both jaws. It is very rare. In other cases, many teeth may be congenitally missing. Commonly affected teeth are permanent third molar, first premolars and lateral incisors
- *Supernumerary teeth*: Very rarely, at birth, one or two teeth are found in the incisal region. This requires extraction. These teeth are called predeciduous dentition. Sometimes teeth are found embedded under tooth of permanent dentition and these are called postpermanent dentition. Mesiodens are found in the midline

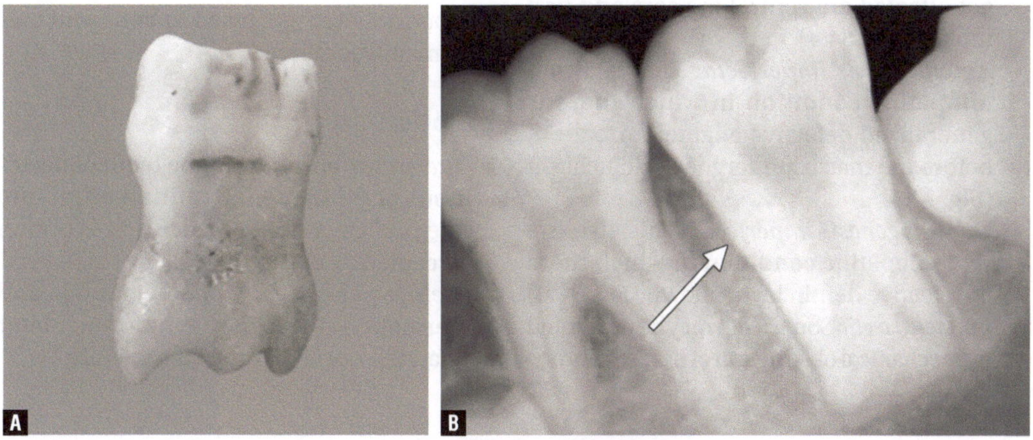

Figs 34.3A and B: Molar showing taurodontism (A) Clinical appearance; (B) Radiographic appearance

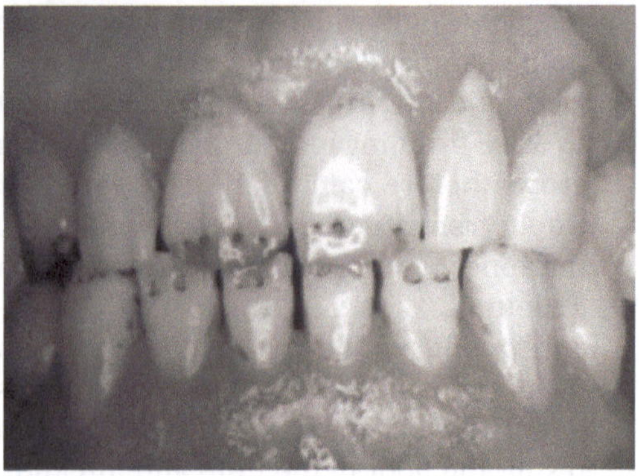

Fig. 34.4: Anterior teeth showing enamel hypoplasia

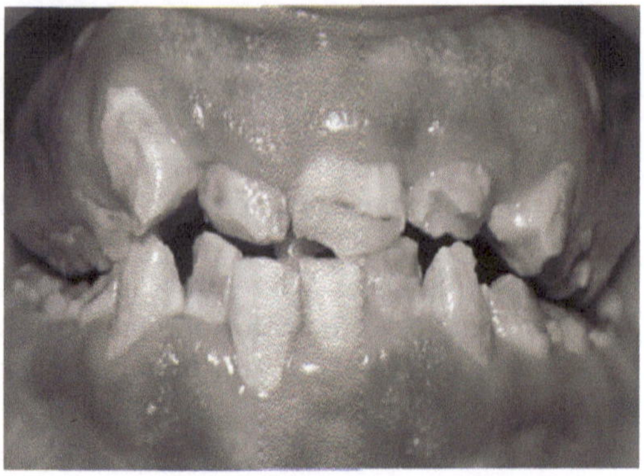

Fig. 34.5: Amelogenesis imperfecta *(For color version, see Plate 11)*

between permanent central incisors. These may be impacted, palatally or labially placed. Another is in permanent first premolar region. To prevent malocclusion and for reasons of aesthetics, extraction of teeth is indicated.

Structure

- *Enamel hypoplasia:* In this, enamel formation of deciduous and permanent dentition is defective or absent. Thin brown-stained enamel chips off easily. There may be small groove pits or fissures on the enamel surface. The disturbance is the result of malnutrition or endemic fever at the time of crown development. Teeth which usually get affected are central incisors and first molars (Fig. 34.4)
- *Amelogenesis imperfecta*: This is a rare idiopathic condition in which there is generalized defective enamel formation, before the matrix undergoes calcification (Fig. 34.5)
- *Dentinogenesis imperfecta*: This also is a rare idiopathic condition in which there is defective dentin laying down (Fig. 34.6)
- *Impacted teeth*: Some teeth may be prevented by mechanical obstruction of bone or fibrous tissue from erupting into the oral cavity. Third molar is invariably impacted
- *Ankylosed teeth*: A few teeth, which are not exfoliated, get fused to bone and may remain submerged.

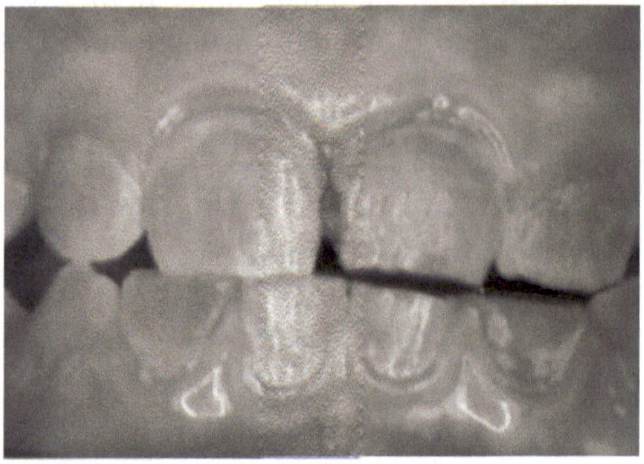

Fig. 34.6: Dentinogenesis imperfecta type I *(For color version, see Plate 11)*

Eruption

- *Premature eruption*: Some teeth of deciduous or permanent dentition erupt into the oral cavity prior to dates of eruption accepted as normal
- *Delayed eruption*: Some deciduous and permanent teeth may erupt much later than the normal eruption schedule.

CHAPTER 35

Fluorosis of Teeth

INTRODUCTION

Fluorosis of teeth is due to presence of excess fluorine in drinking water. It is specially affected by ingestion of fluoride containing drinking water during the time of tooth formation. Normally, water contains fluorine, at a level of 0.8–1 ppm. If it is more than 1 ppm, it may lead to fluorosis; affected teeth appear chalky white on eruption and later turn brown.

ETIOLOGY

The unaesthetic appearance of permanent teeth (adult teeth) is of important concern in dental fluorosis. From birth of child up to 6 years of age, permanent teeth are at highest risk of developing fluorosis, though some research states that first 2 years of life of child is most crucial. Despite the high amount of fluoride intake, after 6–7 years of the age, most of the permanent teeth (except third molar) would have completed their development, so risk of developing fluorosis is insignificant. The factors determining the severity of fluorosis are amount of fluoride exposure, age of the child during exposure, individual response, genetic factors, weight, nutrition, degree of physical activity and bone growth.

Overexposure to fluoride may occur through various sources, some of which include fluoride containing dentifrices or mouthrinses which children are at risk to swallow, bottled or untested package of drinking water for its fluoride content, improper use of fluoride supplements, and public water fluoridation. Consumption of natural water with fluoride well above the recommended level, brick tea, or pollution from high fluoride coal can lead to severe fluorosis.

HISTOPATHOLOGY

During enamel maturation, an excess of fluoride ions in the extracellular matrix alters the rate of enzymatic breakdown of enamel matrix proteins—amelogenin—and the rate of removal of breakdown products. This results in the formation of less calcified enamel which has altered optical properties and appears opaque and lusterless relative to normal enamel.

Traditionally, severe fluorosis is considered as enamel hypoplasia; however, hypoplasia is not a result of fluorosis. The defects in enamel seen as pits, bands and loss of some areas of enamel seen are the results of hypomineralized, brittle and fragile enamel after eruption of teeth in mouth.

STAGES

The stages of Dean's fluorosis of teeth have been given in Figure 35.1 and Table 35.1.

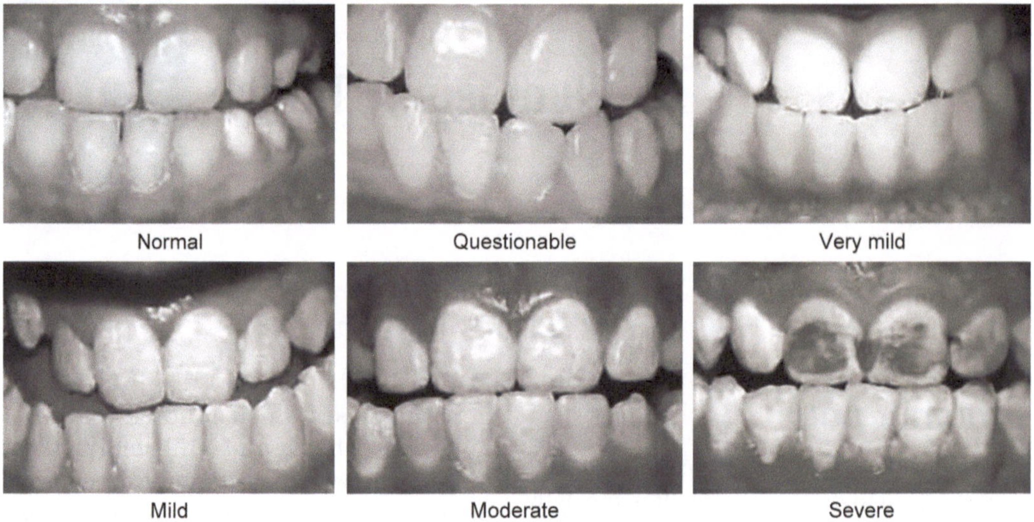

Fig. 35.1: Stages of Dean's fluorosis index

Table 35.1: Dean's fluorosis index

Classification	*Criteria—description of enamel*
Normal	Smooth, glossy, pale creamy-white translucent surface
Questionable	A few white flecks or white spots
Very mild	Small opaque, paper white areas covering less than 25% of the tooth surface
Mild	Opaque white areas covering less than 50% of the tooth surface
Moderate	All tooth surfaces affected; marked wear on biting surfaces; brown stain may be present
Severe	All tooth surfaces affected; discrete or confluent pitting; brown stain present

TREATMENT

- Mottled enamel is frequently stained in an unsightly brown color. For cosmetic reasons, it has become the practice to go for bleaching the affected teeth
- For decreasing the intake of fluorine, defluoridation of water can be done
- Cosmetic rehabilitation by artificial crowns and veneers.

Attrition, Abrasion and Erosion

CHAPTER 36

ATTRITION

Dental attrition is a type of physiological tooth wear at the incisal or occlusal surfaces caused by tooth-to-tooth contact, resulting in loss of tooth tissue. It is a physiological process and commonly seen as a normal part of aging. But excessive wear leading to loss of tooth surface can be pathological in nature. The reason for pathological wear of the tooth surface is bruxism, which is clenching and grinding of the teeth. If the attrition is severe, the enamel gets completely worn out leaving underlying dentin exposed. This leads to an increased risk of dentin hypersensitivity and dental caries (Fig. 36.1).

Clinical Appearance

Attrition occurs as a result of contact of opposing tooth. Mainly affects cuspal, incisal and proximal surface of teeth.

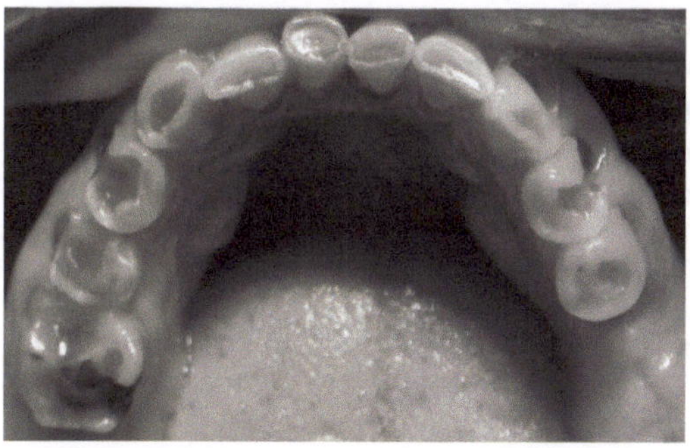

Fig. 36.1: Attrition *(For color version, see Plate 11)*

Sign and symptoms of attrition can include:

- *Loss of tooth anatomy:* Enamel of occlusal table of molar teeth may appear thin and flat, but teeth may appear the same height when in occlusion, though. It may also lead to altered occlusion due to decreased vertical height
- *Sensitivity or pain:* Attrition may be entirely asymptomatic, or there may be dentin hypersensitivity. It can also cause tenderness of the periodontal ligament due to occlusal trauma
- Tooth discoloration due to enamel wear
- Loss in posterior occlusal stability
- Mechanical failure of restorations.

Etiology

The main reasons for wear of retained natural teeth in elderly people can be attrition, abrasion, erosion or a combination of these. The number of teeth with incisal or occlusal wear increases with age. This tooth wear can be physiological or pathological; caused by several other factors such as bruxism or clenching, developmental defects, hard or rough-textured diet, and absence of posterior teeth support. Similarly, attrition of incisors is seen when an edge-to-edge class III incisal relationship is present.

In addition to these factors, independent variables such as male gender, bruxism, edge-to-edge relation of incisors, loss of molar

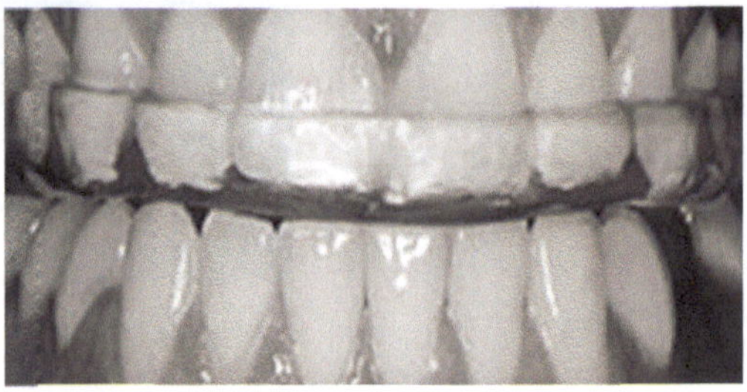

Fig. 36.2: Patient wearing occlusal splint

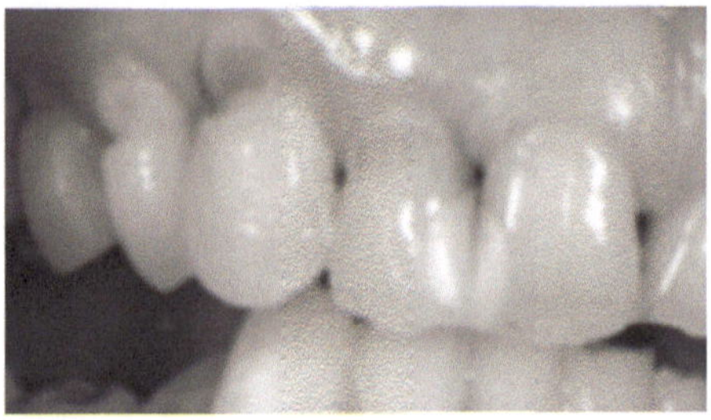

Fig. 36.3: Abrasion *(For color version, see Plate 11)*

occlusal contact, and unilateral buccolingual cusp-to-cusp relation are also responsible for occlusal wear.

In patients with attrition due to bruxism, wearing a full-coverage acrylic occlusal splint is recommended to prevent bruxism and further attrition (Fig. 36.2). Patients must be monitored closely, with clinical photographs after interval of 6–12 months to evaluate whether the tooth surface loss is being prevented or not.

ABRASION

Abrasion is loss of tooth structure due to contact with external foreign object. At the cementoenamel junction, the progression of tooth loss can be rapid since enamel is very thin in this region of the tooth. When the enamel is lost abrasion leads to quick destruction of the softer dentin and cementum of the tooth (Fig. 36.3).

Common causes of this wearing of tooth are toothbrushes, toothpicks, floss, and any dental appliance frequently set in and removed from the mouth. The appearance of abrasive defect when caused by hard tooth brushing is commonly described as V-shaped; where it is typically seen at cervical necks of the teeth, as a deep ridge on the buccal or labial surfaces. The surface is shiny rather than carious, and sometimes the ridge is deep enough to expose pulp chamber.

The teeth most commonly affected are premolars and canines.

EROSION

Erosion is the loss of tooth substance as a result of chemical action on the tooth surface. The smooth lesions exhibit no chalkiness and are common on the palatal and lingual surfaces of the teeth.

Etiology

Extrinsic Acidic Sources

Consumption of acidic drinks and foods with low pH level causes the teeth to demineralize leading to dental erosion. This includes fruit juices like orange and apple juice, alcoholic and carbonated drinks such as colas, lemonades. Erosion can also be seen in infants using feeding bottles containing fruit juices.

Intrinsic Acidic Sources

Dental erosion can also occur by nonextrinsic factors. People with diseases such as gastric acidity, and gastroesophageal reflux disease often suffer from this, where gastric juice from the stomach comes into contact with the teeth causing erosion. It is seen in the industrial workers involved in the use of acids (Fig. 36.4).

TREATMENT

- *Attrition:* Treatment is psychological. Restoration is given to protect dentin and

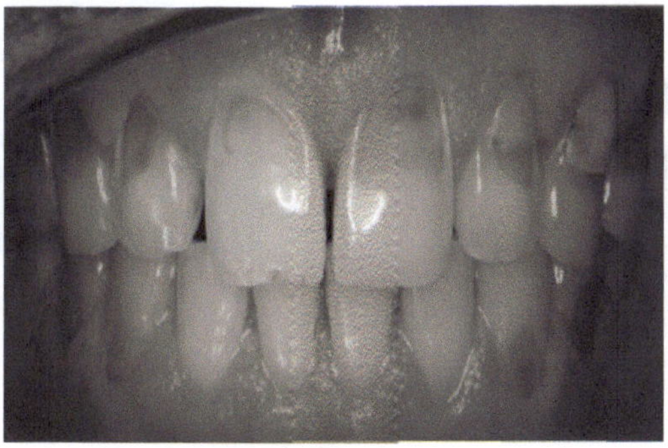

Fig. 36.4: Erosion

pulp. Dentures, crowns and occlusal splints restore vertical height and lost tooth structure

- *Abrasion:* Faulty habits must be corrected. Enamel and dentin margins to be restored by conservative treatment
- *Erosion:* A change of profession is suggested. Alkaline toothpastes are prescribed. Conservative treatment is done to preserve pulp and restore aesthetics.

Oral Manifestation of Systemic Disease

CHAPTER 37

INTRODUCTION

Oral manifestations can be seen in many systemic diseases. The oral cavity is a mirror to the general body health because oral cavity presents significant signs of systemic diseases. Diagnosis of these oral manifestations helps the patient to receive appropriate medical treatment and referral. The lesions of the oral cavity and its associated structures, facial skeleton, extraoral skin, etc. caused by some of the more common systemic diseases are highlighted.

HEMATOLOGIC DISEASES

Anemia

The most common hematologic disorder is the iron deficiency anemia. Its oral manifestations are atrophic glossitis, mucosal pallor and angular cheilitis. Atrophic glossitis shows loss of the tongue papillae resulting in a smooth and erythematous tongue which may appear sometimes as migratory glossitis, also known as geographic tongue. It has unknown etiology which affects 1–2% of the population.

Atrophic glossitis does not have a white keratotic border and the area of the lesion increases in size instead of changing their position. However, the tongue may be tender in more severe cases.

Another lesion known as angular cheilitis occurs at the corners of the lips, caused by *Candida albicans* infection. It symptoms include reddening, cracking, and discomfort to the patient.

Various oral complications associated with sickle cell anemia involve mandibular osteomyelitis which results in areas of osteoporosis and erosion, preceded by osteosclerosis. In addition, anesthesia or paresthesia of the mandibular nerve and asymptomatic pulpal necrosis can also be seen.

Dysphagia due to pharyngoesophageal ulcerations is also seen in patients suffering with iron deficiency anemia.

Leukemia

It is a blood disease of white blood cells leading to immature production of cells. It may be myeloid involving granulocyte series or lymphoid involving lymphocyte series or monocyte involving monocyte series. Oral manifestations of leukemia frequently include gingival hypertrophy, petechiae, ecchymosis, mucosal ulcers, and hemorrhage. The gingival hemorrhage is due to ulceration of the sulcus epithelium and necrosis of the underlying tissues. Rapid loosing of teeth is due to necrosis of the periodontal ligament. In some cases, destruction of the alveolar bone is also observed.

Bacterial infections of the oral tissues are common in these patients which require early management. Treatment of leukemia with chemotherapeutic agents can result in reactivation of herpes simplex virus and oral mucositis.

Polycythemia

In this disorder, there is abnormal increase in the number of red blood cells. The oral mucous membrane appears deep purplish-red, the gingival and tongue being most prominently affected. The cyanosis is due to excess of reduced hemoglobin. The gingiva is often engorged and swollen and bleed upon slightest provocation. Submucosal petechiae are also common, as well as ecchymosis and hematoma.

Thrombocytopenic Purpura

It is defined as a purplish discoloration of the skin and mucous membrane due to the spontaneous extravasation of blood and, in itself, is a symptom rather than a disease entity. It may be thrombocytopenic purpura or non-thrombocytopenic purpura.

In majority of cases, that is severe and often profuse gingival hemorrhage which may be spontaneous and usually arises in the absence of skin lesions. Petechiae also occur on the oral mucosa, commonly on the palate and appear as numerous tiny, grouped clusters of reddish spots only a millimeter or less in diameter. Ecchymosed lesions may enlarge to form such mucosal hematomas, which present as large dark tumors.

Blood Dyscrasias

The various elements of the blood as well as its liquid portion, i.e. serum, play extraordinary role in many physiologic mechanisms and processes in the human body. The oral lesions of these diseases are similar to the other lesions of oral cavity, which occur due to irritation of infection. However, these lesions vary in severity as per the disease.

Hemophilia, Christmas Disease, Pseudohemophilia

Deficiency of antihemophilic globulin (AHG) leads to hemophilia, deficiency of Christmas factor leads to Christmas disease (Hemophilia VIII) and deficiency of plasma thromboplastin antecedent leads to pseudohemophilia (also called von Willebrand's disease). These diseases present similar clinical features, except hemophilia which is a sex linked and occurs only in males.

Oral manifestations are spontaneous bleeding or persistent bleeding following minor trauma. The most important difference between purpura and hemophilia is that in purpura, bleeding time is increased but clotting time is normal while in hemophilia, clotting time is increased but bleeding time is normal.

SYPHILIS

It is also known as "lues" disease and is caused by spirochete, *Treponema pallidum*. It may be either acquired or congenital (mother). The organism can infect the person through mucous membrane or abraded skin or through sexual intercourse with a syphilitic person. It may also result from kissing. Cases have been reported where dentist got syphilis in the nail bed through saliva. The clinical course of syphilis is divided into three stages, i.e. primary, secondary and tertiary. The various manifestations of these stages are mentioned in the section below (Fig. 37.1).

Primary Stage

After incubation period of about 1 month, the syphilitic chancre develops at the site of infection. Extragenital chancre is found on the lips, tongue and palate. These chancres may appear as small abrasions or resemble the penile chancre. These usual primary lesions are elevated, ulcerated nodule showing local indurations and producing regional lymphadenitis. Such a lesion on the lip may have a brownish, crusted appearance.

The intraoral chancre is an ulcerated lesion covered by a grayish white membrane, which may be painful because of secondary infection.

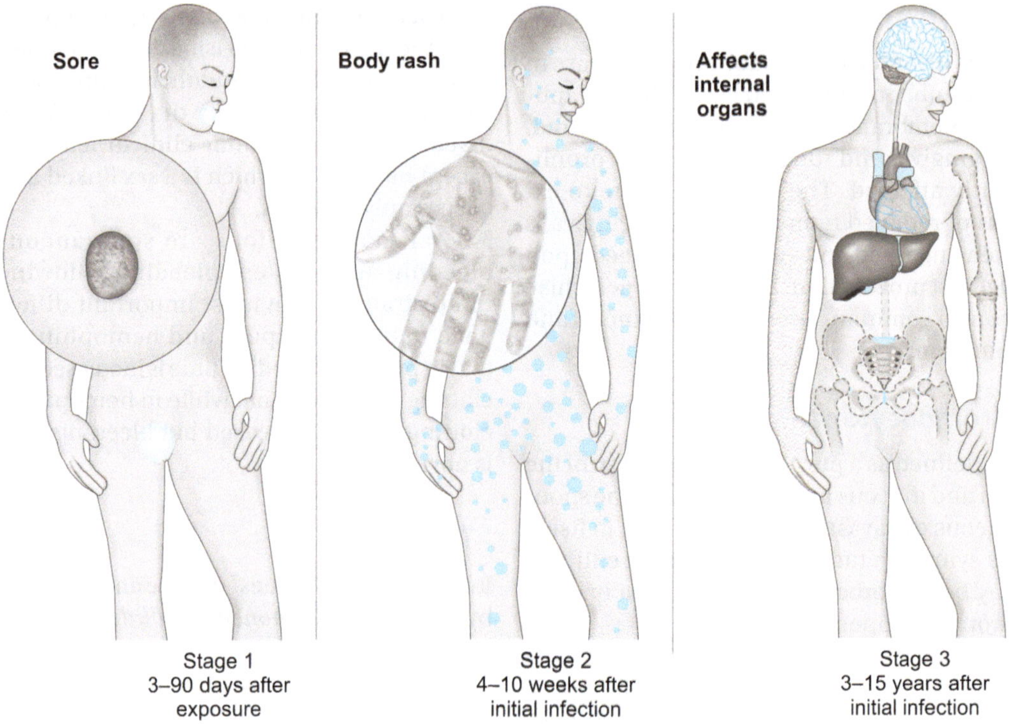

Fig. 37.1: Symptoms of different stages of syphilis

These chancre contain highly contagious spirochetes, which are clearly visible by dark-field examination. An enlarged lymph node is always found along the lymphatics draining the area of the chancre.

Secondary Stage

It is also called as metastatic stage, which commences about 6 weeks after the primary lesion. In this stage, there are diffuse eruptions on the skin and mucous membrane. On the skin, macules or papules may be there. This stage is most infectious. The clinical features are malaise, low-grade fever, headache, lacrimation, sore throat, weight loss, myalgia, arthralgia and generalized lymphadenopathy. They are often ovoid or irregular in shape and are surrounded by an erythematous zone. The patches coalesce to form so called "snail-track ulcers". The patches are highly contagious and the serological reaction is always positive.

Tertiary Stage

These lesions usually do not appear for several years and involve chiefly cardiovascular system, the central nervous system and certain other tissues and organs. The gumma is the chief localized tertiary lesion and occurs mostly on the skin, mucous membrane, liver, testes and bone. The lesion varies from a millimeter to several centimeters in diameter. The tonsils, soft palate, hard palate and tongue may be affected. It is initially yellow, homogeneous mass of rubber-like consistency, which undergoes degeneration and produces ulceration. These ulcers have soft edge with depressed base and discharge yellow fluid. Bone of hard palate and nose may be affected leading to necrosis and perforation of hard palate and collapse of nasal bridge. Tongue may be involved either by small gummas or coalescing to form large gumma. The most frequent lesion on the tongue is the development of chronic superficial glossitis in which it is divided into many lobules by fissures. There may be leukoplakia due to involvement of skin, which becomes edematous.

Congenital Syphilis

It is transmitted to the offspring only by infected mother and is not inherited. There are a number of stillbirths due to congenital syphilis. Person with this disease manifests a variety of lesions including high palatal arch, saddle nose, relative protuberance of mandible, rhagades and saber shin. In the classical disease the Hutchinson's triad, hypoplasia of the incisor and molar teeth, 8th nerve deafness and interstitial keratitis is present.

DIABETES

This disease is due to disturbances of insulin secretion by pancreas. It is characterized by loss of weight, fatigue, marked thirst, marked hunger and polyuria.

Oral features are dryness of mouth (xerostomia) and sweet taste in mouth. Tongue is red and painful with marginal indentations and coating on the dorsal surface. There is diffuse erythema of oral mucosa. In these individuals, there is tendency of formation of supragingival calculus with gingiva which is spongy, purplish and bleeds easily. There is pocket formation and more incidences of gingival and periodontal abscess resulting in loss of tooth.

TUBERCULOSIS

Oral lesions in tuberculosis are rare. Oral tuberculosis, however, is always a secondary lesion and occurs in patients affected with advanced pulmonary tuberculosis.

An increased incidence of gingivitis and chronic destructive periodontal disease as well as alveolar bone changes characterized by enlargement of the cancellous spaces has been reported in some cases, but are not confirmatory. The sites most frequently involved with ulcers are pharynx, tonsils, tongue, and hard and soft palate. They may occur on the buccal mucosa and at the commissures of the lips.

VITAMIN DEFICIENCIES

Vitamin A

- Source: Fish liver oil, milk, egg yolk and butter
- Dosage: Adult 5000 IU/day; 4–6 years 2500 IU/day; pregnancy 6000 IU/day
- Lactation: 8000 IU/day, in deficiency 5000–10000 IU/day.

Oral Manifestation Due to Deficiency of Vitamin A

It is believed that deficiency may cause atrophy of enamel-forming cells to a nonspecified stratified epithelium which results in enamel hypoplasia and poor mineralization of dentine.

There is keratinized metaphase of epithelium and thus increased susceptibility to infection. There are disturbances in bone growth shape and texture. Gingiva shows epithelial hyperplasia and hyperkeratinization with proliferation of the epithelial attachment. Subgingival calculus formation is also there.

It is believed that pocket formation does not occur in vitamin A deficiency if local deposits are not there but when local irritants are present, pockets are deeper than in nondeficient animals and present associated hyperkeratosis.

Vitamin B Complex

Deficiency signs may be due to the deficiency of one of the following components which make vitamin B complex, i.e. thiamine (B1), riboflavin (B2), nicotinamide, pyridoxine (B6), pantothenic acid and cyanocobalamin (B12).

Thiamine

- Source: Outside bran coats of grain and rice and yeast, others are ripe peas and beans, etc.

- Requirement:
  - Infants 100–200 IU (0.3–0.6 mg) in deficiency
  - Adults 10–25 mg, massive dose 25–100 mg.

The following oral disturbances have been related to thiamine deficiency:

- Hypersensitivity of oral mucosa
- Minute vesicles on buccal mucosa, under the tongue or the palate
- Erosion of oral mucosa.

It has been postulated that the activity of the oral flora is diminished in thiamine deficiency.

Riboflavin

- Source: Yeast and liver of vertebrates
- Requirement: Adult 2.3 mg.

Deficiency symptoms include glossitis and cheilosis. Glossitis is characterized by magenta discoloration and atrophy of papillae. Disappearance of the papillae of tongue varies and depends upon the severity of deficiency and the dorsum presents patchy atrophy. Cheilosis is one of the most frequent changes. It begins as a tiny, raw, painful area at the commissure of the lips, at the mucogingival junction. In severe cases, multiple fissures develop. The lesion tends to spread to lower lip causing fissuring but characteristically spares the upper lip.

Nicotinic Acid

- Source: Yeast, whole cereals, liver, eggs
- Requirements: 15–25 mg, in deficiency 100–500 mg can be given.

The oral changes include glossitis, which is the earliest clinical sign. In acute form, there is hyperemia, enlargement of papillae and indentation of the margin, followed by atrophic changes and resultant glazed surface. The tongue in acute stage is "beefy red", painful with burning. In chronic cases, there is fissuring of the tongue.

Pantothenic Acid

- Source: In animals' liver and kidney and in plants the storage organs such as rice husks
- Requirements: 50–200 mg/day.

Deficiency signs have been noticed in animals but not in human beings.

These include angular cheilitis, hyperkeratosis with ulceration and necrosis of the gingival and oral mucosa, proliferation of the basal cell layer of oral epithelium, and resorption of the crest of alveolar bone.

Pyridoxine

- Sources: Yeast, rice polishing, seeds, grams, covering of cereals such as wheat and maize
- Requirement: Little is known. In few cases, daily doses of 10–100 mg have been given. In deficiency, edematous magenta tongue has been noted.

Folic Acid

- Source: Occurs widely in animals and green vegetables
- Requirement: 5–20 mg.

In deficiency, there is soreness and burning sensation of the tongue accompanied by the atrophy of the filiform papillae. Necrotic changes in gingival, periodontal ligament and alveolar bone without an inflammatory response attributed to granulocytopenia associated with deficiency.

Cyanocobalamin

- Source: Liver, egg, fish and meat.

The deficiency results in pernicious anemia and these patients have glossopyrosis (burning of tongue with a sore) red tongue and baldness of the dorsum due to atrophy of lingual papillae. In severe cases, there may be atrophic changes of the oral mucosa.

Vitamin C

- Source: All living plants are excellent sources but it is abundant in citrus fruits,

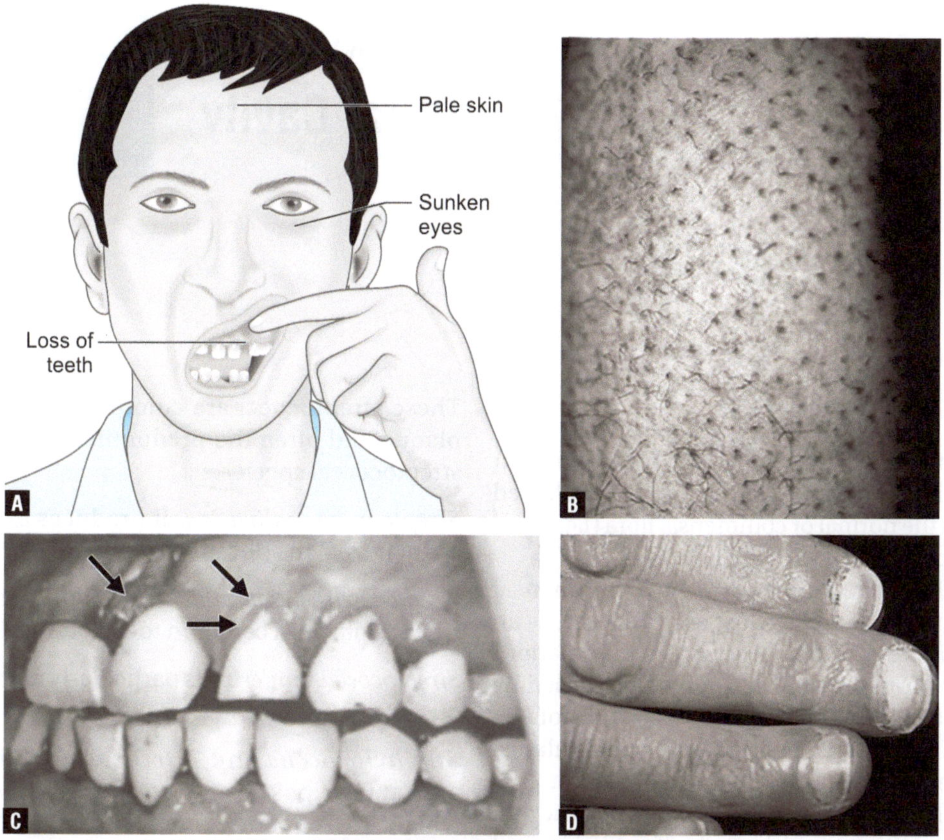

Figs 37.2A to D: Symptoms of scurvy

berries, apple, pears, etc. Considerable amount is present in human milk but is less in cow's milk

- Requirement: 50–100 mg/day.

In extreme deficiency "scurvy" (Figs 37.2A to D) results in which there are hemorrhage tendencies and retardation of wounds healing. There is failure of formation and maintenances of intercellular substances in tissues of mesenchymal origin and osteoporosis. Weakened vessels are responsible for petechiae, ecchymoses and delayed wound healing. Other symptoms include dry and pale skin, hair and tooth loss, small bleeding around the hair also known as corkscrew hair.

Gingiva is hemorrhagic, bluish-red, enlarged and friable. Alveolar bone loss results from ascorbic acid deficiency. There may be chances of hemorrhages in the periodontal ligament.

Vitamin D

- Source: Liver oil of fish, egg yolk and butter
- Requirement: For babies, children and adolescents is 400 IU. Adults require little less.

Its deficiency will cause disturbances in calcification of bones and teeth. There is osteoporosis of alveolar bone and reduction in the width of periodontal ligament. The rate of cementum formation is normal but calcification is defective. Resorption of cementum has been noted in individuals with rickets.

CHAPTER 38

Bacteriology and Virology of Oral Cavity

INTRODUCTION

Group of microorganisms that reside at particular surfaces of the body are referred to as the normal or commensal flora (i.e. living in cooperation with the host).

The interaction between the commensal normal flora and its host is considered as an ecosystem. As in all ecosystems, this relationship is often fragile and can be disturbed by minor shifts in the balance of a variety of factors. In humans, a normal ecological balance is necessary for maintenance of health.

The topographical arrangement of the oral cavity with its varied terrain of teeth, gingival crevices or pockets, buccal and lingual sulci, lips and tongue has great influence on the physical parameters of bacterial colonization.

Microflora of oral cavity consists of various bacteria (rods, cocci, aerobic, anaerobic).

GRAM-POSITIVE COCCI

Streptococci: About 90% of streptococci have been found in plaque and isolated.

Streptococcus mutans: It is the principal etiological agent of human dental caries. These produce both soluble and insoluble extracellular glucose polymers (glucans/mutans) from sucrose and levans (polymers of fructose) which form the matrix of dental plaque.

Streptococcus sanguis: It is also capable of producing extracellular glucans from sucrose. These streptococci are common in dental plaque and often the predominant plaque streptococcal species.

Streptococcus salivarius: It produces extracellular fructans (levans) from sucrose.

Streptococcus mitior (mitis): It include α-hemolytic streptococci common to the oral cavity.

Streptococcus milleri: It is particularly numerous in gingival crevice.

Staphylococcus and *Micrococcus:* They are catalase positive, Gram-positive cocci which are frequently isolated from the oral cavity.

Staphylococcus salivarius: It is a commensal of dorsum of tongue.

Peptostreptococcus and *Peptococcus:* These are anaerobic Gram-positive cocci which are commonly isolated from the oral cavity.

GRAM-NEGATIVE COCCI

Neisseria species are common isolates in the mouth and are characteristically aerobic or facultative, oxidase positive, Gram-negative proportion of the organisms which initially colonize clean tooth surfaces probably due to presence of an extracellular slime or capsular material. Anaerobic counterpart of *Neisseria, Veillonella* species are also common in mouth, often relatively high in numbers.

GRAM-POSITIVE RODS AND FILAMENTS

Six Gram-positive genera are typically pathogenic in humans. Two of these are *Streptococcus* and *Staphylococcus* which are sphere-shaped called cocci. The remaining organisms are bacilli which are rod-shaped and can be subdivided on the basis of their ability to form spores. The non-spore formers are *Corynebacterium* and *Listeria* (a coccobacillus), whereas *Bacillus* and *Clostridium* produce spores. The spore-forming bacteria can again be categorized based on their respiration: *Bacillus* is a facultative anaerobe, while *Clostridium* is an obligate anaerobe. Gram-positive bacteria are capable of causing serious and sometimes fatal infections in newborn infants.

Other anaerobic rods and filaments that have been isolated from the mouth include *Leptotrichia buccalis, Arachnia, Propionibacterium, Eubacterium* species.

GRAM-NEGATIVE RODS AND FILAMENTS

Hemophilus species are Gram-negative aerobic and facultative rods that have been shown to be frequently present in saliva and on oral mucosal surfaces and may be present in dental plaque.

Fusobacterium and *Bacteroids* species are anaerobic Gram-negative filaments and rods, which are commonly isolated from dental plaque, especially in subgingival region.

Capnocytophaga is the predominant Gram-negative facultative rod in the gingival sulcus of the aged.

OTHER MICROORGANISMS

Spirochetes are common inhabitants of the gingival crevice. Three distinct species, which may be present, are *Treponema denticola, Treponema macrodentium,* and *Treponema oralis.*

Yeasts, particularly *Candida albicans,* are also common oral isolates from healthy individuals.

Protozoa, including *Entamoeba gingivalis, Trichomonas, Selenomonas* species are often seen.

Most viruses are considered as transients; however, herpesvirus hominis (HSV) is carried by many people. Likewise, *Epstein-Barr* and *Varicella zoster* viruses are often considered as normal oral flora and hepatitis B virus (HBV) and *Cytomegalovirus* may be found in oral cavity in the caries state.

Actinobacillus actinomycetemcomitans, Porphyromonas gingivalis and *Bacteroides forsythus* have been found to be major periodontopathogens.

VIROLOGY

Classification of Viruses

Viruses are mainly classified by phenotypic characteristics, such as morphology, nucleic acid type, mode of replication, host organisms, and the type of disease they cause. Currently, two main schemes are used for the classification of viruses: the International Committee on Taxonomy of Viruses (ICTV) system and Baltimore classification system, which places viruses into one of seven groups. Accompanying this broad method of classification are specific naming conventions and further classification guidelines set out by the ICTV.

Viral classification starts at the level of order and continues as follows, with the taxon suffixes given in italics:

- Order (*-virales*)
- Family (*-viridae*)
- Subfamily (*-virinae*)
- Genus (*-virus*)
- Species

Species names generally take the form of *(disease) virus.*

CLINICAL PRESENTATION OF COMMON ORAL VIRAL INFECTIONS

Herpes Simplex Virus Type 1

Primary Herpetic Gingivostomatitis

Herpes simplex virus (HSV) is divided into two types, HSV-1 and HSV-2. Primarily, mouth, (Fig. 38.1) throat, face, eye, and central nervous system infections are caused by HSV-1. HSV-2 causes primarily anogenital infections. But both these herpes simplex viruses can affect any area.

Most of HSV infection are subclinical and generally affect children, teenager and young adults. Herpes infection can affect the face and mouth and called orofacial herpes (Fig. 38.2), genitalia called genital herpes, or hands called herpetic whitlow. The virus in its serious forms may infect and damage eye known as herpes keratitis, or invade the central nervous system, damaging the brain called herpes encephalitis. In immunocompromised patients [undergoing chemotherapy for organ transplantation or people with (AIDS) or leukemia], intraoral ulcers may appear at any site and may last for several weeks or months, if untreated. Usually, HSV is never removed from the body by the immune system. The virus penetrates the nerves at the site of primary infection subsequent to which, it migrates to the cell body of the neuron, and becomes latent in the ganglion. As a sequela of primary infection, the immune system creates antibodies to the particular type of HSV involved, which in turn avoids a subsequent infection of that type at a different site.

Many people infected with HSV-2 are asymptomatic or having subclinical herpes.

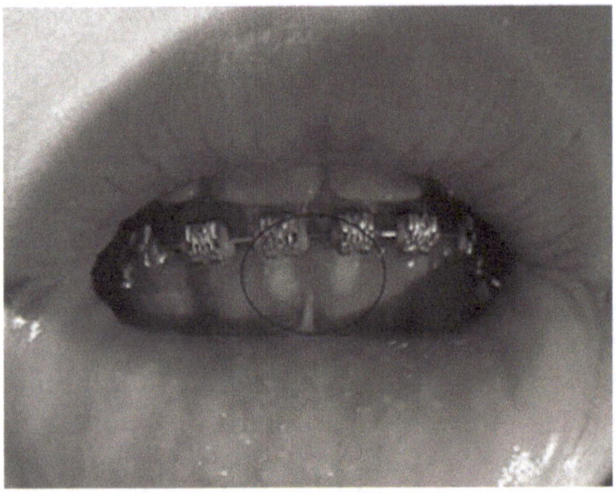

Fig. 38.1: Herpetic gingivostomatitis

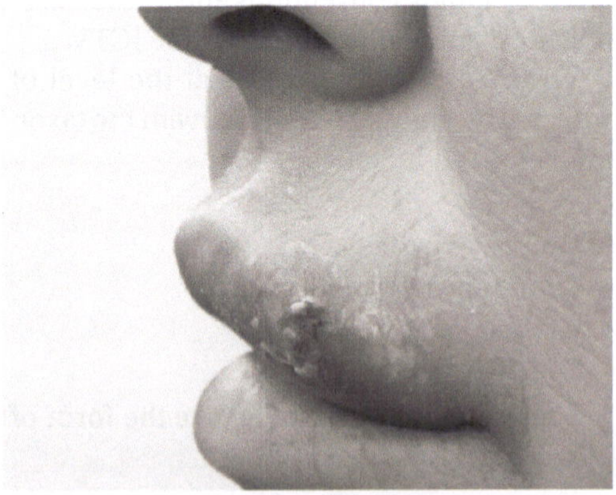

Fig. 38.2: Herpes labialis

Coxsackievirus

These are ribonucleic acid (RNA) enteroviruses and named after the city in New York where they were discovered first. These viruses are separated in two groups A and B. Group A has 24 types and group B has 6 types.

Group A coxsackieviruses infect the mucous membranes and skin. Three clinical types of oral infection are: herpangina, hand-foot-and-mouth disease, and acute lymphonodular pharyngitis can develop.

Herpangina is a common mouth infection in childhood characterized by sore throat, fever followed by multiple small round ulcers mainly in soft palate and tonsillar pillars caused by coxsackievirus. The oral lesions in herpangina are smaller than HSV and heal without treatment in one week.

Verruca Vulgaris (Common Wart)

This is the most common human papilloma viruses (HPV) lesion found on the skin. The lesions found in the mouth are usually in the areas of heavy keratinization such as lips, hard palate and less common in the gingiva. Common wart can grow anywhere on the skin.

Hand-foot-and-mouth disease is a highly contagious disease affecting children under the age of 10 years being spread by oral and fecal-oral routes. The incubation period is 3–6 days followed by malaise, cough, abdominal pain, low-grade fever, difficulty to eat and sore mouth. Oral lesions are found in buccal mucosa, tongue and hard palate which resolve in one week. Following oral lesions, elliptical exanthematous rashes appear in hand and foot.

Human papilloma viruses (HPVs) are small DNA viruses. Most HPV infections cause no symptoms and resolve spontaneously. Papillomas, condylomata, focal epithelial hyperplasia, and warts are the common examples of HPV infection.

Human Immunodeficiency Virus and Acquired Immune Deficiency Syndrome

What is AIDS?

- AIDS stands for acquired immune deficiency syndrome, and represents the clinical consequence of being infected by human immunodeficiency virus (HIV)
- HIV is primarily a blood-borne virus.

Transmission

- Transmission occurs via blood and semen
- Transmission probably requires repeated blood-blood or blood mucosa contact
- In the general population, transmission is related to promiscuity and mainly occurs during (anal) sexual intercourse usually in promiscuous homosexuals or bisexuals
- Transmission also occurs
  - Via transfusion with contaminated blood products
  - Antenatally from mother to child
  - By use or sharing of dirty needles.
- There is no evidence of transmission by bedding, clothing, and food or by aerosol
- The main hazard to dental workers arises from needlestick injuries.

High-risk Groups

- Homosexual or bisexual men, especially who change their partners frequently
- Intravenous drug abusers who share injection equipment
- Hemophiliacs and other recipients of unscreened blood
- Infants born to infected mothers.

Sign and Symptoms

- Usually symptomless
- Sometimes, glandular fever-like symptoms lasting from 3–14 days
- Signs may include:
  - Bilateral lymphadenopathy
  - Hepatosplenomegaly
  - Rashes or candidiasis (oral thrush).

Oral Manifestations

- Candidiasis (thrush) can be angular, oral and/or esophageal; is the commonest oral lesion; rubbing off leaves a raw bleeding surface
- *Oral viral leukoplakia:* Hairy, corrugated or fatty smooth leukoplakia occurs mainly on the tongue, unilaterally or bilaterally, and is unable to rub off
- *Kaposi sarcoma:* A rare vascular tumor seen as a localized red or purple, flat or raised lesion on the hard palate or skin. Mostly seen in homosexuals and is the first presenting symptom
- Herpes simplex virus "cold sores" occur intraorally and nasolabial, can occur in other organs also. They are troublesome, recurrent and spread with disastrous results
- Squamous cell carcinoma occurs in younger people without predisposing causes of smoking, alcoholism and poor nutrition

- Lymphoma is limited to the brain and non-Hodgkin type. Untoward lesions in the mouth require biopsy
- *Papilloma:* HPVs produce oral lesions on the gingiva as known as condylomata acuminata. These can be excised and should be examined histopathologically
- Xerostomia and recurrent oral ulceration: Increase with poor general health, lack of oral hygiene and with mouth breathing.
- Recurrent aphthous ulceration
- Erythema multiforme is common in sick patients with following symptoms:
  - Major weight loss
  - Unexplained diarrhea
  - Fever
  - Severe thrush.
- Incubation time between HIV infection and AIDS varies from 15 months to 14 years. Maximal precautions against patient positive with hepatitis B and suspected/ diagnosed with AIDS.

Advance Preparation

- Use hand pieces, contrangles and water syringes that can be sterilized
- Treat the patient in a separate enclosed room, and keep all materials needed for surgery ready to prevent contamination with traffic
- Use disposable materials wherever possible
- Disinfect and drape all surfaces, which are as follows:
  - Entire dental chair
  - Control switches
  - Instrument tray, support for hand pieces, suction and air water syringe
  - Halogen light/lamp handle, X-ray head and controls.
- The patient should be seen preferably at the end of the day to allow time for preparation and clean up.

Protection of the Dental Personnel

- Wear a disposable paper gown or cloth gown that can be sterilized
- Cover the hair with the cap
- Wear safety glasses with a side shield that can be disinfected
- Wear two pairs of surgical gloves
- Wear two surgical ties on masks.

Patient Preparation

- Cover hair with disposable cap
- Use a disposable drape over clothing
- Provide protective glasses.

Protection during Treatment

- Touch only draped or covered areas
- Avoid procedures that have a high-risk of injury to hands
- Avoid high-aerosolization procedures
- Use a disposable radiographic holder
- Submerge the exposed plastic film in iodine scrub diluted with alcohol (1 for 30 minutes), rinse and dry before processing.

Post-treatment Procedures

1. Place all instruments and reusable linen in the sterilizer; after sterilization clean and sterilize a second time.
2. Keep all disposable covers and materials in a bag for direct incineration. Sterilize first.
3. Soak.
   - Prosthetic appliances
   - Rubber base impressions
   - Other appliances.

Iodine surgical scrub diluted 1:1 in alcohol for 30 minutes. Alginate impressions should be handled with gloves.

Disinfect all surfaces which have been touched but not draped with iodine surgical scrub diluted 1:1 with alcohol, or 0.5% hypochlorite and kept wet for few minutes. Then wash with alcohol or water.

Post-exposure Prophylaxis

On exposure to a needlestick injury, the individual should report to district medical officer. He will send the patient for HIV testing and start 2-drug post-exposure prophylaxis (PEP)

Table 38.1: Percutaneous injuries

Exposure	*Source*		
	Low-risk	*High-risk*	*Unknown*
Not severe	2 PEP	3 PEP	2 PEP
Severe	3 PEP	3 PEP	2 PEP

Abbreviation: PEP, Post-exposure prophylaxis

Table 38.2: Mucous membrane and non-intact skin exposure

Exposure	*Source*		
	Low-risk	*High-risk*	*Unknown*
Small volume (drops)	2 PEP	2 PEP	No PEP/2 PEP
Large volume (blood splash)	2 PEP	3 PEP	No PEP/2 PEP

Abbreviation: PEP, Post-exposure prophylaxis

Table 38.3: Recommended regimens

Category	*Drug regimen*
3 drug PEP/Basic regimen	Zidovudine/azidothymidine 300 mg BD and Lamivudine 150 mg BD for 28 days
3 drug PEP/Expanded regimen	Zidovudine + Lamivudine as above plus Indinavir 800 mg TID/Nelfinavir 750 mg TDS for 28 days

Abbreviation: PEP, Post-exposure prophylaxis

regimens. When HIV status is not known, the first dose of antiretroviral therapy (ART) to be started immediately and if the serum report is negative, the PEP can be discontinued (Tables 38.1 to 38.3).

Exposure

- Percutaneous
  - Not severe: Solid needle superficial scratch
  - Severe: Large bore needle, needle in artery and vein, deep injury.
- Mucosa and non-intact skin exposure
  - Small volume: Droplets
  - Large volume: Major blood splash.

Status of Exposure

- Low-risk: Asymptomatic HIV, viral load <1500 c/mL
- High-risk: Symptomatic HIV, high viral load, AIDS patients
- Unknown: consider the case as risky and 2-drug PEP should be started
- Start PEP immediately
- Advise individual to practice safe sex or avoid sex, avoid breastfeeding
- Avoid donation of blood, body fluids or organs until serology is negative for 6 months post-exposure
- Greatest risk is at 6–12 weeks after the exposure
- Single serology is not confirmatory. Repeat at 6 weeks, 3 months and 6 months.

Hepatitis

There are presently five forms of hepatitis (Fig. 38.3). They are:

- Hepatitis A (Infectious)
- Hepatitis B (Serum)
- Hepatitis C
- Hepatitis D
- Hepatitis E.

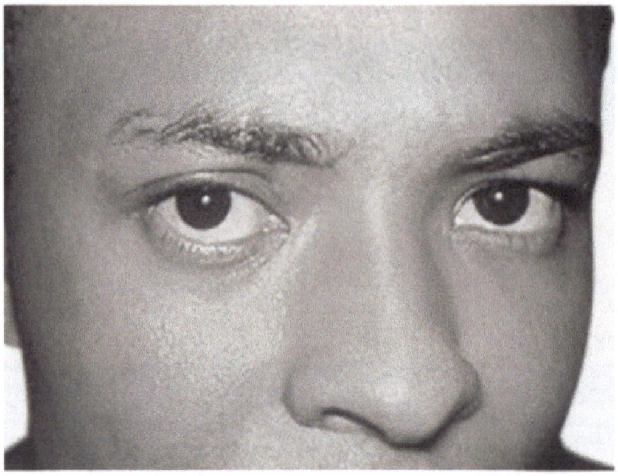

Fig. 38.3: Jaundiced eyes

Of this, HBV infection is considered an occupational risk for dental professional and other healthcare workers. It is a risk that includes the possibility of dental personnel getting HBV from an infected patient and the potential transmission of HBV to susceptible patients from infected dental personnel. The usual symptoms of hepatitis A, B and C may include fatigue, nausea. Poor appetite, mild fever or yellowing of skin or eye (Fig. 38.3).

Infectious Hepatitis (Type A)

- Hepatitis A is transmitted through contaminated blood and water and as a result of poor hygiene
- The virus multiplies in the intestinal tract and then invades the bloodstream subsequently localizing in the liver
- Laboratory tests are available to detect hepatitis A. These specific tests include the detection of immunoglobulin M antibodies to hepatitis A, which indicate active disease and immunoglobulin G antibodies to hepatitis A, which indicates convalescence or immunity
- Although hepatitis A is not considered a major health hazard for dental personnel, a consultation with physician is indicated for all dental patients with a history of hepatitis.

Serum Hepatitis (Type B)

The prevalence of hepatitis B is particularly high amongst people whose occupation, illness brings them into contact with infected blood, blood products, saliva and semen. They include dentists, surgeons, gynecologists, anesthetist, pathologists, hygienists, dental operation room assistants and occupational therapists.

Humans are only reservoir, and infected carriers are the means of spread in the community.

- Hepatitis B is commonly thought to be transmitted through instruments contaminated with blood. However, the virus is found in all body fluids, including saliva of an infected individual. Thus, it can be transmitted by anything with saliva, including handpiece spray
- The incubation period is from 2 months to 3 months. In some patients, there is no clinical illness, but only abnormalities in the chemistry of liver function
- In others, the symptoms may include anorexia, nausea, vomiting, jaundice, fever, weakness, malaise, and abdominal discomfort in the upper right quadrant, joint pain and urticaria. The average minimum length of disability with the disease is 7 weeks
- If the dental surgeon suspects that a patient has hepatitis B, or is a carrier, he may order a hepatitis blood profile to be performed before treating the patient. These include tests for hepatitis A, hepatitis B surface antigen (HbsAg) and antiHbsAg tests to detect hepatitis B
- HBsAg is the surface antigen coating of the HBV. A positive HbsAg test implies that the whole virus as well as virus surface antigen particles is being formed in the person's infected liver and that the person's blood can transmit the disease. Thus, a patient with a positive HbsAg test is considered a potential carrier
- A test can also be performed for anti-HbsAg, the antibody to the surface antigen of hepatitis B. Anti-HbsAg is protective against infection and a positive test indicates that the person is immune to hepatitis B infection
- Heptavax B engerix is a vaccine recommended for all dentists, auxiliaries and

dental technicians. One dose is given initially, a second dose a month later and final dose 6 months after the first. A booster is recommended after 5 years

- The hepatitis B vaccine will protect only against hepatitis B. Protection is about 80% at 1 month, 82% after 2 months, 87% at 3 months and 95% after the third dose. If an individual is exposed during this period to an infectious carrier, receiving immunoglobulin will not interfere with the effectiveness of safety of the heptavax B vaccine.

Prior to immunization, personnel may be tested to determine if they already have been infected with the HBV. An HbsAg positive test indicates that the person is already immune. Anyone who tests as being already immune does not need the heptavax B vaccine.

Hepatitis C Virus

Hepatitis C virus (HCV) causes a slow progressive chronic infection. Transmission of HCV infection occurs largely during blood to blood transmission. The groups at risk of HCV infection are people who receive blood transfusion, drug addicts, prisoners and people born in countries with a high prevalence of HCV infections. Chronically infected patients can have a variety of problems relating to long-term infection with HCV. More than 20–25% patients develop cirrhosis of liver after about 20 years of the initial infection.

Hepatitis D Virus

Around 4% of persons with acute HBV infection are concomitantly infected with hepatitis delta virus (HDV). It was discovered in 1977 and is regarded a defective blood-borne virus requiring the presence of HBV to replicate. Patients coinfected with HBV and HDV have substantially higher mortality rates than those infected by HBV alone. Because HDV infection depends upon the presence of HBV for replication, immunization to prevent HBV infection, through either pre- or post- exposure prophylaxis, can also prevent the HDV infection.

Hepatitis E

Hepatitis E is a viral hepatitis (liver inflammation) caused by infection with a virus called hepatitis E virus. It is one of the five known human hepatitis viruses: A, B, C, D, and E. It is a positive-sense single-stranded non-enveloped RNA icosahedral virus.

Hepatitis E, similar to hepatitis A virus, spreads via the fecal-oral route. The infection is acquired when a person consumes water or food that has been contaminated with feces containing hepatitis E. Hepatitis E, henceforth, can be transferred if a person eats food prepared by an infected person who has not washed their hands after using the bathroom.

Special Precautions While Treating Patients with Hepatitis

- Because of the serious threat posed by hepatitis B, special precautions must be taken to protect both personnel and other patients from the spread of the disease
- Wear disposable gloves even when taking radiographs. Wipe saliva from film packets and place them on a paper towel. Open packets and process films. Keep all debris on the paper towel and throw away. Remove gloves and throw them away
- Wear safety glasses, a mask and gloves during all procedures
- While still wearing gloves, remove soiled instruments by picking them up on a paper towel
- Sterilize instruments before scrubbing them, wrap instruments in the towel label "Hepatitis" and autoclave
- After the instruments have been autoclaved, scrub them (wearing heavy household gloves). Repackage and autoclave again
- Toss all disposables into a lined trash can (so they will not be handled again)
- Disinfect everything touched during treatment.

CHAPTER 39

White Lesions of Oral Cavity

INTRODUCTION

White lesions found on the oral mucosa have a white coating. They require differential diagnosis because they may indicate trauma, infection, or a cancerous process. The various white lesions of oral cavity have been described in Table 39.1.

Table 39.1: White lesions of oral cavity

Lesions	*Clinical features*	*Causes*
Leukoderma	Most commonly seen on buccal mucosa along posterior occlusal plane, bilaterally. Clinically resembles leukoplakia	Unknown
Leukoplakia (Fig. 39.1)	Asymptomatic white patch which cannot be wiped off. Males are more affected. Common sites involved are buccal mucosa, floor of mouth, tongue, lips	Unknown. May be related to tobacco and alcohol use
Black hairy tongue (Fig. 39.2)	The filiform papillae elongate with black or brown discoloration, giving a black and hairy appearance, it is asymptomatic	Opportunistic. Epstein-Barr virus infection
White sponge nevus	Asymptomatic, bilateral, dense, shaggy, white or gray, generalized opacification of buccal mucosa. Sometimes, other membranes may also get involved	Hereditary, autosomal dominant
Focal (frictional) hyperkeratosis	Asymptomatic white patch, commonly seen on edentulous ridge, buccal mucosa and tongue. Does not rub off	Chronic irritation from snuff or chewing tobacco
Mucosal burns	Painful white fibrin exudates covering superficial ulcer with erythematous ring.	Chemicals (Aspirin). Heat and electrical burns
Geographic tongue	White annular lesions with atrophic red centers, pattern migrates over dorsum of tongue, varies in intensity and may spontaneously disappear. Occasionally painful	Unknown
Lichen planus (Fig. 39.3)	Bilateral white striae (Wickham) asymptomatic except when erosions are present. Seen in middle ages. Buccal mucosa is most commonly affected	Unknown. May be precipitated by stress, hyperimmune condition
Candidiasis (Fig. 39.4)	White patches that scrap off with some difficulty leaving bleeding bases. It may form fissures or ulcers, radiating from the angle of the mouth in elderly persons. Erythematous type forms smooth and red patches on the hard palate, buccal mucosa or dorsal surface of the tongue. Candidiasis is associated with poor oral hygiene, debilitating diseases, and prolong antibiotic and anticancer therapy. An early indication of HIV and AIDS infections in young individuals	Opportunistic fungus *Candida albicans*
Oral submucous fibrosis	Areas of opacification with loss of elasticity. Oral lesion is found commonly in buccal mucosa, tongue	Chronic irritation from gutka or chewing tobacco.

Abbreviations: HIV, human immunodeficiency virus; AIDS, acquired immune deficiency syndrome.

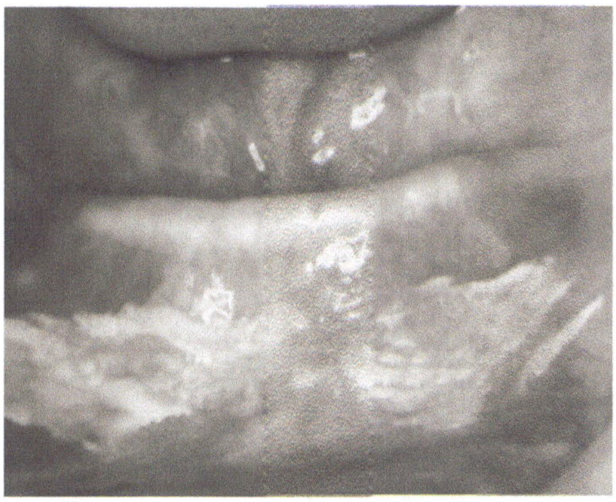

Fig. 39.1: Leukoplakia *(For color version, see Plate 11)*

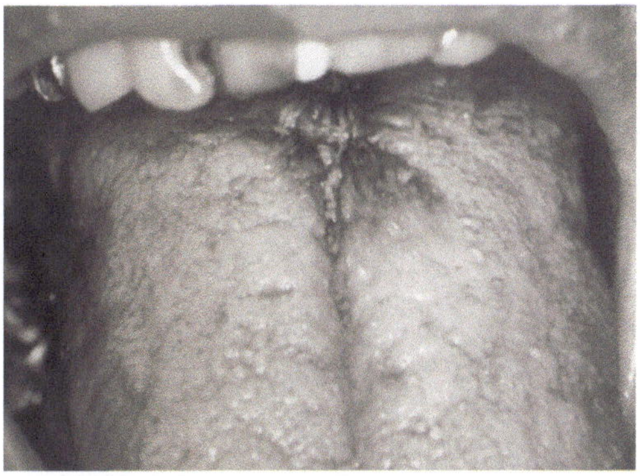

Fig. 39.2: Black hairy tongue *(For color version, see Plate 11)*

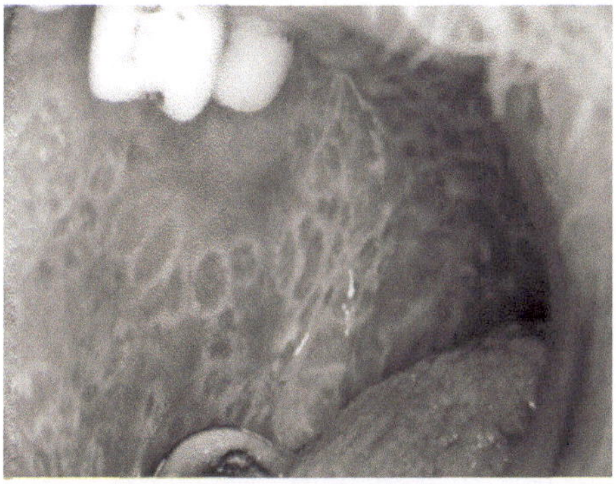

Fig. 39.3: Lichen planus

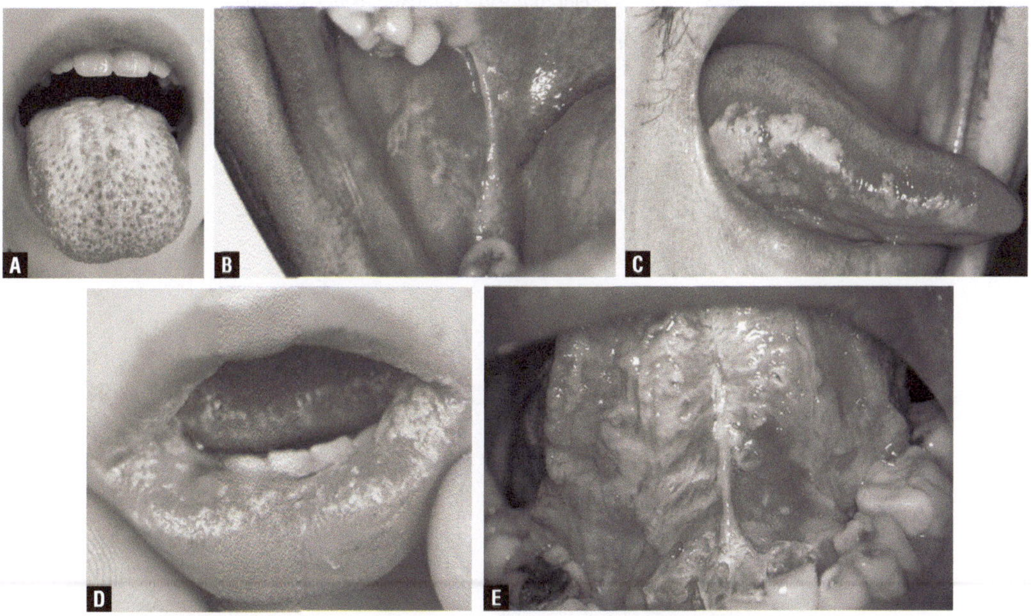

Figs 39.4A to E: Candidiasis of the oral cavity *(For color version, see Plate 12)*

SUMMARY OF WHITE LESIONS OF ORAL CAVITY

White lesions are common findings in the oral cavity and may be benign, pre-malignant or malignant. Early diagnosis can minimize progression of oral cancers. Flowchart 39.1 summarize various kinds of oral white lesions.

Flowchart 39.1: White lesions of oral cavity

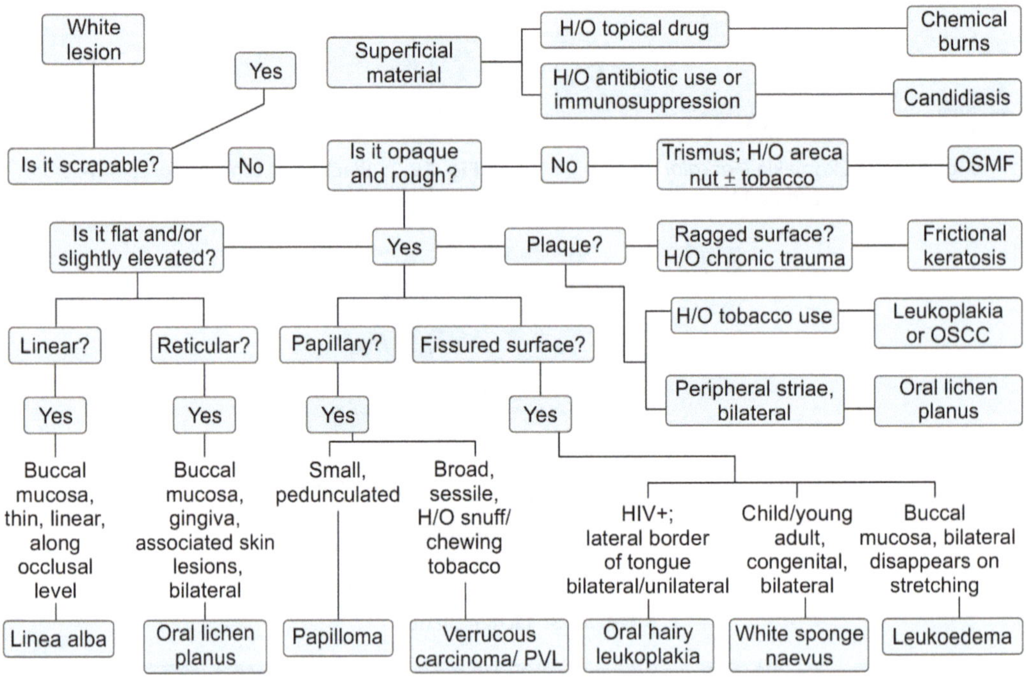

Abbreviations: OSCC, Oral squamous cell carcinoma; OSMF, Oral submucous fibrosis; H/O-History of; PVL, Proliferative verrucous leukoplakia; +, Positive.

Oral Malignancy

CHAPTER 40

INTRODUCTION

Tumor is simply a swelling of the tissue. In the strict sense, the word does not imply a neoplastic process.

NEOPLASM

A neoplasm is often considered as an independent, uncoordinated new growth of tissue which is potentially capable of unlimited proliferation and which does not regress after removal of the stimulus which produced the lesion.

Types of Tumors

- Benign
- Malignant.

Benign Tumor

It remains compact, localized and increases in size slowly. Benign tumor is encapsulated, which forms a clear boundary between them and the surrounding healthy tissue. It only harms the patient by its bulk and its position which may obstruct an important structure.

Malignant Tumor

This type of tumor, on the other hand, is noncapsulated. It is invasive in nature and the tumor grows at the expense of tissue in which it lies. There is ulceration. It is very painful and causes death of the patient. There is evidence of spread by metastasis. Normally, the basement membrane is broken. It spreads into surrounding tissues and the boundary is indefinite. It appears as a diffuse swelling. It is fixed to the surrounding tissues due to deep infiltration. Lymph nodes are enlarged due to secondary growth. The patient becomes anemic and debilitated.

Table 40.1: Differences between carcinoma and sarcoma

Carcinoma	*Sarcoma*
Epithelial origin	Connective tissue origin
Stroma formed by host cells	Formed by tumor cells
Common after 40 years of age	Common in young
Skin ulcerates due to growth	Ulcerates due to pressure involvement
Metastasis by lymphatics	Metastasis by blood stream

Malignant tumors can be broadly categorized into two types:

1. *Carcinoma (Cancer)*: It is a malignant tumor of epithelial origin.
2. *Sarcoma:* It is a malignant tumor arising from mesen-chyme or its derivatives (Table 40.1).

ORAL CANCER

This type of tumor arises from the oral epithelium. The most common location for oral cancer is tongue followed by lip and the least common location is palate. The male/female ratio is 2:1.

Classification

- Squamous cell carcinoma
  - Carcinoma in situ
  - Well-differentiated
  - Moderately differentiated
  - Poorly differentiated
  - Undifferentiated.
- Adenoid squamous cell carcinoma
- Basaloid squamous cell carcinoma
- Clear-cell squamous cell carcinoma
- Spindle cell squamous cell carcinoma
- Lymphoma
- Melanoma.

Etiology

The cause of oral cancer is not known at the present time. Little evidence has been found for a genetic role. However, several factors have been found to be associated with the development of oral cancer. These are called predisposing factors. There is increasing evidence that human papillomavirus and herpes simplex virus play a significant role in the etiology of oral cancer.

Predisposing Factors

- Age of the patient
- Tobacco use (Cigarettes, pipes, cigar, smokeless tobacco)
- Excessive alcohol intake
- Nutritional deficiencies (iron, vitamin A, zinc, copper)
- Syphilis
  - Tertiary syphilis
  - Arsenic compounds used to treat syphilis.
- Poor oral hygiene
- Chronic physical (sharp teeth) and thermal trauma causing nonhealing ulcer
- Defective immune system (congenital, acquired)
- Viruses: Human papillomavirus, Epstein-Barr virus
- Gastroesophageal reflux disease.

Clinical Presentation

Signs

- Squamous cell carcinoma forms a small ulcer which fails to heal, and bleeds
- An exophystic mass/ulceration
- A granular-type raised lesion or combinations of these lesions
- Ulcerated lesions often will have raised margins that are indurated on palpation
- White lesions with areas of erythematous to have a higher incidence of being cancerous than do homogenous white lesions
- In case of tongue involvement, if it involves the deeper structure, and involves the hypoglossal nerve, if the patient is asked to protrude the tongue, will deviate towards the involved side. Carcinoma of palate can involve the glossopharyngeal and/or vagus nerves, resulting in unilateral paralysis of the soft palate and loss of the gag reflex on the involved side. This can be associated with hidden head and neck tumors in the nasopharynx and pharynx.

Symptoms

- Tend to develop late in the course of the disease
- Sore when they do not heal; there is a change in its size and they bleed easily. Thickening skin or lump in the cheek can also be the symptom of this cancer
- Large lesion in the posterior portion of the oral cavity may interfere with the passage of food and air; the patient may complain of weight loss and difficulty in breathing
- Other symptoms include pain, hoarseness, dysphagia, intractable ulcers, bleeding, numbness, loosening of teeth and change in the fit of a denture.

Laboratory Findings

The diagnosis of oral cancer is dependent on a microscopic examination by an oral or general pathologist. Tissue is taken from the involved site and is given for histopathological examination.

System of Classification and Staging of Oral Carcinomas

T: Size of primary tumor
- TIS - Carcinoma in situ
- T1 - Lesion less than 2 cm in diameter
- T2 - Lesion 2–4 cm in diameter
- T3 - Lesion greater than 4 cm in diameter
- T4 - Massive lesion with deep invasion

N: Regional lymph node involvement
- N0 - No palpable nodes
- N1 - Single node, homolateral, 3–6 cm or multiple nodes homolateral, none over 6 cm
- N2 - Single/multiple homolateral nodes, one greater than 6 cm in diameter, or bilateral nodes or contralateral nodes

M: Metastasis
- M0 - Not known distant metastasis
- M1 - Distant metastasis - PUL (pulmonary), OSS (osseous), HEP (hepatic), BRA (brain).

Staging of Oral Cancer

According to International Agency for Research on Cancer, staging of oral cancer is depicted in Table 40.2.

Management of Oral Cancer

- Surgical
- Medical
  - Radiation
  - Chemotherapy.

Table 40.2: Staging of oral cancer

Stages	*Classification*		
0	Tis	N0	N0
I	T1	N0	M0
II	T2	N0	M0
III	T1,T2, T3	N1 N0,N1	M0
IVA	T1,T2,T3 T4a	N2 N0,N1,N2	M0
IVB	Any T T4b	N3 Any N	M0 M0
IVC	Any T	Any N	M1

Dental Management

- Early detection of the lesion by dental surgeon
- Head and neck including intraoral soft tissue examinations
- A patient who comes in with a lesion that appears clinically to be cancerous, or a patient who has a less hard, fixed and/or matted lymph node, should be referred directly to a cancer treatment center or to head and neck surgeon
- Dental treatment planning for the patient with oral cancer begins when the lesion has been found and a diagnosis established
- Before radiotherapy, the following things are to be followed:
  - Non-restorable teeth are to be extracted
  - Periodontal mobile teeth are to be extracted. Nonvital teeth should be treated endodontically
  - Chronic inflammatory lesions in the jaws should be examined and treated. To allow healing, extractions of teeth should be done at least 2 weeks before the start of radiotherapy
  - To avoid osteoradionecrosis, teeth are to be extracted minimum 3 weeks before starting of radiotherapy.

Dental Caries

CHAPTER 41

INTRODUCTION

Dental caries is a disease of hard dental tissue, caused by specific types of bacteria. These bacteria produce acid which destroys the tooth's enamel and the layer beneath referred as the dentin. Dental caries, in layman terms, is called as tooth decay or cavity.

Oral cavity is full of different strains of bacteria. A sticky film called dental plaque is build up over tooth surface. This plaque contains various bacteria along with saliva proteins, food and other natural ingredients. Plaque are most commonly seen at, fissures and grooves in the back teeth, near the gum margin and proximal surfaces of the teeth.

Acids are produced due to the interaction between the bacteria and carbohydrate in the food products. These acids dissolve and destroy minerals (calcium) in the enamel. This leads to erosion and destruction of the enamel surface of the teeth which gradually enlarges and develops into a cavity.

If the decay is not removed and cleaned at this stage, bacteria will continue to grow and invade dentin further down and eventually will get into the tooth's inner layer called as dental pulp tissue. This contains blood vessels and sensitive nerve fibers.

A tooth root exposed by receding gums is also a potential site to develop decay. As the root's outer layer, cementum, is not as thick as enamel, acids from the dental plaque can dissolve it rapidly, leading to caries of the root surface.

ETIOLOGY

There is no universally accepted opinion about the etiology of dental caries. Over the years, three principal theories of cariogenesis have been suggested.

1. *Proteolytic theory:* According to this theory, the organic portion of enamel or dentin is first destroyed by proteolytic enzymes produced by plaque bacteria. Thereafter the unprotected calcified portion is destroyed, possibly by acids. This theory seems more rational in caries of cementum or dentin where the organic portion is moderately high. This theory is not relevant in enamel caries, where the mineralized portion makes up some 96% of the total teeth matter.
2. *Proteolysis-chelation theory:* Chelation is a chemical process where metallic ions are lost from complex molecules because they are attracted to other complex molecules. This process does not depend upon acidity and can take place at neutral or even alkaline pH. According to the proteolysis-chelation theory, the protein element of the tooth is first broken down by the proteolytic enzymes of plaque into amino acids. The amino acid then chelate with calcium ions of the calcium hydroxyapatite, gradually decalcifying the tooth substance.
3. *Acidogenic theory:* In 1882, WD Miller culminated a hypothesis in which he stated, "Dental decay is a chemicoparasitic process consisting of two stages, decalcification of

enamel, which results in total destruction and decalcification of dentin followed by dissolution of the softened residue".

The sugar of diet is converted into acids by the action of the plaque bacteria and the acids subsequently destroy the calcified materials of the tooth.

Bacteria: Various bacterial strains are capable of converting sugar into acids. They are *Streptococcus mutans, Lactobacillus acidophilus, Streptococcus sanguinis* and *Streptococcus salivarius.*

Sugar: Refined pure carbohydrates are more caries producing than complex ones. The sucrose is worst in relation to causing caries. Polysaccharides are less easily fermented by plaque bacteria than monosaccharides and disaccharides.

Acids: Dental plaque has a resting pH which is fractionally on the acidic side of neutral (approximately 6.8 pH) and roughly 10 minutes after exposure to sugar, it reaches its lowest pH in the region of 5 before slowly returning to normal over a period of 30–60 minutes. A number of acids are produced by the action of plaque bacteria on sugar and the most significant is lactic acid. It is seen that calcium hydroxyapatite will begin to dissolve when pH is 5.5 or less and this is referred to as the critical pH.

Secondary Factors

Secondary etiological factors are those which are not directly involved in causing a disease but influence the disease to a greater or lesser extent. These factors are numerous as follows:

Poor Oral Hygiene

It is an obvious feature that caries tends to be more prevalent in dirty mouth than clean one. More the plaque is allowed to accumulate on teeth; the more is the acid build up and attack on the tooth surface. Tooth brushing will remove foodstuff lodged between teeth, thus preventing release of sugar into saliva over a long period.

Diet

The diet has been shown to affect the caries rate in various ways.

- *Composition:* The quantity of sugar consumed has less effect than type of sugar. Sucrose is particularly harmful. The consumption of fluorides in normal quantity in water is a known preventive method in the reduction of dental caries
- *Consistency:* Soft sticky foodstuff cling to the teeth and remain in the mouth for longer period than others food. They are then able to release sugars into the plaque over a long period. The fibrous food does not remove plaque to any significant extent from the teeth and although they may be preferable to sweet sticky foods, they are no substitute for normal tooth brushing
- *Frequency:* More frequently the sugar is consumed, the greater is the period during which acid is available to attack the tooth surface.

Saliva

More the viscosity of saliva there is greater difficulty with oral hygiene and more chances of caries. The rate of salivary flow varies throughout the day and is minimal during sleep. This is the reason for stressing the importance of cleaning the teeth before going to bed. In patients with xerostomia there is a risk of increased caries rate.

Pregnancy

In relation to dental caries, there was a proverb—"A tooth for a baby", is an old saying meaning there by with each child birth the mother looses one tooth due to calcium depletion from the tooth surface However this is not acceptable because in no way calcium from enamel can be resorbed into the bloodstream once the tooth has erupted.

Teeth

The teeth themselves can influence the caries rate in several ways:

- *Form:* Teeth with deep developmental pits and fissures are more likely to be prone to caries. The fissure of teeth narrows to an extent where they cannot be made plaque free by tooth brushing
- *Position:* Crowding and malalignment make oral hygiene much more difficult. This will tend to cause an increase in both periodontal disease and caries
- *Structure:* Areas of hypocalcification may be more prone to caries and of course teeth with reasonable fluoride content are much less susceptible to caries. The critical pH of calcium hydroxyapatite is 5.5 and that of calcium fluorapatite is near 4.5.

Iatrogenic Factors

Iatrogenic factor means those that are caused by humans. Even well-designed dentures and orthodontic appliances are at risk because of trapping dental plaque. The margins of best restoration are liable to secondary caries.

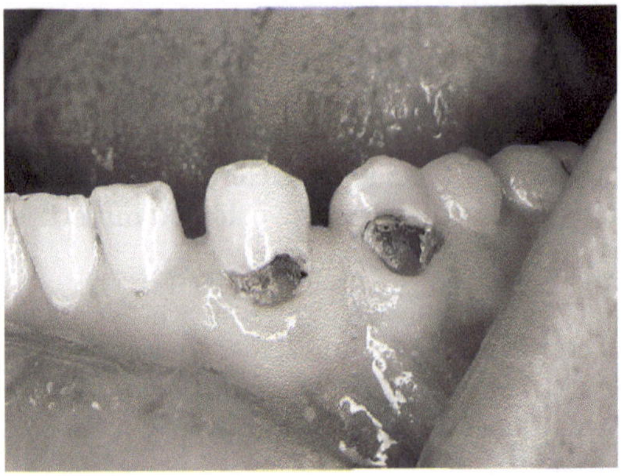

Fig. 41.1: Smooth surface caries *(For color version, see Plate 12)*

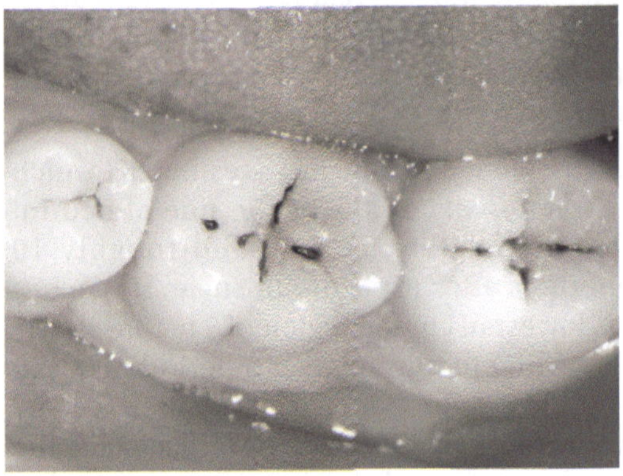

Fig. 41.2: Pit and fissure caries *(For color version, see Plate 12)*

CLINICAL PICTURE

Caries attack the enamel, cementum and dentin gradually eating into and destroying the tooth. The clinical picture varies with the site and the extent of the lesion. Following types of caries are found:

- *Smooth surface caries:* It is found most commonly at the interproximal contact points but it can occur on any smooth surface of the tooth (Fig. 41.1). It appears as a chalky white area which gradually becomes roughened due to breakdown of the enamel. Eventually, an open cavity is formed. As dentin is softer than enamel, the caries destroys it more quickly undermining the enamel. The caries is visible through translucent enamel as bluish-white area. In the next stage, the caries spreads in the dentin and it leaves a progressively larger area of enamel unsupported and eventually the enamel collapses leaving an open carious cavity. The caries at the base may be either soft and creak colored or hard and dark. With the continuing spread of the lesion, the pulp eventually becomes involved and infected producing pulpal inflammation known as pulpitis. The extension of pulpitis through the apical foramen into the periodontal ligament is known as apical abscess
- *Pit and fissure caries:* As the name suggests, this type of cavity develops initially in fissures or developmental pits of the teeth (Fig. 41.2). The first indication of the trouble is appearance of small black pit where probe gets caught. This is the initial break in the enamel and extends as far as the

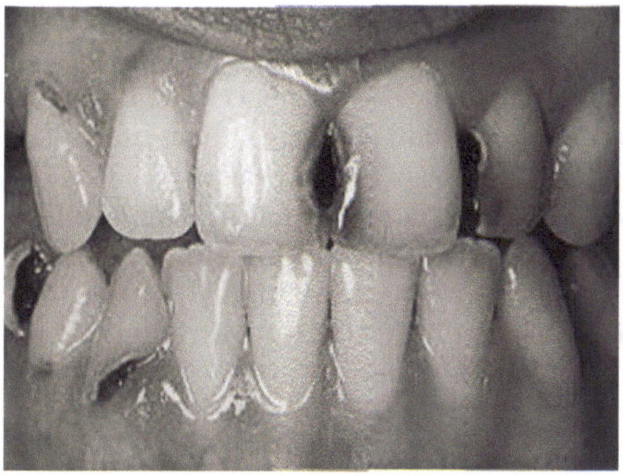

Fig. 41.3: Cervical caries

dentinoenamel junction. Thereafter, caries destroys the dentin which is softer, and in this process, it undermines the enamel. The caries shows through the translucent enamel as blue-white area surrounding the caries' initial pit. After this stage, the caries spreads similar to smooth surface caries

- *Cervical caries:* The cervical caries attacks the areas of exposed dentin; hence, the first two stages described in smooth surface caries is not there. The dentin begins to breakdown forming an open cavity from the outset. This type of caries tends to occur much more commonly in old subjects (Fig. 41.3).

Pain

The degree of pain in a carious lesion varies from extreme pain to none at all. The pain felt at each stage is as follows:

RADIOGRAPHIC APPEARANCE

Small, interproximal cavities are difficult to diagnose because the closed contact between adjacent teeth makes it impossible to see or probe them. Hence, the radiograph will show up as dark areas in the tooth. Similarly, apical abscess presents as dark area in the bone surrounding the apex of the root.

- The small pit and the bluish-white area completely painless
- Deep carious lesions because of the exposed dentin is generally painful with heat and cold, occasionally with sweets.

PREVENTION OF DENTAL CARIES

Dental research workers are making steady progress but no measures have yet been discovered which will completely prevent dental caries. However, there is no doubt that the methods recommended today are of considerable value in this respect. The effectiveness of all but a few of these methods depends on the thoroughness with which instructions of the dentist are carried out.

Such control methods include:

- Regulation of the consumption of refined carbohydrate
- Regular oral hygiene
- Regular dental care, including prophylactic fillings
- Fluoridation of domestic water supplies.

It is appropriate, before these measures are discussed, to emphasize the importance of the care of the expectant mother. As has been already described, the tooth germs for the deciduous teeth and for nearly all permanent teeth are developed during pregnancy. The final stage of mineralization or calcification of deciduous teeth also occurs during this period so that the crowns are nearly completed by the time the child is born.

Therefore, the teeth, together with the rest of the growing baby, are dependent on the mother for all the essential nutrients for development from the earliest days of pregnancy. Hence, the diet of the mother should be a balanced diet.

REGULATION OF REFINED CARBOHYDRATE CONSUMPTION

For the initiation and development of dental caries, it is necessary that fermentable carbohydrates should be present in the mouth. Thus, the diet has an importance related to its local, as well as its general or systemic effect.

The aim, therefore, is to prevent bacteria in mouth, by reducing their main source of food, namely fermentable carbohydrates, thereby preventing the formation of the enzyme and acids that destroy tooth structure.

Diet is the total oral intake of substances that provide nourishment and/or calories. Nutrition is the absorption of nutrients.

- Sugars in diet have main role in causing dental caries
- There is direct relationship between excess consumption of refined, easily fermentable carbohydrate and incidence of dental caries
- Fats and proteins have shown no role in the etiology of dental caries
- Fluoride is an essential nutrient and its presence in drinking water (less than 1 ppm) helps in prevention of dental caries
- Fibrous diet is known for reducing the incidence of dental caries.

CHAPTER 42

Infection Control Protocol in Dental Practice

INTRODUCTION

- An aggressive approach called standard precautions that treat all human blood and body fluids as potentially infectious for human immunodeficiency virus (HIV), hepatitis and other blood-borne pathogens is routinely followed
- Dental instruments are categorized into three categories:
  - Critical instruments that invade sterile tissues or enter vascular system, for example, forceps, scalers, chisels, surgical burs, probe, etc.
  - Semicritical instruments which come in contact with mucous membranes but do not invade tissues, like dental mirror, restorative instruments, handpiece, impression trays, etc.
  - Noncritical instruments are those which contact intact skin only, e.g., medicament jars, glass slabs, etc.

PROTOCOL FOR INFECTION CONTROL

Critical materials are autoclaved or heat sterilized. Semicritical materials are preferably autoclaved/heat sterilized. Heat sensitive are treated with a high level sterilization for 10 hours with 2% glutaraldehyde, 0.5% sodium hypochlorite or as recommended by the manufacturer. Noncritical materials can be disinfected with an intermediate to low level disinfectant.

- All dental healthcare personnel should be immunized against hepatitis B virus and tetanus
  - History taking is specific to identify HIV, hepatitis B and tuberculosis patients. This includes nondietary weight loss of 10 lb in 6 months and sores in mouth that may be recurring
  - Protective barriers like surgical and utility gloves are used consistently, and to be replaced after each patient
  - Masks to protect face, oral and nasal mucosa are used and changed after each patient or after 20–60 minutes
  - Regular eyewear with side shields to protect against splatter and spray should be used.
  - Protective clothing like aprons, lab coats, gowns, head covers, and shoe covers/slippers are used
  - Preprocedural mouth rinse with 0.2% chlorhexidine is done for each case except in routine examination cases
  - Aerosol is minimized using high volume suction. Sudden jerky movement of chair and talking to patient when his mouth is open is discouraged
  - Sharps are handled using needle recapper or one-handed scooping technique or with one-handed technique
  - Hand washing with 4% chlorhexidine or 3% parachlorometaxylenol (PCMX) with scrubbing for 15 seconds is followed
  - Used instruments pass through a procedure of precleaning, corrosion control,

drying, lubrication, packaging, sterilization, drying and cooling, storage and distribution before being used again, if of a critical/semicritical category

- Sterilization monitoring is done daily with chemical strips and weekly with biological monitoring
- Surface and equipment asepsis is done by surface covers (especially of light handles, chair switches, X-ray machine switch, etc.) or by precleaning and disinfection (spray-wipe-spray technique)
- Any prosthesis or impression taken out of the oral cavity is disinfected with 2% glutaraldehyde or 0.5% hypochlorite for 10 minutes before use
- Gloves, plexiglass shields, eyewear and air suction more than 20 ft/min is used in the laboratory while handling infective material
- Surface covers or 10 minutes of 2% glutaraldehyde immersion and washing maintains radiographic asepsis
- Antiretraction valves and water line flushing for 10 seconds is done after each patient
- Aspirators are flushed with a disinfectant cleaner. Suction bottles have 30 mL of 2% glutaraldehyde or 60 mL of 2% hypochlorite
- Bacterial waterline filters are maintained on unit waterlines. Dental unit water reservoirs are kept dry at the end of the day and disinfectant cleaner filled and kept overnight once a week
- Heat labile instruments are autoclaved at 121°C, 151 lb/psi for 15–30 minutes or alternatively 136°C, and 30 lbs/psi for 35 minutes except surgical carbide burs and dental mirrors, which are preferably heat sterilized in a hot air oven at 160°C for 1 hour. Glass bead sterilization is done for endodontic instruments at 210–230°C for 30 seconds. Hand pieces are autoclaved after alcohol wiping, lubrication and packing. These are lubricated with two separately labeled oil cans for presterilization and poststerilization
- Manufacturer's recommendations are followed closely in disinfecting or sterilizing instrument/equipment.

CHAPTER 43

Sterilization and Disinfection

INTRODUCTION

Sterilization is the process of removal and killing of all microorganisms which includes highly resistant bacterial spores. Sterilization is an absolute term, meaning the absence of all microorganisms.

Disinfection is the process of killing most of but not all microorganisms. The number of organism is reduced to a level so that they cannot cause infection; in this process, most of the organisms are killed but some resistant spores may survive.

Disinfectants are the chemicals which are used for disinfection. They should be used only on inanimate objects.

Antiseptics are disinfectants in their mild form that are used externally on living tissues to kill microorganisms, e.g. on the mucous membrane and skin.

Uses of Sterilization

- *For surgical procedures*: Gloves, aprons, surgical instruments, syringes, etc. are to be sterilized
- Sterilization of microbiological works such as preparation of culture media, reagents and equipment, where a sterile condition is to be maintained.

Background of Sterilization and Disinfection

There has never been a greater need for infection control not just in hospitals or general medical and dental surgeries, but in other work environments such as veterinary practices, chiropody, professional beauty clinics, tattoo artistry, acupuncture, hair dressing, and laboratories in the food and water industries, schools, and colleges.

Visual or verbal identification that patient or client is free from infection should not be relied upon. They may be reluctant to advise you or they may not even know that they are infected. Visually, they may appear perfectly normal; however, many blood-borne viruses like hepatitis B and HIV, e.g. may not display any outward signs or symptoms. Infection control procedures should be practiced wherever and whenever there is a potential for exposure to viruses or bacteria.

How is an Infection Transmitted?

There are a number of ways by which infection or disease can be transmitted from one individual to another:

- Contaminated instruments
- Aerosol or airborne
- Personal contact
- Contaminated food and water.

Many bacteria are harmless or may cause only minor discomfort. However, some bacteria can cause serious ailments, which could ultimately be fatal. The introduction of an infection control policy and procedures can be designed to give maximum protection against transmission by any or all of the above routes.

What is Infection Control?

Infection control is the total discipline that provides for a safer working environment for both practitioner and patient. It can include:

- The wearing of suitable protective clothing, for example, gloves, masks, eyewear
- Maintaining a clean and tidy treatment area, ensuring only essential equipment is kept in the area
- Ensuring equipment and work surfaces are regularly cleaned and disinfected between patients
- Immunization of staff
- Identification of high-risk patients enabling appropriate infection control procedures to be implemented in preparation for their treatment
- Sterilization of all instruments that are used in the course of treatment immediately after use and for some procedures immediately before use
- Regular training of all staff in infection control techniques, including emergency procedures when cross infection is suspected (i.e. needlestick injury).

The adoption of an effective control policy is of paramount importance. Advice should be sought from your local health authority or infection control officer on policy and procedure recommendations for your particular professional discipline.

Do I Sterilize or Disinfect?

The short answer is "If it can be sterilized, sterilize it."

Sterilization is the complete destruction of all microorganisms, including the most resistant bacterial spores.

Disinfection is "the killing of pathogenic organisms, but not usually of bacterial spores."

Chemical disinfection may not destroy the agents responsible for harmful or life-threatening disease such as hepatitis B or HIV. In practical terms, disinfectants are used on such items as work surfaces, treatment room furniture and equipment. For instruments used in the course of treatment, especially those which may come into contact with blood or mucous, sterilization should be the standard required within your infection control policy. Particular attention should be paid to hollow instruments or those made up from components, such as dental headpieces, where in the course of treatment, blood and mucous can migrate inside the instrument. Unless proper and effective sterilization is carried out between patients, contaminated blood and mucous can be transferred to the next patient. Remember, sterilization provides the greatest of safety.

How can I Sterilize my Instruments?

There are a number of ways to sterilize instruments some more advantageous than others. In the first instances, you should establish with the manufacturer their recommendations on suitable methods for sterilization of each particular item.

For instruments other than "sharps", cleaning should be carried out after use to remove solid debris, blood, and other matter. Failure to clean could result in contaminated material being "backed" onto the instrument. Particular attention should be paid to the cleaning of hollow instruments, such as dental handpieces, where contaminated materials may be out of sight. Instrument with sharp edges, particularly from high-risk patients, should be sterilized prior to the cleaning process to avoid danger during handling, and then resterilized for use.

In any sterilization process, the most important features the equipment should exhibit are:

- Controlled cycle where the physical conditions required to achieve sterilization are present and controlled automatically, thus removing potential for user error
- Lid lock, where access to the items during a sterilization cycle is prohibited by means of locking system, thus preventing items being added or removed before the cycle has been completed.

METHODS OF STERILIZATION

Autoclave

An autoclave uses steam under pressure for a specific period of time to sterilize. Autoclaving is the preferred method of sterilization by healthcare professionals worldwide, including the World Health Organization (WHO) and the Centers for Disease Control and Prevention (CDC), because it is a rapid, simple and effective process. Also, as it does not use chemical, it is safer and more environmentally friendly. Autoclaving is also more cost-effective than other methods, and with fully automatic equipment can give the most reliable and reproducible in practice of sterilization process (Fig. 43.1). There are three types of autoclaving process which are discussed in the section below.

For Unwrapped Instruments and Utensils

These may be portable or transportable which do not require connection to mains steam, water, or drainage. They also run on standard mains electricity supply. They should be fully automatic in operation and achieve one (or more) of the temperature/time standard listed in Box 43.1. Autoclave for unwrapped instruments is not suitable for the sterilization of wrapped or porous loads.

Box 43.1: Recommended sterilization temperatures and times for autoclaves

- 134°C for 3 minutes
- 126°C for 10 minutes
- 121°C for 15 minutes

Sterilization is effected by moist heat, the condensation of steam onto surfaces of the instrument releases latent heat. Instruments should, therefore, be loaded in the autoclave so that all their surfaces are exposed to steam.

Nonelectric steam sterilizers (Fig. 43.1) work on the same principle as the unwrapped instrument autoclave.

But rely on an independent heat source (gas or liquid fuel burner) for use where there is no mains electricity available.

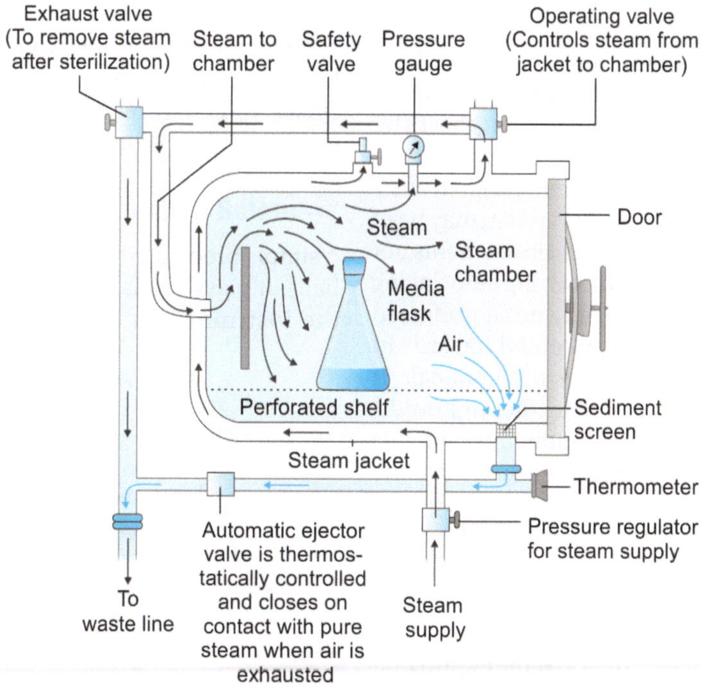

Fig. 43.1: Steam sterilization method by autoclave

For Porous Loads

This autoclave has prevacuum and postdrying cycles. When sterilizing wrapped instruments or surgical packs (cloth), it is necessary first to remove all the air from the chamber and packs by means of a vacuum pump and steam purge stage. This ensures that there are no air pockets, which could prevent steam penetration and therefore, sterilization. Secondly, the load must be dried in the chamber at the end of the cycle to ensure that there are no microbes retained in the pack, which could compromise the sterility of the pack when stored.

For Fluids

These autoclaves may have variable cycle parameters (temperature and time) for the different conditions suitable for sterilizing liquids and media. In addition, many have a post-sterilization cooling stage and pressure ballasting with sterile air to reduce the cycle time and prevent bottles or bags exploding in the chamber or during unloading.
Other methods of sterilization are:

Cold Chemicals

This method involves the immersion of the instrument in a chemical sporicidal solution. Depending on the type or strength of the chemicals used and the instrument(s) to be sterilized, sterilizing time can range from 7 hours to 12 hours. While this system may be of value in sterilizing unwrapped instruments not suited to those methods involving autoclaving temperatures, it is generally not a preferred method because of the potential hazards in using and disposing of the toxic chemicals. It cannot be used to sterilize textiles or liquids. After removal from the solutions, instruments must be rinsed using sterile water and therefore cannot be stored sterile. Many systems do not have lid locks or controlled cycles, which can lead to user error and ineffective treatment.

Chemical Vapor

This uses a chemical sporicidal solution, which is vaporized within the sealed chamber of the equipment. Again a useful system for sterilizing delicate instruments, but it can be more expensive than other methods due to the cost of special chemicals, and instruments are dried before starting a cycle. There are also potential hazards in using and disposing of the chemicals used. This cannot be used for sterilizing cloth or liquids.

Gas

This method uses toxic gases, e.g. ethylene oxide or formaldehyde with low temperature steam as the sterilizing agent. Whilst the method can be effective, particularly for very delicate instruments, the process requires very specialized equipment, installation, and handling of the toxic used. It is, therefore, not a system suited to general practice applications.

Dry Heat

Involves the application of very high temperatures for long periods, which makes the method unsuitable for many instruments, particularly those for which a rapid turnaround is required. Hot air cannot be used for plastics, rubber or textiles. Modern dry heat sterilizers have door interlocking devices, controlled cycles and chart recorders that have greatly increased their cost (Fig. 43.2 and Box 43.2).

Steel Ball or Glass Bead

A simple process, which involves heating steel balls or glass beads in a chamber into which the instrument is inserted. Temperatures

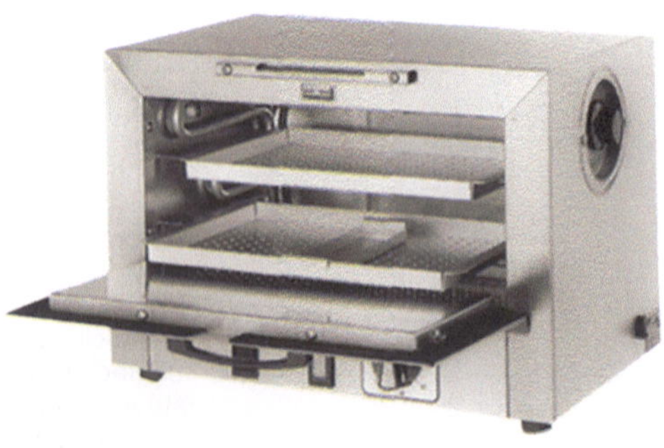

Fig. 43.2: Dry heat sterilizer

Box 43.2: Recommended sterilization temperatures and times for dry heat

- 175°C for 20 minutes
- 165°C for 40 minutes
- 155°C for 120 minutes

required are similar to that for dry heat sterilizers. However, the method is only suitable for very small instruments, and only those parts in contact with the balls or beads are sterilized. This method is not suitable for hollow instruments.

Radiation

Two general types of radiation used for sterilization are ionizing radiation and non-ionizing radiation. In ionizing radiation short wavelength, high-intensity radiation is used to destroy microorganisms. Commonly employed ionizing radiations are gamma rays or X-rays that react with DNA resulting in a damaged cell. Nonionizing radiation uses longer wavelength and lower energy. So, it can only be used for sterilizing surfaces. The frequently used nonionizing radiation for sterilization is ultraviolet light, which possesses multiple applications.

One industrial use of nonionizing radiation is the breakdown of ozone (O_3). Though ozone is mixed with water in order to kill bacteria, it also destroys process media. Hence, it must be broken down so that water can be used for its designated purpose. Water stream is passed under ultraviolet bulbs which breaks the oxygen-oxygen bonds and consequently causes safety to the water processed.

UNACCEPTABLE METHODS OF STERILIZATION

Water Boilers

Immersion of instruments in boiling water does not achieve sterilization as many bacterial spores can withstand boiling. As a method of disinfection only, it can be useful; however, the lack of lid locks or controlled cycles on most types of this equipment can lead to ineffective disinfection. Cross infection from contaminated water (containing bacterial spore not killed by boiling).

Domestic Pressure Cookers

Although pressure cookers operate on a similar principle to autoclaves, they are designed for cooking, not sterilizing. There is no guarantee that a domestic pressure cooker will reach a high enough temperature or, without a controlled cycle, maintain temperature for the required length of time to achieve sterilization. Domestic pressure cookers should not be used for sterilization.

INDICATORS OF STERILIZATION

There are three types of indicators, which are widely used:

1. Biological indicators: These are the only direct methods of validating sterilization as they show destruction of microbiological life. Unfortunately, they do not provide an instant result as following the sterilization process. They must be incubated or processed to determine "pass" or "fail". Their reliability depends on strict quality control during manufacture and decreases during storage. Manufacturer's instructions for use must be followed at all times. Biological indicators are available for all forms of sterilization.
2. Chemical indicators: These do not verify sterilization, but confirm the item has been exposed to the physical conditions required to effect sterilization. They can monitor the conditions of time, temperature, moisture or gas depending on the sterilization method being used. When used with gaseous processes, they will indicate quantitatively the presence of the sterilant but must be located throughout the chamber and load to measure penetration. Chemical indicators will give an instant result.

3. Mechanical indicators: These include temperature measuring devices with gauges or light-emitting diode (LED) displays (time and temperature) and chart recorders/ printers. They indicate that required parameters have been reached during the cycle. Should any one of the parameters fall to reach the minimum within the cycle requirements, it should be assumed that the items are not sterile. The use of chart recorders or printers allows data to be kept with practice records or the sterilizer service history.

ANTISEPTICS, GERMICIDE AND DISINFECTANTS

The term antiseptic, germicide and disinfectant are often confused and sometimes used synonymously.

Antiseptic

It is the drug which inhibits or arrests the growth of microorganisms but does not necessarily destroy them. These are used on living tissue.

Germicide

An agent capable of destroying microorganisms.

Disinfectant

It is a substance which kills pathogenic microorganism. These are used on nonliving substances, instruments, etc.

Mechanism of Action

The action ranges from simple precipitation of proteins by silver (Ag), nitric oxide (NO), or other heavy metals to complex actions interfering with enzymatic processes, which are essential for multiplication and survival of microorganisms. The phenol coefficient is used as a test for the evaluation of effectiveness, but it has its limitations also. Some of these drugs may prove highly irritant on the skin or oral mucosa, or may be corrosive on metal instruments.

Desirable Properties

- The essential property is that the drug should destroy microorganisms rapidly and completely without being toxic to hot cells. So, efficacy as germicide must be balanced against injury to tissues
- The drug must penetrate well. To achieve this, the drugs are formulated so as to have low surface tension, which allows spreading
- The drug must be active in presence of organic material and not be inhibited by it
- It should have a pleasant odor, taste and should not stain
- It must be stable so that it should not be prepared again and again each time.

In dentistry, the antiseptics and disinfectants have two general uses:

1. Disinfection of instruments.
2. Treatment of accessible infections.

Most of the drugs and methods used fall short in one or more of the desirable properties mentioned above; hence, there are numerous drugs in use and the selection of a suitable one is often difficult.

MAINTENANCE OF INSTRUMENTS

All equipment should be maintained in accordance with the manufacturer's instructions and the recommendations contained within health authority publications on the use of sterilizers in practice. Full records should be kept of the service history.

Training

Operators should be fully trained in the use of sterilizing equipment. The manufacturer's operating instructions should be kept with the equipment at all times. Records of cycles completed, together with a note of any irregularity or failure should be kept.

Biomedical Waste Management

CHAPTER 44

INTRODUCTION

Biomedical waste has been defined in Gazette of India as "any waste, which is generated during the diagnosis, treatment or immunization of human beings or animals, or in research activities, or in production or testing off biological". The various hazard symbols, have been illustrated in Figures 44.1A and B.

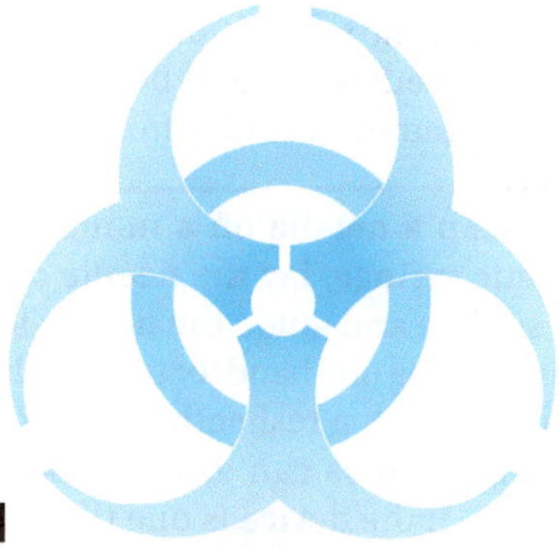

A

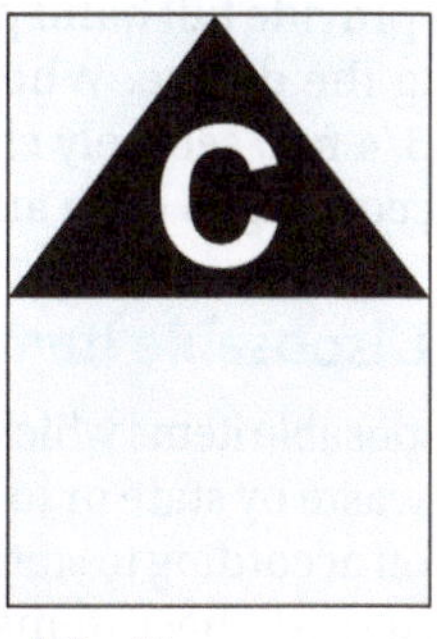

B

Figs 44.1A and B: Management of biomedical waste: (A) Biohazard symbol; (B) Cytotoxic hazard symbol

HAZARDS

Biomedical waste can adversely affect human health by three methods:

1. Hazards for patients attending health care.
2. Hazards for healthcare workers.
3. Hazards for community at large.

In healthcare settings:

- About 85% of generated waste: Nonhazardous
- About 15% of generated waste: 10% infectious hazardous and 5% noninfectious hazardous waste.

STEPS IN BIOMEDICAL WASTE MANAGEMENT

Management of biomedical waste has been described in Table 44.1:

- *Waste survey:*
  - Differentiate the type of waste
  - Quantify the waste generation
  - Determine the point of generation and disinfection.
- *Categorization of waste:* Tissue waste, chemical, instrument, sharp items, liquids, medicines, etc.
- *Segregation and safe storage:* Sharps/nonsharps, chemical/cytotoxic
- *Choice of bins and receptacles:* Plastic, metal bins
- *Handling and treating:*
  - Labeling of bins and waste
  - Disposable items have to be shredded/mutilated

Table 44.1: Summary of waste category, color coding and its disposal

Category	Type of waste	Type of container	Color	Treatment and disposal
1	Human anatomic waste (human tissues, e.g. teeth, gingival, mucosa)	Plastic bags	Yellow	Incineration/deep burial
2	Waste sharps (Needles, syringes, scalpel, blades, glass capable of causing cuts)	Plastic bags/ puncture proof containers	Blue/white/ transparent	Disinfectant/autoclave/ microwave/shredding
3	Discarded medicines and cytotoxic drugs (Outdated, contaminated drugs, medicines)	Plastic bags	Black	Incineration/Disposal in land fills
4, 5	Soiled wastes (Blood, fluid, soiled dressings, cotton, plaster, linen, bedding/tubing, catheters, intravenous administration sets)	Disinfected container and plastic bags	Red or blue	Incineration/ Autoclave/microwave/ shredding
6, 7	Liquid waste and chemical waste	Plastic bags	Black	Disinfectant/discharge in drain/landfills

- Extreme care while handling sharp items
- Disposable items should be dipped in disinfectant
- Liquid waste should be treated with chemical disinfectant
- Mercury, amalgam should be kept in sulfide solution
- Needle tips to be put in disinfectant and shredded or burnt.

INFECTIOUS DISEASE HAZARD (BIOHAZARD) COMMUNICATION

Containers of regulated medical waste are to be labeled and/or identified in compliance with local regulations. These containers involve contaminated sharps containers, contaminated reusable sharps containers (i.e. pans used for holding contaminated instruments), bags of contaminated laundry, specimen containers, and storage containers.

Handling and Disposing Sharps

Place needles and other disposable sharps like scalpel blades, orthodontic wires and broken glass into a puncture-resistant, leak-proof, color-coded container which can be closed and labeled with the biohazard symbol. It must be located in close proximity to the point of use for immediate disposal. It should be noted that one should not cut, bend, break or remove needles by hand before disposal, and do not remove needles from disposable syringes.

To re-cap a needle on a nondisposable anesthetic syringe, lay the needle cover on a firm surface and guide the needle into the cover only using one hand, or use one-handed resheathing with a resheathing device, self-sheathing needles can also be used as an alternative. If the device is one that is hand-held, it must provide full hand protection for hand holding the device. When the sharps container is 3/4 full, securely close and treat or dispose according to state and local laws.

Nonsharp Disposable Items

Nonsharp disposable items which are regarded as regulated waste by state or local laws must be disposed-off according to state and/or local regulations. At least, these items must always be placed in leak-proof, labeled containers. Though disposable items may include the body fluids of patients, they are not subject to medical waste regulations like gloves and patient bibs. Thus, should be placed in a linen trash receptacle. Nonregulated waste should not be disposed-off in red bags. Definite requirements of the local regulatory agency (usually state or country health departments) should be regularly checked for disposal.

OCCUPATIONAL SAFETY AND HEALTH ADMINISTRATION HAZARD COMMUNICATION STANDARD

Occupational Safety and Health Administration's (OSHA's) Hazard Communication Standard (HCS) was first adopted in 1983 for the manufacturing sector of industry. This organization then expanded its scope of coverage to all industries where employees are potentially exposed to hazardous chemicals. It warrants the need of chemical manufacturers and importers to evaluate the hazards of the chemicals they produce or imports. The rule provides definition of health and physical hazards to utilize as the criteria for determining hazards in the evaluation process. The information about the hazards and protective measures is then required to be conveyed to downstream employers and employees by putting labels on containers and preparing and distributing safety data sheets. All employers with hazardous chemicals in the workplaces are needed to have a hazard communication program, which includes container labels, safety data sheets, and employee training.

Ensuring that hazard and protective measure information is available in workplaces through hazard communication programs aids employees' design and implement appropriate controls for chemical exposures. Employers must have the right to know the hazards and identities of the chemicals. In addition, they should be allowed to participate actively in the successful control of exposure which in turn can reduce the potential adverse effects. The information transmitted under the HCS requirements provide the foundation upon which a chemical safety and health program can be built in the workplace.

TEST YOURSELF

Expected Theory Questions

- What is acute inflammation? Write the various steps involved in acute inflammation.
- Define necrosis. Describe various types of necrosis.
- Write a short note on immunity and its types.
- What is an anomaly? Elaborate its classification according to size, number, form, structure and eruption.
- What is dental caries? Write about its various methods of prevention.

Expected Viva Questions

- What are the components of vitamin B complex?
- What is the dosage of vitamin C for adults?
- What are the characteristics of severe fluorosis according to Dean's Fluorosis Index?
- What is the difference between carcinoma and sarcoma?
- What are the special precautions taken while treating a hepatitis patient?

SECTION

5

Dental Radiology

SECTION OUTLINE

Dental Radiography

CHAPTER 45

INTRODUCTION

Radiographs are the pictures produced by X-rays coming in contact with an appropriate film, in a similar manner to the production of photographs by light rays. They are sometimes referred to as roentgenographs. Dental radiographs are taken by passing X-rays through the teeth and jaws and recording the resultant shadow on an X-ray film.

Radiographic exposure techniques are warranted for an accurate diagnostic and treatment procedures. The dental specialist should be able to appropriately position the patient, the tube head, and the X-ray film for intraoral or panoramic film exposures. He must also be able to read and to follow manufacturers' instructions carefully.

When a photographic camera is pointed at a scene and the shutter release is pressed, light enters through the lens and records an image on the film. If, by some misfortune, your hand happens to be in front of the lens at the time of shooting, a shadowy image of this appears on the film. If instead of your hand you held a more transparent object in front of the lens, such as a glass rod, the shadow would not be so dark. In a similar way, X-rays emitted from an X-ray machine and directed at an X-ray film will record the shadow of anything in the path of the rays. X-rays are useful because they can penetrate many objects without leaving a shadow, but the denser a substance is, the more likelihood there is of it casting a shadow on the film. The denser an object is, the more complete will be the shadow; for e.g. the enamel of a tooth will produce a more marked shadow than will dentin and an amalgam restoration will have an even more marked shadow than enamel.

A large number of terms used in radiography have the prefix "radio", such as radiopaque, which describes an object through which X-rays cannot pass and which therefore casts a shadow on the film, and radiolucent, which describes an object through which X-rays can pass and which therefore does not cast a shadow on the film.

PRODUCTION OF X-RAYS

Primary rays are produced in the X-ray machine when a stream of electron strikes a target area made of tungsten. The electrons are produced somewhat in the same way as the action inside a television set, with a very high voltage occurring through conversion from the normal house current. The electrons are emitted from a glass tube, which is usually suspended in oil for heat absorption. The primary rays are highly penetrating and these produce the required image on the film. However, some rays are reflected from more solid objects which they cannot penetrate and may be scattered in different directions. These rays are called secondary rays and are an undesirable feature of an X-ray examination (Fig. 45.1).

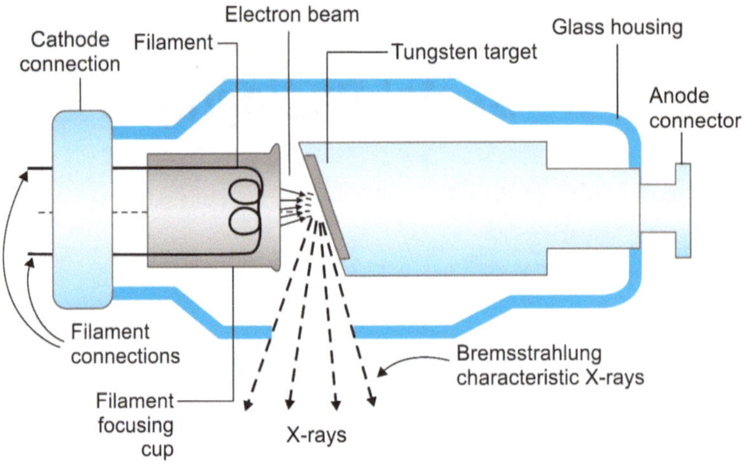

Fig. 45.1: Production of X-ray from dental X-ray tube

PROTECTION OF THE PATIENT AND THE OPERATOR

- Distance rule of six feet and the proper angle of the operator with respect to the X-ray tube must be followed
- An angle of 135° is recommended as a safer zone
- The operator should never hold films in patient mouth
- The tube should never be held by the operator
- Protective guards especially around gonads should be used by both operator and the patient
- Wall of the operatory room should be sufficiently thick or covered with black papers so that someone occupying the adjacent room should not receive radiation
- Personnel waiting in X-ray department should be kept informed of various newer materials and equipment and also of various protective devices.

Primary Considerations

- Take a radiograph of the patient, if clinically necessary
- The radiation protection supervisor (RPS) shall ensure that all staff understand and observe the local rules
- Only a trained and competent operator should use the X-rays equipment.

X-ray Room and Environment

- Room size should be large enough to provide safe accommodation for those persons who have to be in the room during exposure. This will be achieved if there is sufficient space to allow the operator to be 2.0 meter or farther from the tube and patient, and well outside the primary beam
- *Additional protective panels:* These may be required if the workload exceeds 150 mA/mm per week for panoramic films or 30 mA/mm per week for intraoral films. This is roughly equivalent to 50 panoramic or 300 intraoral films
- A dental surgery or any other room should not be used for other work (or as a passageway) whilst radiography is in progress
- *Radiation warning sign:* If the room door opens directly into an area where the instantaneous dose rate is greater than 7.5 μSv/h, a radiation warning sign should be displayed
- *Automatic warning signal:* If the controlled area extends to the room entrance, an automatic warning signal indicating emission of radiation is required to warn against entry
- Persons in all occupied areas outside the X-ray room should be adequately protected.

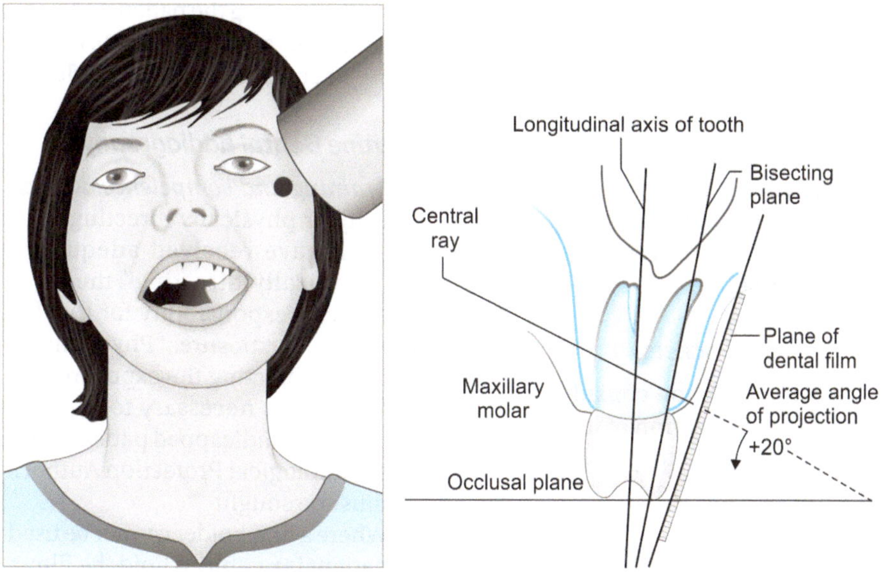

Fig. 45.2: Periapical X-ray exposure

INTRAORAL RADIOGRAPHY

Usually, dental radiographs are made on intraoral film which is made with the film held in the mouth during exposure. They are taken by keeping the film in closer contact to the object, hence it gives more detail in comparison to the extraoral radiographs, which are taken from outside your mouth and possesses less superimposition of shadows.

Types of Intraoral Radiography Films and their Purposes

Periapical

The periapical film offers details concerning the entire tooth and adjacent tissues (Fig. 45.2).

Bitewing (Interproximal)

The bitewing film aids in the detection and determination of depth of caries or other defects of the coronal two-thirds of the crown portion of the opposing teeth and the surrounding alveolar crest (Figs 45.3A and B).

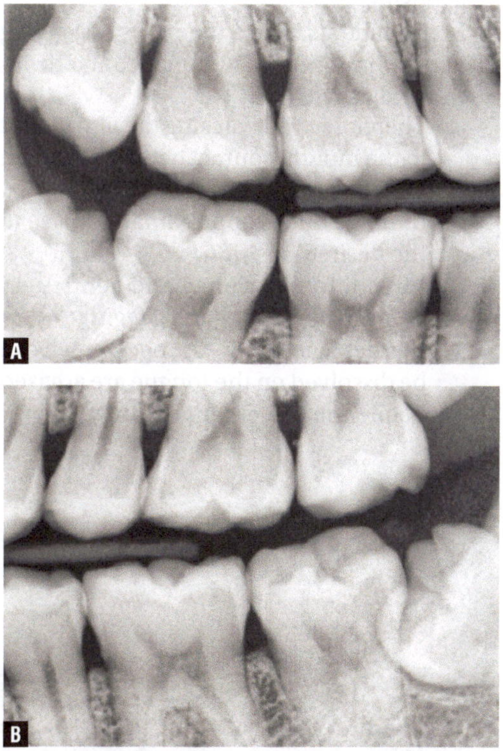

Figs 45.3A and B: Bitewing dental X-rays (A) Right side, (B) Left side

Occlusal

These types of radiographs allow examination of large areas of the jaws from a particular angle which is not possible with other intraoral methods. It is used in diagnosing fractures, salivary duct stones, and impacted teeth. However, occlusal radiographs are used much less in comparison to periapical and interproximal radiographs (Fig. 45.4).

Placement of Film Packets

Various factors should be considered while placement and stabilization of intraoral film packets to attain satisfactory results:

- Confirm that the film is appropriately placed
- Center the film lingual to the tooth/teeth except the bicuspid during radiography
- Do not cause movement of the film during exposure
- Many patients have a tendency of gagging when film is moved along in contact with the oral tissues
  - Therefore, while placing the film packet in the mouth, contact between the film and the oral tissues should be avoided until the film is approximately close to the desired position
  - In addition, patience and gentleness helps in alleviating the gagging
  - Besides, anesthetic lozenges which can be dissolved on the tongue are advised before the placement of film
  - Instructing the patient to breathe deeply through the nose can also act beneficial in controlling the gag reflex.

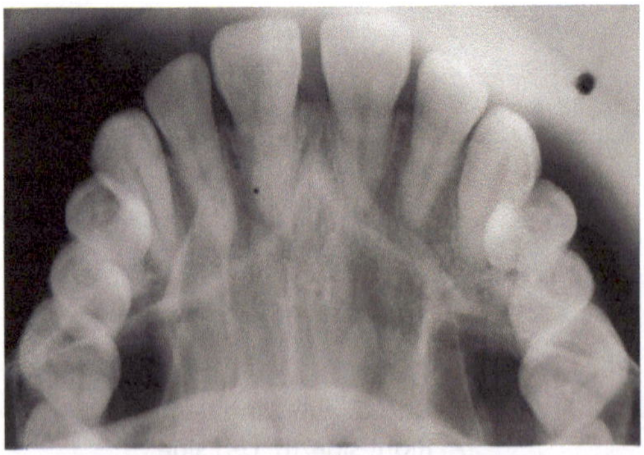

Fig. 45.4: Occlusal radiograph

Routine Dental Radiography

- *Training and competence:* A person clinically or physically directing an exposure shall have received adequate training ("Clinically directing" means having a clinical responsibility for the decision to affect an exposure. "Physically directing" means affecting the exposure)
- Where it is necessary to support a small child or handicapped patient, the advice of a Radiological Protection Authority (RPA) must be sought
- Where a film holder cannot be used and the patient is unable to hold the film, a person assisting must observe adequate protective measures in accordance with the advice of an RPA
- Exposure values should be checked before using the X-ray machine, particularly if changing between long and short cone techniques
- *Attenuation of beam:* Since the beam is not fully absorbed by the patient, it should be considered as extending beyond the patient until it has been attenuated by distance or intercepted by shielding such as a brick wall.

Panoramic Radiography

It is also called panoramic X-ray, is a two-dimensional (2D) X-ray,examination that captures the entire mouth in a single image, including the teeth, upper and lower jaws, surrounding structures and tissues. The jaw is a curved structure similar to that of a horseshoe.

Precautions

- It is a form of focal plane tomography. Image of multiple planes are taken in this radiography to make up composite panoramic image (Fig. 45.5)

- *Automatic warning signal:* Where the controlled area extends to the entrance of the X-ray room, an automatic warning signal indicating when the equipment is in the ready state and radiation is being emitted should be provided at the room entrance

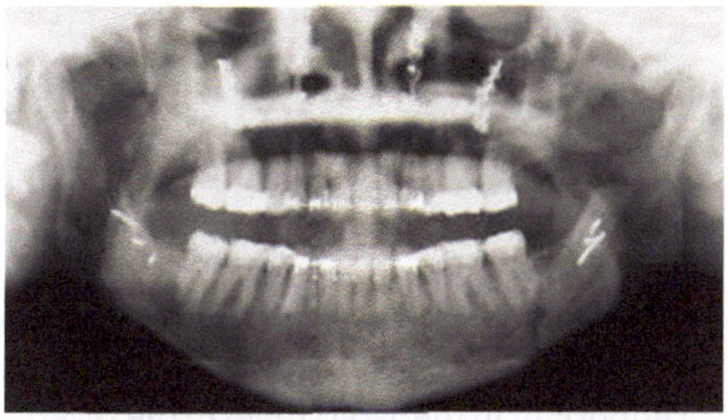

Fig. 45.5: Panoramic radiograph

- *Rotation faults:* The irradiation switch should be released immediately if the rotational movements fail to start or stop before the full arc is covered.

Cephalometry

- It is the measurement of the bony structure of the head using reproducible lateral and anteroposterior radiograms used primarily for orthodontic treatment planning
- Cephalometry should not be carried out without prior consultation with an RPA (Figs 45.6A and B)
- Ordinary dental X-ray equipment operating at less than 60 kV should never be used for cephalometry. Equipment operating at or above 60 kV may be suitable if used with specially designed auxiliary equipment.

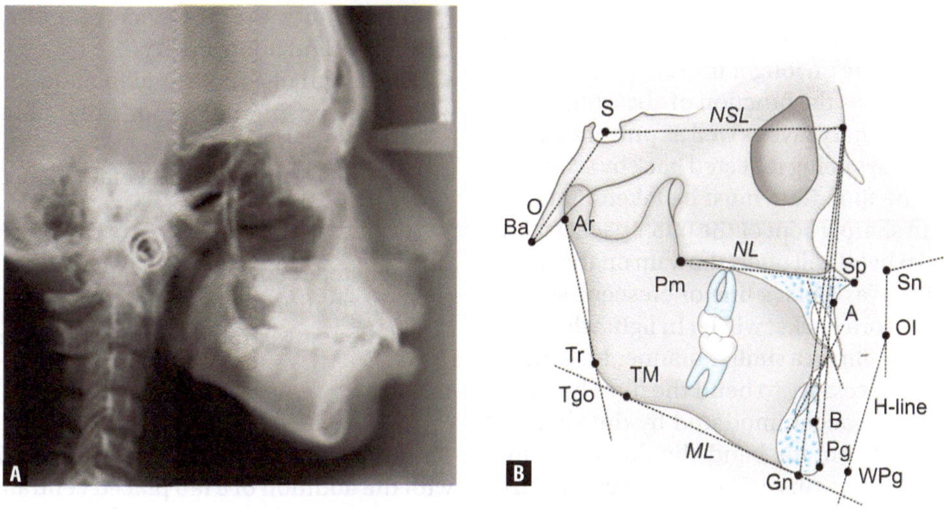

Figs 45.6A and B: Cephalometry of the face

CHAPTER 46

Dental Films and their Uses

INTRODUCTION

Dental films are supplied as film packets of various sizes. Each packet is, in fact, a light sealed envelope of a soft paper material containing a film, a sheet of black paper protecting against light leakage, and a sheet of lead foil. Any rays striking the lead foil have already passed through the subject and the film and are therefore no longer useful. Thus, the lead foil performs the function of absorbing these excess primary rays as well as preventing secondary rays being reflected back by scattering on to the film. Care must be taken that films are not sharply bent or the outer packets torn. A sharp bend will often show up on the developed film as a black line or crescent-shaped mark. A torn packet will let in light which will affect the film in a similar manner to X-rays. It may be necessary to bend the film; however, for it to be accommodated by the shape of the mouth, but the bend should be no more than a gentle curve. There are several sizes and types of dental films.

PERIAPICAL FILMS

The most usual size, called standard, is 3.2 × 4.1 cm (1.1/4 × 1.5/8 inches). There is a smaller size, 2.2 × 3.5 cm (7/8 × 1.1/4 inches), often called child size, but this is frequently used for taking radiographs of adult anterior teeth.

The periapical film shows the entire tooth, and usually the lengths of 3–4 teeth are accommodated on a standard film. They are useful for detecting:

- The state of the alveolar bone supporting the teeth. Periapical views are particularly important in the assessment of the severity of chronic periodontal disease
- Changes around the apex of a tooth. This may denote the presence of a chronic abscess and abnormality
- The length of a root canal in endodontics and the position of a root canal filling in relation to the apex
- Fractures of the roots and retained root tips
- Missing or unerupted teeth
- Supernumerary teeth
- Impacted teeth
- Malformation of the roots which may make an intended extraction more complicated.

BITEWING FILMS

These may be the same as periapical films with the addition of a tab placed centrally on the face, towards the tube, so that the patient holds this between the teeth (hence bitewing) and the X-ray beam is directed along the axis of the tab.

There is a longer film (no. 3 bitewing), 5.4 × 2.7 cm (2 × 1 inch). This covers all the posterior teeth, but distortion is possible.

Bitewings show only the crowns and cervical portion of the roots of the teeth, but have the advantage of showing both upper and lower teeth at the same time. This means that, if the radiographs are being taken to examine the crowns (e.g. for interproximal caries), one bitewing will show the same area as two periapicals, that is only half the amount of exposure to X-ray as needed. Bitewings, therefore, are mainly used for full-mouth surveys to check for caries or early periodontal disease.

OCCLUSAL FILMS

These are somewhat larger, 5.7 × 7.6 cm (2.1/2 × 3 inch), and are placed between the teeth in the occlusal plane. Their purpose is to show all or a large part of the mandibular arch or the maxilla in one film. They may be used to detect abnormalities such as salivary duct calculi in the floor of the mouth, or to localize a tooth or an object in another plane of the jaw. They are often taken to record the position of buried teeth such as upper canines or lower third molars. It is possible to discover and identify the shape and extent of cysts, fracture lines in the jaws and other abnormalities of the bones such as tumors, both benign and malignant.

ORTHOPANTOMOGRAPHS

These are the most common extraoral radiographs with which the dental hygienist will come in contact. They are larger films, measuring 30 × 15 cm, placed in a curved cassette and designed to give a pan-oral picture of the entire dentition on the one film. The film is placed on one side of the head and the X-ray source is set on the other side. The source moves around in an arc, exposing a thin line of the film as it does so. In this way, a flattened out view of the entire dentition and the surrounding structures is produced. These films are extremely useful in making an overall assessment of the patient's dentition, but they have the disadvantage of lacking the clarity of detail found in periapical views. The radiation dosage involved in taking an orthopantomograph is only 80% of that involved in a full-mouth periapical survey.

OTHER EXTRAORAL FILMS

There are many other extraoral films used in dentistry, especially in oral surgery and orthodontics. However, the dental hygienist probably will not be very involved with any of these views. It is unlikely that the hygienist would be required to take such views and they are unlikely to contain the sort of information which the dental hygienist would wish to have. If further information is required about these views, the student is referred to standard texts on dental radiography.

EXPOSING THE FILM

Little is to be gained by detailed written descriptions of the techniques of using dental X-ray machines. Practical skills are best taught by demonstration and practice under supervision.

However, it is necessary to know the factors which influence the density of the image on the film and to understand the principles behind the two basic techniques for taking periapical radiographs.

Density of the Image

This means the darkness of the pictures on the film. This is influenced by the following factors:

- *Kilovoltage*: The greater the kilovoltage, the denser the image
- *Current*: The greater the current, the denser the image
- *Time:* The longer the exposure, the denser the image
- *Film*: The faster the film, the denser the image
- *Distance*: The nearer the film to the source, the denser the image.

BASIC TECHNIQUES FOR PERIAPICAL RADIOGRAPHS

Periapical films may be exposed by either the bisecting angle technique (short cone technique), or the paralleling technique (long cone technique).

Bisecting Angle Technique

This technique is used in areas where the parallel technique is impossible due to poor access, making the angle between the tooth and film more than 15°. A true image of the tooth length and width is obtained by using this technique (Fig. 46.1).

Principle

In any 90° arc, there is one angle that will allow an X-ray beam to cast an accurate shadow of the tooth on the film. For this to work, three angles are measured.

1. Angle 1 is the long axis of the tooth.
2. Angle 2 is the angle of the film.
3. Angle 3 is the angle that bisects the angle 1 and 2. Then beam is then directed at 90 to angle.

It is based on a geometric theorem, Cieszynski's rule of isometry. The film is positioned as close as possible to the lingual surface of the teeth resting the palate or the floor of the mouth.

The most common method which is used to hold the film is to use the patient's forefinger to support the film from the lingual surface, though it has disadvantages of bending the film and resulting in distorted image, slippage

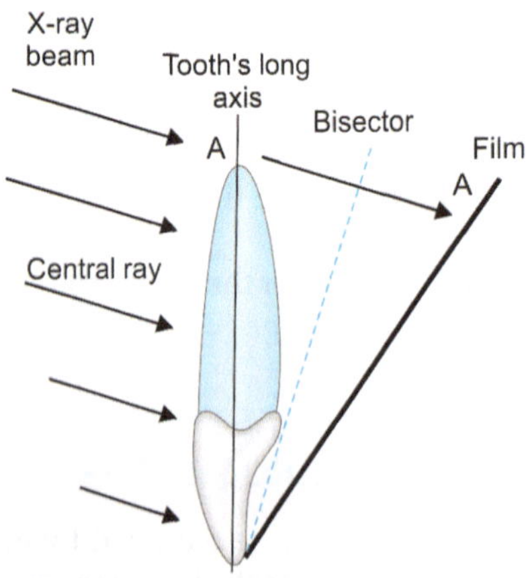

Fig. 46.1: Bisecting angle technique

Table 46.1: Angulation guidelines for bisecting projections

Projection	*Maxilla*	*Mandible*
Incisors	+40 degrees	-15 degrees
Canines	+45 degrees	-20 degrees
Premolars	+30 degrees	-10 degrees
Molars	+20 degrees	-5 degrees

of film, cone cut image, etc. The patient head should be upright with sagittal plane vertical and occlusal plane horizontal. The film is positioned behind the area of interest with the apical end against the mucosa on the lingual or palatal surface. The occlusal or incisal edged should be against the teeth with the edge of the film extending just beyond the teeth. This is a better technique which decreases exposure time (Table 46.1).

Paralleling Technique

If the film is, in fact, placed parallel to the long axis of the tooth, either by interposing a cotton wool roll between them, or by using special paralleling device holders, the central ray of the beam can be directed perpendicularly to both film and tooth, producing a more accurate picture. Since, the film and tooth are further apart, the source must be placed further away from the film, hence the long cone.

Angulation

It is not possible in this text to detail all the angulations and film positions for the numerous different views. Some excellent illustrations and directions for the techniques of film placement can be obtained from the X-ray supply companies, especially Kodak and (for long cone) Rinn.

HELPFUL HINTS

- A few patients gag badly when the film is placed in the mouth, especially on the posterior part of the palate. To overcome this, some operators apply topical anesthetic to the mucosa of the palate for a few minutes. (No topical anesthetic is of value unless it is given time—at least 2 minutes to work). But the best method by far is to spray the side of the film which is placed against the tissues with ethyl chloride. The thin film may then be placed in position with no reaction

- When placing the film in the patient's mouth, make sure that the embossed dot on the edge of the film is placed occlusally. Then, when the film is being clipped to a hanger for processing, it can be clipped near the embossed dot with the knowledge that no important part of the radiograph is being damaged. Alternatively, some dentists like the film to be placed with the dot always at the lower edge. In this way, there is never any doubt about whether the film is of upper or lower teeth, which lets the inexperienced orientate the film without the help of anatomical landmarks
- When a periapical film is being taken for a lower molar tooth, patients often have some difficulty holding the film packet in place. If the occlusal edge of the film is clamped by artery forceps, these can be held by the patient so that the film is in the correct position, either with the hand, or by closing the teeth gently onto the handle. Special flanged forceps can be obtained for this purpose.

PROCESSING THE FILM

Once again, it is not the purpose of this text to detail the stages involved in processing a film. These can be learned adequately only by practice. However, the hygienist should have grasped the theory of developing and processing prior to practicing the techniques.

Developing

Once the film has been exposed to the X-rays, it contains an invisible, latent image, which is covered into a visible one by the developing solution. The emulsion of the film contains silver salts and the developer acts on those which have exposed to the X-rays, precipitating the silver. The density of the image is affected by the following:

- *Temperature:* The warmer the solution, the darker or denser the image
- *Time:* The longer the film is in the developer, the darker it gets
- *Concentration:* The stronger the development solution, the darker the image it produces
- *Age of the solution:* The developer will eventually become "worked out" if used for too long and the image will be pale and weak.

Various manufacturers of developer give tables of recommended times and temperatures for using their products. The solution should be mixed according to the instructions and the times and temperatures carefully adhered to.

Fixing

the fixing solution serves two purposes—it dissolves off the unused emulsion, thus clearing the film, and it fixes the image permanently on the film, so that it is no longer affected by exposure to light.

The time and temperature of fixing are not as critical as they are for developing. Once the film has been cleared, it can be viewed briefly in the daylight, without harm, but it should be kept in the fixer for the full recommended time before being finally washed and dried. Films can be left in the fixer for longer than recommended time, but should not be left longer than 1 hour, or the density of the image may be reduced.

Washing

Thorough washing after processing is essential to remove all chemicals from the film, because if they are left they will cause staining. This can only be done adequately in running water.

TYPES OF PROCESSING

Following are the types of processing:

- Manual
- Semiautomatic
- Fully automatic
  - Without replenisher
  - With replenisher.

Manual processing: The manual processor uses the standard time-temperature method and small containers of the different processing solutions. The dental personnel should be familiar with the manual processor, if the automatic processor is unavailable (Fig. 46.2).

The *automatic X-ray processor* is a machine for developing and fixing dental X-ray films without user contact between insertion of the exposed film and receipt of the developed film into the wash-tank for collection at the termination of the process.

The film is unwrapped in the dark room and directly loaded into the automatic processor after exposure. The unit is composed of rollers and compartments filled with chemical solutions through which the film advances. The film is released at the end of the processing cycle. The cycle varies from 4 minutes to 6 minutes.

- *The preventive maintenance*: Preventive maintenance is vital for keeping this machine operational. The operator must adhere to the daily, weekly, and monthly maintenance schedule as prescribed by the manufacturer
- *Operation:* Market has several automatic processors. Each machine has a marginally different design as well as maintenance and operational requirements. Hence, one must consult the operators' manual so as to avoid damage to a very expensive piece of equipment.

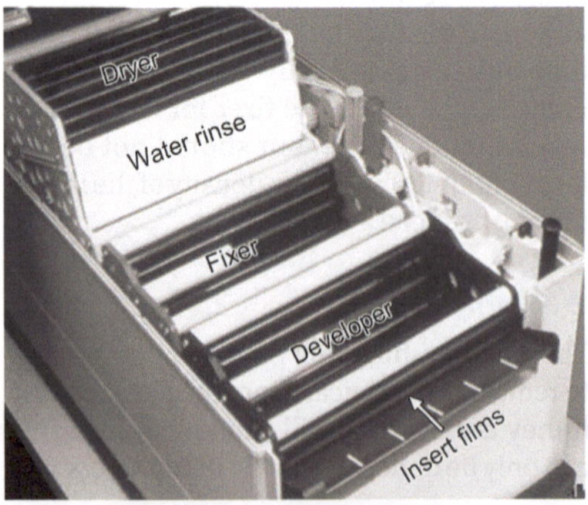

Fig. 46.2: Manual processor

Rapid processing solutions are used for emergencies in cases where time is crucial. The film is developed for 15-20 seconds and fixed for a similar period of time. The films do not possess the similar amount of contrast and will discolor with time; therefore, they must be fixed and washed correctly to minimize the discoloration.

DIGITAL RADIOGRAPHY

Digital radiography is a form of X-ray imaging which uses digital X-ray sensors in place of traditional photographic film. It is currently available in most dental practices with current technology—scanners and/or digital cameras. Its advantages include that their density, contrast and magnification can be manipulated on the computer screen to help in the diagnosis. The images can also be readily stored and can aid in the education of client, referral opinions, or letters, etc. The digital files can easily be transferred from computer to computer by both desk and internet (Fig. 46.3).

There are four ways through which radiographs can be converted to digital image, which are as follows:

1. *Digital cameras*: Digital photography is an inexpensive method of converting conventional radiographs to digital images. The radiograph is placed on a view box or window looking into blue sky and the photograph is taken which is further transferred to a computer for editing and storage. Usually, the digital image should be converted to black and white format to avoid discoloration caused by artificial lights. Digital photography and scanning

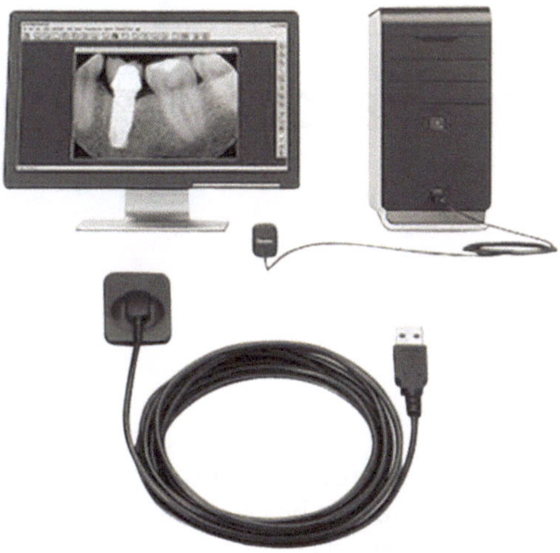

Fig. 46.3: Digital dental radiography equipment

are the cost effective methods of attaining digital radiographs.

2. *Scanning:* This method needs a scanner hooked up to computer which must be available to backlight the radiograph.
3. *Phosphorus sensor*: This technique uses an image plate which differs in the size from small periapical films to larger panoramic sizes. These plates can be further reutilized. The plate is placed in scanner and transmitted to a computer after exposure with a conventional dental radiograph unit. The image captured can be easily transferred. It has less radiation per image in contrast to conventional radiology. However, computer image is not instant and must be scanned to view and needs more steps than charge coupled device (CCD) or complementary metal oxide semiconductor (CMOS) technology.
4. *CCD/CMOS sensor:* This technique utilizes a sensor plate attached to a computer. Its advantage includes that the image is directly displayed on the computer. The disadvantage is that the sensors are not cost effective and currently is available only in periapical film size no. 2.

Hazards of Radiation

CHAPTER 47

INTRODUCTION

X-rays are a boon to mankind if used carefully and sensibly. Repeated and excessive exposure of the same regions of the body to the X-rays will eventually bring about changes which are cumulative (i.e. they add up) and may thus do a great deal of damage. The X-rays themselves do not "add up" in the body but the slight changes that excessive exposure produces in the affected cells remain, and eventually the cells may be irreversibly altered. The taking of dental radiographs is relatively safe, since the amount of radiation used in dental radiographs is much less than that used in most medical views. It is the operator who is principally at risk, rather than the patient, since the operator may be repeatedly exposed to small doses.

HAZARDS OF RADIATION FROM DENTAL RADIOGRAPHY

- Somatic effect is that which occurs in exposed individuals
- Genetic effect is manifested in the future generation of the exposed individual
- Stochastic effects for which the probability of an effect occurring rather than its severity is regarded as a function of the dose without threshold such as carcinoma
- Nonstochastic for which the severity of the effect varies with the dose for which a threshold may therefore occurs such as cataract, infertility.
- Effects of radiation both somatic and genetic can also be classified into:
  - Acute effects
    - ◊ Large area of the body
    - ◊ Small area of the body.
  - Chronic effects
    - ◊ Large area of the body
    - ◊ Small area of the body.

Acute effects: It will be manifested within few hours to few days of acute irradiation and the severity of the effect will depend on the dose and the dose rate.

Chronic effects: They are mainly due to low level or chronic irradiation.

Acute radiation affecting large area of body: They are only possible in nuclear accident and atomic bombardments. With large amount of radiation, following effects are seen such as minor hematological changes, vomiting; death can occur within 6 weeks.

Acute radiation affecting limited area of the body: Such type of effects is seen in cases of malignant tumors. Large doses are administered in short span of 3–10 days. This results in death of irradiated cells. Acute reaction occurs with skin erythema and even bone marrow depression.

Chronic radiation to large areas of the body: This type of hazard is usually seen in workers who are exposed to continuous radiation, e.g. radiographers.

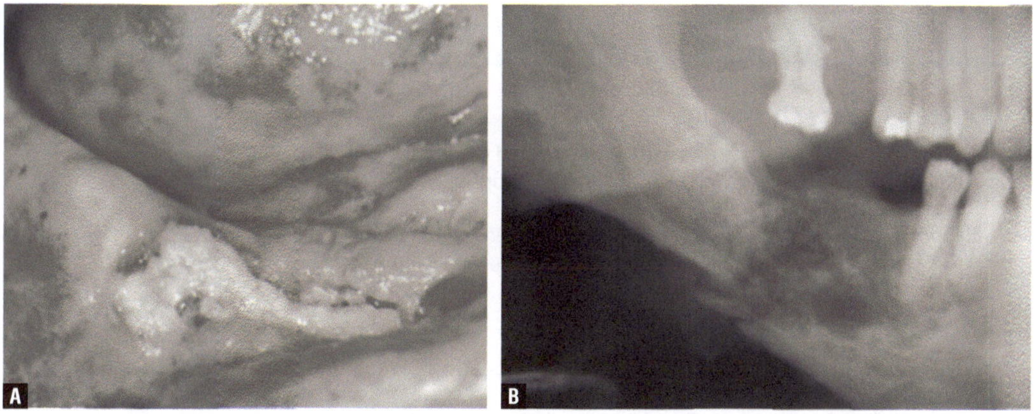

Figs 47.1A and B: Sequelae of osteoradionecrosis. (A) Prolonged exposures of bone intraorally; (B) Pathologic fracture of mandible *(For color version of Fig. 47.1A, see Plate 12)*

Maximum permissible dose (MPD): 0.3 rem/week
Total accumulated dose should not be more than 5 rem/year
MPD = (N-18) × 5 rems (N: age in years).

Chronic radiation to small areas of the body:
- *Radiation burns:* Seen in cases where operator holds the film in patient's mouth. The radiation received every day causes erythema like sunburns:
  - Skin becomes dry and slightly discolored, and patient feels burning sensation
  - Nails become fragile with broken ends
  - Cuticle around the nail is also affected.
- Slight change in blood supply to sebaceous and sweat glands
- Loss of hair (alopecia)
- Cataract
- Effect on oral mucous membrane: Area of redness and inflammation with repeated exposure pseudomembrane are formed because of breakdown of mucous membrane. Secondary infection by *Candida albicans*
- Effect on salivary glands
- *Effect on taste buds:* Loss of taste sensation and alteration in saliva
- *Effect on teeth:* If radiation precedes calcification of teeth, tooth may be destroyed after calcification; if radiation continues, malformation can result. Root development is retarded
- *Effect on the bones:* Loss of vascular and hematopoietic elements, e.g. osteoradionecrosis (Figs 47.1A and B).
- *Radiation caries:* Decrease in salivary flow, pH and buffering capacity of saliva lead to rampant caries. Topical application of 1% sodium fluoride can reduce it.

WHOLE BODY RISK

- Damage to blood cells
  - Anemia
  - Infection
  - Hemorrhage.
- Gastrointestinal effects
- Developmental anomalies
- Cancer
- Leukemia
- Gene mutation.

TEST YOURSELF

Expected Theory Questions

- Explain the production of X-rays with a well-labeled diagram.
- What is bisecting angle technique? Explain its principle.
- Explain the processing of an X-ray film.
- Elaborate in detail the hazards of radiation.
- Write a short note on periapical and bitewing radiographic films.

Expected Viva Questions

- What is the optimum distance between the operator and X-ray tube?
- What is the standard size of periapical films?
- What is the maximum permissible dose of radiation per week?
- What is stochastic effect and nonstochastic effect of radiation exposure?
- What are the effects of higher temperature of developing solution on the radiographic image?

SECTION

6

Gingival and Periodontal Diseases: Classification and Management

SECTION OUTLINE

Gingival and Periodontal Diseases

CHAPTER 48

INTRODUCTION

The word "perio" means "around" and "dontal" refers to teeth. Periodontal diseases are infections of the structures around the teeth, which include the gums, the cementum that cover the root, periodontal ligament and alveolar bone. The first signs of periodontal diseases usually begin with gingivitis (inflammation of the gums). The gums appear reddened at margins, slightly swollen and bleed when gently proved.

Untreated periodontal diseases like gingivitis and periodontitis can eventually lead to tooth loss and other health problems.

Gingival diseases are divided into:

- Acute gingival disease
- Chronic gingival diseases.

The American Academy of Periodontology (AAP) in 1999 has classified the periodontal diseases and conditions which are now adopted in most parts of the world.

Gingival Diseases

- *Dental plaque-induced gingival diseases:* These diseases may occur on periodontium with no attachment loss or someone with attachment loss that is stable and not progressing.
  - *Gingivitis associated with dental plaque only:*
    - ◊ Without local contributing factors
    - ◊ With local contributing factors.
  - *Gingival diseases modified by systemic factors:*
    - ◊ Associated with endocrine system:
      - ▸ Puberty-associated gingivitis
      - ▸ Menstrual cycle-associated gingivitis
      - ▸ Pregnancy-associated gingivitis
      - ▸ Pyogenic granuloma
      - ▸ Diabetes mellitus-associated gingivitis.
    - ◊ Associated with blood dyscrasias:
      - ▸ Leukemia-associated gingivitis
      - ▸ Others.
  - *Gingival diseases modified by medications:*
    - ◊ Drug-influenced gingival diseases:
      - ▸ Drug-influenced gingival enlargements
      - ▸ Drug-influenced gingivitis: Oral contraceptive-associated gingivitis, others.
  - *Gingival diseases modified by malnutrition:*
    - ◊ Ascorbic acid deficiency gingivitis
    - ◊ Others.
- *Non-plaque-induced gingival lesions:*
  - Gingival diseases of specific bacterial origin:
    - ◊ *Neisseria gonorrhoeae*
    - ◊ *Treponema pallidum*
    - ◊ Streptococcal species
    - ◊ Others.

- Gingival diseases of viral origin:
  - ◊ Herpes virus infections
    - ▸ Primary herpetic gingivostomatitis
    - ▸ Recurrent oral herpes
    - ▸ Varicella-zoster.
  - ◊ Others.
- Gingival diseases of fungal origin:
  - ◊ *Candida* species infections; generalized gingival candidiasis
  - ◊ Linear gingival erythema
  - ◊ Histoplasmosis
  - ◊ Others.
- Gingival lesions of genetic origin:
  - ◊ Hereditary gingival fibromatosis.
  - ◊ Others.
- Gingival manifestations of systemic conditions:
  - ◊ Mucocutaneous lesions:
    - ▸ Lichen planus
    - ▸ Pemphigoid
    - ▸ Pemphigus vulgaris
    - ▸ Erythema multiforme
    - ▸ Lupus erythematosus
    - ▸ Drug induced
    - ▸ Others.
  - ◊ Allergic reactions:
    - ▸ Dental restorative materials, e.g. mercury, nickel, acrylic, others
    - ▸ Reactions attributable to tooth-paste's or dentifrices, mouthrinses or mouthwashes, chewing gum additives, foods and additives
    - ▸ Others.
- Traumatic lesions (factitious, iatrogenic, or accidental):
  - ◊ Chemical injury
  - ◊ Physical injury
  - ◊ Thermal injury.
- Foreign body reactions
- Not otherwise specified (NOS).

Chronic Periodontitis

- Localized: Less than 30% of sites involved
- Generalized: More than 30% of sites involved
- Slight: 1–2 mm clinical attachment loss
- Moderate: 3–4 mm clinical attachment loss
- Severe: More than 5 mm clinical attachment loss.

Aggressive Periodontitis

- Localized slight, moderate or severe
- Generalized.

Periodontitis as a Manifestation of Systemic Diseases

- Associated with hematological disorders:
  - Acquired neutropenia
  - Leukemias
  - Others.
- Associated with genetic disorders:
  - Familial and cyclic neutropenia
  - Down syndrome
  - Leukocyte adhesion deficiency syndrome
  - Papillon-Lefévre syndrome
  - Chediak-Higashi syndrome
  - Histiocytosis syndrome
  - Glycogen storage disease
  - Infantile genetic agranulocytosis
  - Cohen syndrome
  - Ehlers-Danlos syndrome (types IV and VIII)
  - Hypophosphatasia
  - Others.

Necrotizing Periodontal Diseases

- Necrotizing ulcerative gingivitis
- Necrotizing ulcerative periodontitis.

Abscesses of the Periodontium

- Gingival abscess
- Periodontal abscess
- Pericoronal abscess.

Periodontitis Associated with Endodontic Lesions

Combined periodontic-endodontic lesions.

Developmental or Acquired Deformities and Conditions

- Localized tooth-related factors that modify or predispose to plaque-induced gingival diseases/periodontitis
  - Tooth anatomic factors
  - Dental restorations/appliances
  - Root fractures
  - Cervical root resorption and cemental tear.
- Mucogingival deformities and conditions around teeth
  - Gingival/soft tissue recession, facial or lingual surfaces, interproximal (papillary)
  - Lack of keratinized gingiva
  - Decreased vestibular depth
  - Aberrant frenum/muscle position
  - Gingival excess:
    - ◊ Pseudopocket
    - ◊ Inconsistent gingival margin
    - ◊ Excessive gingival display
    - ◊ Gingival enlargement.
  - Abnormal color.
- Mucogingival deformities and conditions on edentulous ridges:
  - Vertical and/or horizontal ridge deficiency
  - Lack of gingival/keratinized tissue
  - Gingival/soft tissue enlargement
  - Aberrant frenum/muscle position
  - Decreased vestibular depth
  - Abnormal color.
- Occlusal trauma:
  - Primary occlusal trauma
  - Secondary occlusal trauma.

GINGIVAL DISEASES

Inflammation of gingival tissue is called gingivitis. Gingivitis can be divided into following types:

- Based on location
  - Marginal gingivitis
  - Interdental gingivitis
  - Diffuse gingivitis.

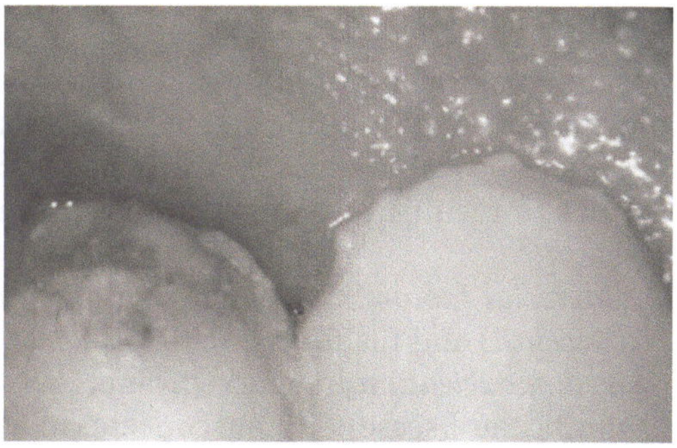

Fig. 48.1: Plaque-induced gingivitis
(For color version, see Plate 12)

- Based on course
  - Acute gingivitis
  - Chronic gingivitis.
- Based on severity
  - Mild gingivitis
  - Moderate gingivitis
  - Severe gingivitis.

Gingivitis (inflammation of gingiva) is the most common type of gingival disease. The role of inflammation in gingival diseases varies in three ways:

1. Inflammation may be primary due to bacterial plaque (Fig. 48.1).
2. Inflammation may be secondary, superimposed on systemically caused gingival disease, e.g. inflammation commonly complicates gingival hyperplasia.
3. Inflammation may be precipitating factor responsible for clinical changes in patients with systemic conditions that themselves do not produce clinically detectable gingival disease, e.g. gingivitis in pregnancy.

ACUTE GINGIVAL DISEASES

Acute Necrotizing Ulcerative Gingivitis

Acute necrotizing ulcerative gingivitis (ANUG) is characterized by punched-out ulcerative lesions of the interdental papillae, gingival bleeding and pain, and sometimes accompanied by gingival edema. It is also known as Vincent's gingiva, Vincent's infection or trench mouth.

Etiology

Exact etiology is not yet fully established or understood. Evidence indicates combination of bacterial, local, systemic and psychogenic factors to result in the occurrence of the disease.

- *Bacterial factors:* Spirochetes (*Borrelia vincentii*) and fusiform bacilli (*Fusobacterium nucleatum* are markedly increased during the disease). Current concepts indicate that particular microorganisms are not the primary etiologic agent but the etiology involves a combination of microorganisms, lowered tissue and general body resistance, which facilitates the pathogenic activity of the bacteria
- *Local predisposing factors:* The factors are as follows:
  - Poor oral hygiene
  - Calculus
  - Impacted food
  - Excessive smoking and consumption of alcoholic beverages
  - Pre-existing gingivitis
  - Periodontal pockets
  - Poor nutrition
  - Poor restorations
  - Areas of malocclusion traumatizing the gingiva.
- *Systemic contributory factors:* ANUG is often superimposed on gingival alteration caused by severe systemic disease
  - Debilitating disease
    - ◊ Syphilis or chronic diseases
    - ◊ Carcinomas
    - ◊ Infections
    - ◊ Ulcerative colitis—gastrointestinal tract (GIT) disorder
    - ◊ Anemia, blood dyscrasias, leukemia and AIDS.
  - Nutritional deficiency
    - ◊ Deficiency of vitamin C and B12 accentuates the severity of the pathologic changes induced by the fusospirochetal bacterial complex.
- *Psychosomatic factors:* Psychological factors appear to be important in the etiology of ANUG, like increase in stressful situations, e.g. final examinations in school and college and induction into armed forces. These conditions demand drastic changes in living style. Correlation is seen to exist between ANUG and two personality traits—dominance and abasement in psychiatric patients
- *Age and gender:*
  - Occurs at all ages; highest incidence reported between 15–35 years
  - Affects both sexes equally
  - More common in children with Down's syndrome
  - Low socioeconomic groups are more commonly affected.

Clinical Features

- *History:*
  - Acute necrotizing ulcerative gingivitis is characterized by sudden onset, sometimes following an episode of debilitating disease or acute respiratory tract infection.
  - Change in living habits
  - Protracted work without adequate rest
  - Psychological stress.
- *Oral signs:* Characteristic lesions are punched out, crater-like depression on the crest of interdental papillae, subsequently extending to the marginal gingiva (Fig. 48.2)

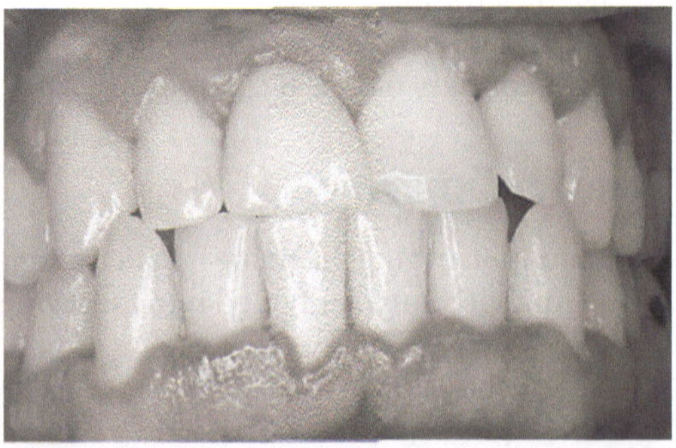

Fig. 48.2: Acute necrotizing ulcerative gingivitis *(For color version, see Plate 13)*

- Surface of gingival craters is covered by a gray, pseudomembranous slough, demarcated from adjacent gingiva by a pronounced linear erythema
- The characteristic lesions progressively destroy the gingival and underlying periodontal tissues
- Spontaneous gingival bleeding on slight provocation is also characteristic sign
- Other signs found is fetid odor and increased salivation
- Acute necrotizing ulcerative gingivitis may affect a single tooth or a group of teeth.

- *Oral symptoms:*
    - Lesions are extremely sensitive to touch
    - Patients complain of a constant radiating, gnawing pain which gets aggrevated by spicy or hot foods and chewing
    - Foul metallic taste
    - Patient complains of excessive amount of pasty saliva.
- *Extraoral signs and symptoms:*
    - Patients are usually ambulatory and have minimum systemic complications
    - In mild and moderate stages of ANUG, local lymphadenopathy and slight fever
    - In severe stages of ANUG, increased pulse rate, high fever, loss of appetite, leukocytosis, and general lassitude is also observed
    - Systemic reactions are more severe in children
    - Also accompanied with ANUG are symptoms like insomnia, constipation, GIT disorders, headache and mental depression
    - In very rare cases as a sequelae to ANUG. Noma or gangrenous stomatitis, fusospirochetal meningitis, pulmonary infections, toxemia and fatal brain abscess may occur.
- *Clinical course:*
    - It is indefinite. The disease may get resolved spontaneously without treatment. Such patients usually give history of repeated remissions and exacerbation
    - If ANUG is left untreated in chronic cases, it leads to progressive destruction of periodontium and denudation of roots. In addition, severity of toxic systemic complications can also occur.
- *Communicability:* ANUG is not seen to be a communicable or contagious disease.

Diagnosis

Diagnosis is based essentially on clinical findings. Bacterial smear is useful only in cases of differential diagnosis because bacterial culture is similar in case of periodontal pockets, pericoronitis, and herpetic gingivostomatitis.

Treatment

- Hydrogen peroxide rinses (3–4 times a day for 2 weeks). Patient is asked to rinse mouth with a glassful of equal parts of 3% hydrogen peroxide and warm water. This rinsing consists of forcefully swishing the solution back and forth in the mouth for 3–4 minutes
- Drugs include penicillin (500 mg) 4 times per day for 5–7 days. It is the drug of choice when systemic complications are present. Metronidazole (400 mg) 3 times a day for 7 days is also effective in controlling the spirochetes
- Thorough scaling and root planing (may require a topical or local anesthetic). Ultrasonic scaling is found to be less traumatic
- Flossing is recommended for interdental cleaning as soon as the acute symptoms have subsided. Interdental stimulation is to be done to remove plaque and facilitate recontouring of the cratered interdental papillae.

Preventive Measures

- Proper oral hygiene technique to be regularly followed
- Nutritional deficiency taken care of by intake of well-balanced diet
- Proper and adequate rest advised

- Avoid stressful situations
- Avoid heavy smoking and alcohol consumption
- Regular professional prophylaxes at recall visits.

Acute Herpetic Gingivostomatitis

Acute herpetic gingivostomatitis is (also known as primary herpetic gingivostomatitis or oral labial herpes) is a combination of gingivitis and stomatitis, or an inflammation of the oral and gingival. Herpetic gingivostomatitis is often the initial stage during the first (primary) herpes simplex infection.

Clinical Features

- *Oral signs:*
  - Diffuse erythematous gingiva (Fig. 48.3A and B)
    - ◊ Edema, gingival bleeding.
  - Initially, discrete spherical gray vesicles are seen. After 24 hours, vesicles rupture forming very painful ulcers with red, halo-like margin.
- *Oral symptoms:*
  - Generalized soreness of oral cavity
    - ◊ Difficulty in drinking and eating
    - ◊ Ulcers are painful and sensitive to touch and thermal changes
    - ◊ Extraoral signs and symptoms.
  - Cervical lymphadenopathy
    - ◊ High fever: 101–105°F
    - ◊ Generalized malaise
    - ◊ Halitosis.

Diagnosis

- From history and clinical examination
- Laboratory confirmatory tests.

Treatment

- Application of topical anesthetic mouth washes
- Local application of antibiotics
- Local application of "acyclovir" ointment
- Plaque, food debris, and superficial calculus to be removed
- Copious fluid intake.

Pericoronitis

Pericoronitis is the inflammation of the gingiva in relation to the crown of an incompletely erupted tooth. Most commonly seen in partially erupted or impacted mandibular third molar region.

Clinical Features

- Gingival flap is inflamed red, with swelling and tenderness
- Pain radiating to ear, throat and floor of mouth
- Foul taste and inability to close the jaws
- Submandibular lymphadenopathy
- Fever, leukocytosis, malaise
- Ulceration at the inner surface of the gingival flap
- It may be complicated to cellulites or abscess formation.

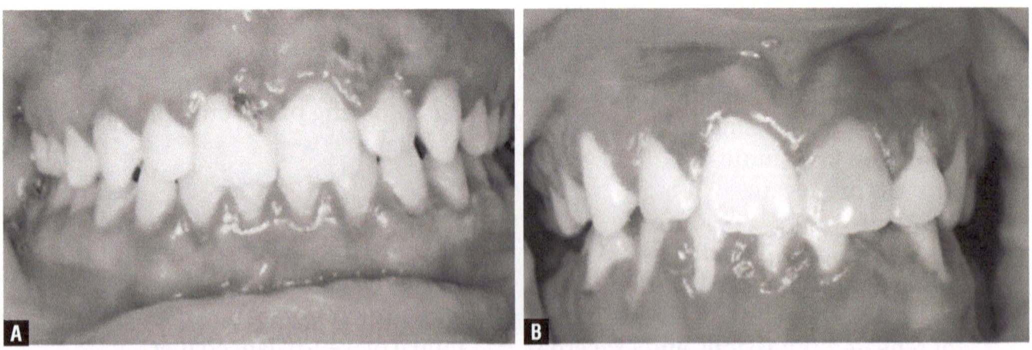

Fig. 48.3A and B: Acute herpetic gingivostomatitis *(For color version of Fig. 48.3B, see Plate 13)*

Management

- Flushing the area with warm water to remove debris
- Irrigating with antiseptic solution after elevating the flap
- Metronidazole and tetracycline are systemically administered as antibiotic therapy
- If abscess formation has initiated, then incision and drainage are established
- Impacted molar, if present, should be surgically extracted
- If the tooth is erupting in normal direction, the pericoronal flap is removed by a procedure known as "operculectomy" with the help of periodontal knives or by electrosurgery.

CHRONIC GINGIVAL DISEASES

Chronic Desquamative Gingivitis

It is characterized by redness and desquamation of the surface epithelium of attached gingiva.

Clinical Features

They vary in severity. They may be mild, moderate or severe.

- *Mild form:* Only diffuse erythema is seen in attached, marginal and interdental gingiva (Fig. 48.4)
- *Moderate form:* Color becomes bright red. Gingiva is soft and slight pitting is seen on applying pressure. Massaging gingiva with a finger results in peeling of the epithelium leading to exposure of underlying bleeding connective tissue surface, burning sensation of mouth, and sensitivity to thermal changes
- *Severe form:* Scattered, irregularly shaped areas where gingiva is denuded and bright red. Surface epithelium is friable, which can be peeled off in small patches. If a blast of air is blown over the gingiva, it causes elevation of epithelium with the consequent formation of a bubble. Extremely painful, burning and drying sensation is felt by the patient. Chronic desquamative gingivitis is commonly associated with skin diseases like lichen planus, pemphigus or mucous membrane pemphigoid, where skin and other mucosal surfaces are also involved.

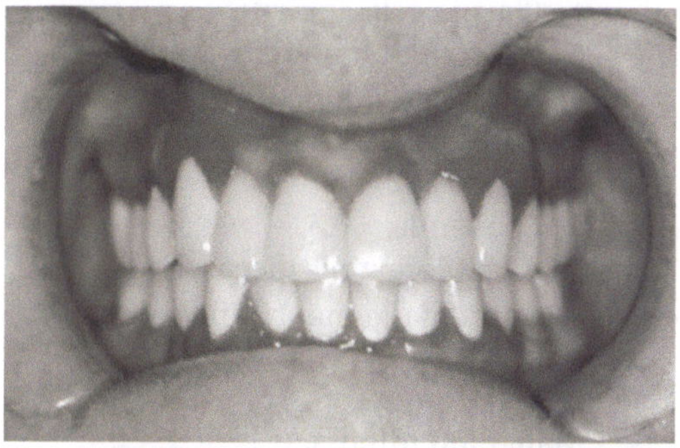

Fig. 48.4: Desquamative gingivitis
(For color version, see Plate 13)

Management

Before treatment is instituted, a proper diagnosis should be made for skin lesions like lichen planus, pemphigus or mucous membrane pemphigoid. Management consists of both local and systemic treatment.

Local therapy:

- Patient is instructed to use a soft toothbrush for proper plaque control
- Hydrogen peroxide mouthwash diluted with water to be used twice daily
- Topical corticosteroid ointment of triamcinolone 1%, fluocinonide 0.05% is applied and gently rubbed on the gingiva several times a day.

Systemic therapy: It constitutes administration of systemic corticosteroid prednisolone 30–40 mg daily.

Chronic Gingival Diseases Due to Nutritional Deficiency, Endocrine, Hematologic, or Immunologic Problems

Gingivitis initiated by bacterial plaque may be aggravated by the systemic conditions.

This is seen in various vitamin deficiencies like vitamin A, vitamin B, vitamin C, thiamin, riboflavin, niacin, pyridoxine, folic acid, cyanocobalamin and protein deficiency.

Gingivitis is seen in various conditions that may produce an imbalance of endocrine system during pregnancy, puberty, diabetes, hyperpituitarism, and use of contraceptives.

Gingivitis is also seen in blood diseases like various leukemias, anemia, thrombocytopenia, agranulocytosis, etc.

Management

The therapy consists of two parts:
1. Systematic therapy.
2. Local therapy.

The systematic condition of the body is corrected. It is due to any vitamin deficiency; the concerned vitamin should be administered in proper doses.

Local therapy: Plaque control should be achieved. Removal of calculus by oral prophylaxis and root planing. Correction of restorative and prosthetic irritational factors, if any.

Antimicrobial therapy is given to prevent the secondary infections. For this purpose, tetracycline and metronidazole may be administered.

Gingival curettage and gingivectomy should be done, if required.

GINGIVAL OVERGROWTH (ENLARGEMENT)

Increase in size of gingiva is a common feature of gingival disease. In past, terms like hypertrophic gingivitis or gingival hyperplasia were used. But, nowadays, this condition is commonly known as gingival enlargement or gingival hyperplasia.

Classification

- Inflammatory enlargement (Fig. 48.5)
  - Chronic
  - Acute.

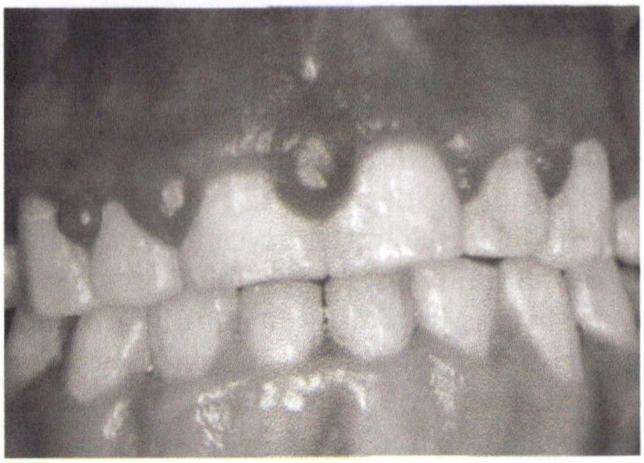

Fig. 48.5: Inflammatory enlargement
(For color version, see Plate 13)

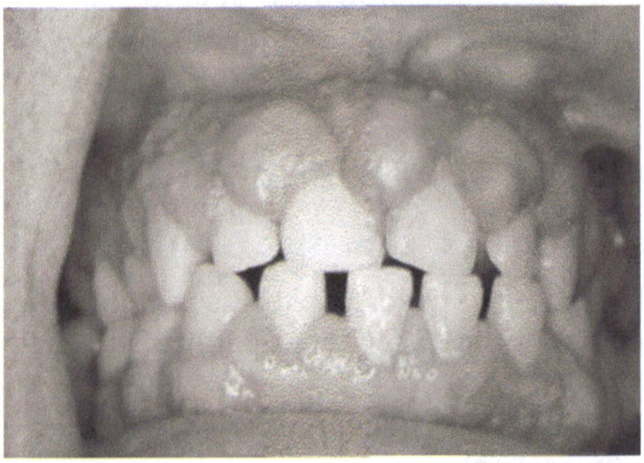

Fig. 48.6: Phenytoin-associated enlargement
(For color version, see Plate 13)

- Drug-induced enlargement (Fig. 48.6)
- Enlargements associated with systemic diseases
  - Conditional enlargements
    - ◊ Pregnancy
    - ◊ Puberty
    - ◊ Vitamin C deficiency
    - ◊ Plasma cell gingivitis
    - ◊ Nonspecific conditional enlargement (granuloma pyogenicum).
  - Systemic diseases causing gingival enlargements
    - ◊ Leukemia
    - ◊ Granulomatous diseases.
- Neoplastic enlargement (gingival tumors) (Fig. 48.7)
  - Benign tumors
  - Malignant tumors.
- False enlargement.

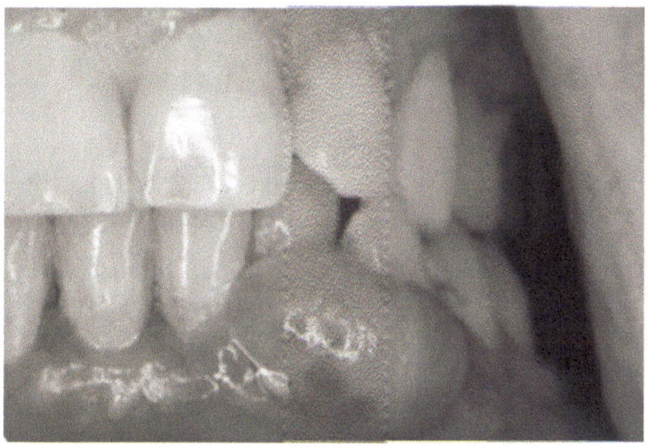

Fig. 48.7: Giant cell granuloma
(For color version, see Plate 13)

Grading

Grade 0: No signs of gingival enlargement
Grade 1: Enlargement confined to interdental papilla.
Grade 2: Enlargement involves papilla and marginal gingiva
Grade 3: Enlargement covers three-quarters or more of crown.

Inflammatory Enlargement

Gingival enlargement may result from chronic or acute inflammatory changes; chronic changes are much more common.

These are commonly secondary complications to any of the other types of enlargement, creating a combined gingival enlargement.

Chronic Inflammatory Enlargement

Chronic inflammatory gingival enlargement shows following characteristics:

Clinical features:

- It originates as a slight ballooning of the interdental papilla and marginal gingiva
- In early stages, it produces a life saver bulge around the involved teeth which increases in size
- It may be localized or generalized and progresses slowly and painlessly, until it is complicated by trauma or infection
- Occasionally, it occurs as discrete sessile or pedunculated mass resembling tumor
- It may be interproximal or on the marginal or attached gingiva
- The lesions are slow growing masses and usually painless
- They may undergo spontaneous reduction in size, followed by exacerbation and continued enlargement
- Painless ulceration, sometimes, occurs in the fold between the mass and the adjacent gingiva.

Histopathology: Lesions that are clinically deep red or bluish-red are soft and friable with a smooth, shiny surface, and they bleed easily. They also have a preponderance of inflammatory cells and fluids, with vascular engorgement, new capillary formation and associated degenerative changes.

Lesions that are relatively firm, resilient, and pink have a greater fibrotic component with an abundance of fibroblasts and collagen fibers.

Management

- *Treatment of chronic inflammatory enlargements:* Scaling and curettage procedures are done for removal of calculus and granulation tissues followed by gingivectomy or flap surgery, as indicated
- Treatment of periodontal and gingival abscess by incision and drainage reduces the swelling and provides relief from pain
- Enlargement due to drugs like phenytoin, cyclosporine, nifedipine requires replacement of drug followed by surgical removal of fibrotic gingival enlargements
- *Leukemic gingival enlargements:* Scaling and root planing is carried out in stages under topical anesthesia
- During pregnancy, irritants such as calculus and plaque are eliminated by scaling or root planing. Use of 0.12% chlorhexidine mouthwash is advised.

PERIODONTAL DISEASES

Periodontal disease is gum disease. The word "periodontal" means "around the tooth." Periodontal disease is a chronic inflammatory disease of the gum and tissues that surround and support the teeth. If left untreated, periodontal disease can lead to tooth loss.

Signs and Symptoms

- Red or bluish-pink gingivae
- Swelling in gingiva or rolled margins of gingivae
- Bad breath or halitosis
- Pus discharge from gingival sulcus or suppuration
- Loose teeth or mobility in teeth
- Dull aching pain in gums
- Bleeding from gums.

Types of Periodontal Diseases Based on Clinical, Radiographic, Histological and Laboratory Characteristics

Chronic Periodontitis

Chronic periodontitis is the most common form of periodontitis usually seen in adults but can occur in children and progresses slowly.

Etiology: It is initiated by dental plaque accumulation that is further facilitated by the presence of local irritants like calculus and faulty restorations, or poor oral hygiene. Presence of systemic diseases like HIV infection and diabetes mellitus may attribute to disease progress.

Clinical features: Gingival inflammation, pocket formation, gingival bleeding, suppuration from pocket, loss of periodontal attachment and alveolar bone, and formation of abscess may also be seen along with tooth mobility in advanced cases. It is usually associated with localized dull pain, hypersensitivity on exposed roots, food impaction, and itching in the gingiva (Fig. 48.8).

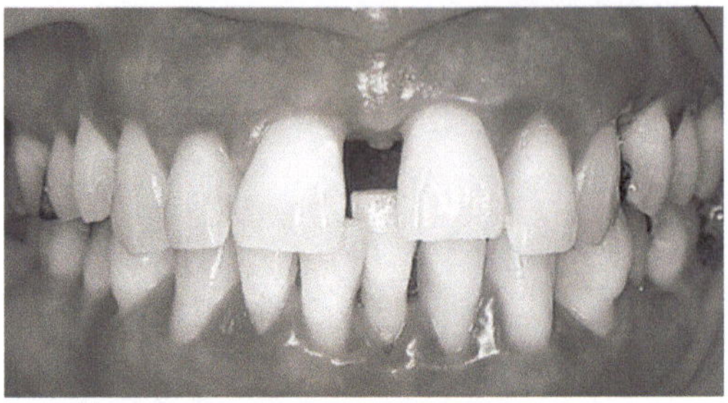

Fig. 48.8: Chronic generalized periodontitis
(For color version, see Plate 13)

Classification: It is classified as:

- Slight: 1–2 mm of clinical attachment loss
- Moderate: 3–4 mm of clinical attachment loss
- Severe: More than 5 mm of clinical attachment loss
- Localized form: Less than 30% of sites involved
- Generalized form: Affecting more than 30% of sites/teeth present.

Aggressive Periodontitis

Usually occurs in otherwise clinically healthy individuals below 30 years and progresses rapidly to produce excessive attachment and bone loss.

Clinical features: Aggressive lesions with deep pockets but locking clinical inflammation of gingival tissues and less plaque or calculus is present. On microbiological analysis, diseased sites are infected with *Actinobacillus actinomycetemcomitans*, other tests may reveal abnormalities in phagocyte function or hyperresponsive macrophages.

In some cases, it may be self-arresting, in others it may not respond to conventional therapy.

Classification: Localized form is circumpubertal in onset; it is localized to first molar or incisor with attachment loss in at least two permanent teeth one of which is a first molar. Usually, prognosis is good and responds well to active therapy.

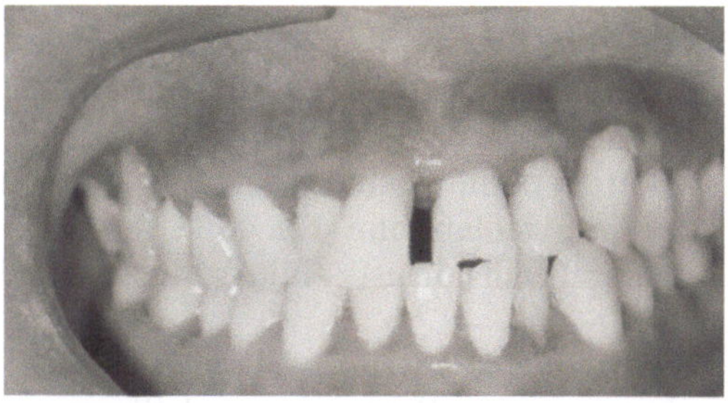

Fig. 48.9: A 21-year-old male with aggressive periodontitis *(For color version, see Plate 13)*

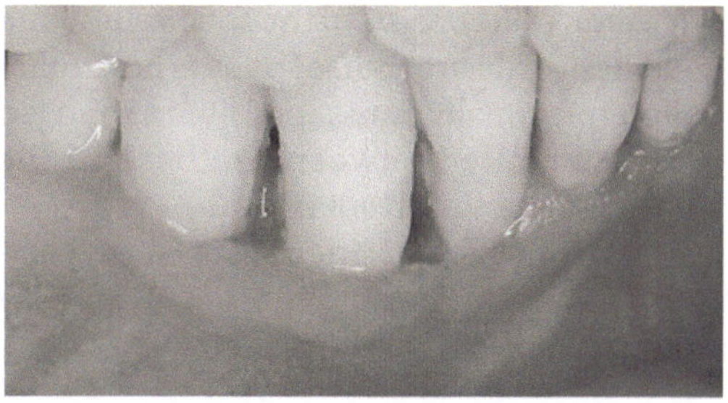

Fig. 48.10: Generalized necrotizing periodontitis *(For color version, see Plate 14)*

Generalized form usually affects persons less than 30 years of age (may be older), associated with proximal attachment loss affecting at least three teeth other than first molars and incisors. This condition is episodic in nature and shows periodontal destruction with poor prognosis (Fig. 48.9).

Periodontitis as a Manifestation of Systemic Diseases

- Hematological disorders
  - *Leukemia:* It is a malignant neoplasm of white blood cell precursors leading to leukemic cell infiltration of gingiva and less frequently alveolar bone, resulting in gingival enlargement, ulceration and infection
  - *Neutropenia*: Destructive generalized periodontal lesions have been seen in children.
- Genetic disorders
  - *Down's syndrome*: Characterized by formation of deep periodontal pockets, more severe in lower anterior region and acute necrotizing lesions (Fig. 48.10)
  - *Papillon-Lefèvre syndrome:* Characterized by hyperkeratotic skin of palms/soles and calcification of dura mater. Leads to severe destruction of periodontium and loss of primary dentition by 6 years and secondary dentition by 15 years of age
  - *Leukocyte adhesion deficiency syndrome:* Affects primary dentition with severe acute gingival inflammation and rapid bone loss
  - *Chediak-Higashi syndrome:* People with this syndrome have light skin and silvery hair (albinism) and frequently complain of solar sensitivity and photophobia. The infections involve mucous membranes, skin, and the respiratory tract.

PERIODONTAL POCKET

The periodontal pocket is defined as a pathologically deepened gingival sulcus. Deepening of gingival sulcus may occur by coronal movement of the gingival margin, apical displacement of gingival attachment or combination of above.

Periodontal pocket may be absolute/true. This type of pocket occurs with progressive pocket deepening leading to destruction of the supporting periodontal tissues and loosening and exfoliation of the teeth.

Absolute pockets are of two types; suprabony pocket and infrabony pocket.

Suprabony Pocket

- Also known as supracrestal or supraalveolar pocket
- Bottom of the pocket is coronal to the underlying alveolar bone (Fig. 48.11A)

- Lateral wall consists of the soft tissue alone
- Pattern of destruction of bone is horizontal
- Interproximally transseptal fibers arranged horizontally (between the base of the pocket and the alveolar bone)
- On the facial and lingual surfaces, periodontal ligament fibers follow the horizontal-oblique course.

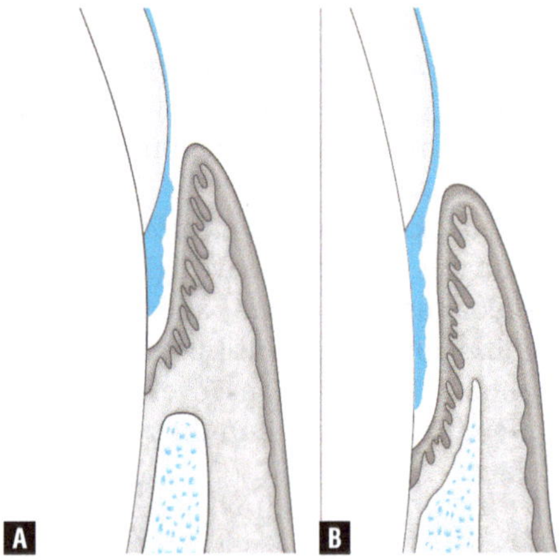

Figs 48.11A and B: Different types of pockets (A) Suprabony pocket; (B) Infrabony pocket

Infrabony Pocket

- Also known as supracrestal or infra-alveolar pocket
- Bottom of the pocket is apical to the crest of the alveolar bone (Fig. 48.11B)
- Lateral wall consists of the soft tissue and bone
- Pattern of destruction of bone is vertical
- Interproximally transseptal fibers are oblique (extent from the cementum beneath the base of the crest of the cementum of the adjacent tooth)
- On the facial and lingual surfaces, periodontal ligament fibers follow the angular pattern.

Other Classification

Simple: Involve one surface of the tooth (Fig. 48.12A).

Compound: Involve more than one surface of the tooth (Fig. 48.12B).

Complex: Originating on one tooth surface and twisting around the tooth to involve one or more additional surfaces (but open into oral cavity on the surface of its origin) (Fig. 48.12C).

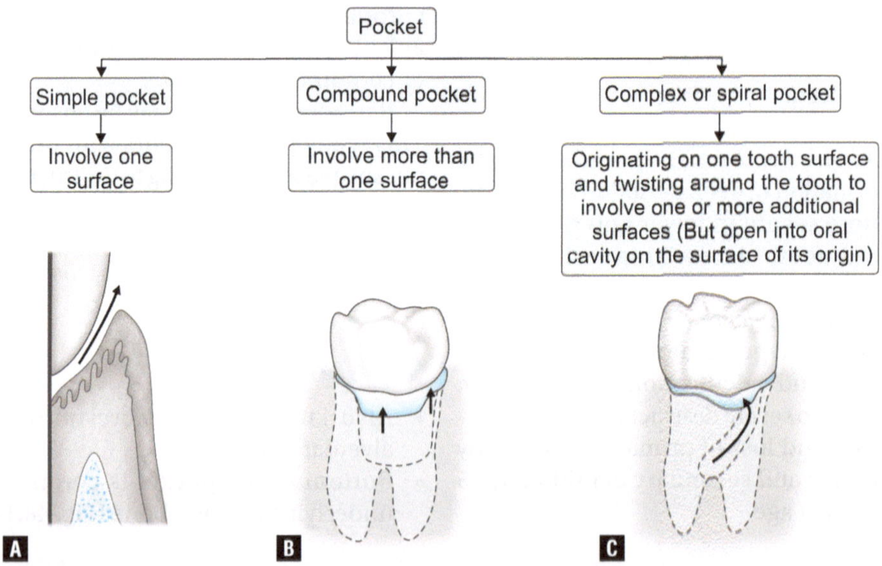

Figs 48.12A to C: Classification of periodontal pockets, (A) simple; (B) compound; and (C) complex

Signs

- A break in faciolingual continuity of the interdental gingiva
- Shiny, discolored, puffy gingival associated with exposed root surface
- Gingival bleeding
- Purulent exudates of the gingival margin or its appearance in response to digital pressure on the lateral aspect of the gingival margin
- Looseness, extrusion and migration of teeth
- Development of diastema where none had existed.

Symptoms

- Localized pain or sensation of pressure after eating, which gradually diminishes
- Foul taste in localized area
- Tendency to suck material from interproximal space
- Radiating pain "deep in bone"
- "Gnawing" or feeling of itching in the gum with relief from the resultant bleeding
- Complains that food "sticks between the teeth", the teeth feel loose
- Preference to eat from the other side
- *Sensitivity to hot and cold:* Toothache in the absence of caries.

DENTAL PLAQUE

Dental plaque is defined as a transparent, tenacious, invisible biofilm adhering to the tooth surface or other hard structures in the oral cavity, including removable and fixed restorations. This biofilm is firmly adherent to the surface it is attached to and cannot be seen by naked eye. Dental plaque is broadly classified as supragingival and subgingival based on its position on tooth surface.

- *Supragingival plaque*: It is found at or above the gingival margin. The supragingival plaque which is in direct contact with the gingival margin is called as marginal plaque
  - *Marginal plaque:* It plays an important role in the development of gingivitis. Though supragingival plaque and tooth-associated gingival plaque are primarily involved in formation of calculus, they do not take part in caries formation. Tissue-associated subgingival plaque is used in soft-tissue destruction characteristics of different forms of periodontitis.
- *Subgingival plaque:* It is found below the gingival margin, between tooth and the gingival sulcular tissue.

Composition

Dental plaque is composed primarily of 70% of microorganisms and 30% interbacterial substances, including extracellular polysaccharides and host cells.

Microorganisms: The types of microorganisms present have been seen to vary with the individual, the site examined and the age of the plaque. Supragingival plaque has been shown to go through the following stages after a thorough cleaning of the tooth surface.

- *Immediately after cleaning:* Within a short time, salivary pellicle is deposited on the teeth
- *After 3–8 hours:* There is colonization by Gram-positive cocci and small rods which include the following:
  - *Streptococcus sanguis:* A common plaque organism found in early plaque and causes bacterial endocarditis
  - *Streptococcus mutans:* When large amount of sucrose is present in diet, it is found in plaque. It produces sticky dextran and mutans and produces lactic acid from glucose or sucrose
  - *Streptococcus mitis* is very common in plaque
  - *Streptococcus salivarius* is found in saliva or dorsum of tongue
  - *Actinomyces viscosus* and *Actinomyces naeslundii* are two Gram-positive rods that are found in early plaque.

- *After 24 hours:* A clinically detachable layer of plaque is formed. Bacteria attached to salivary pellicle grow and form microcolonies. At the end of 24 hours, the flora becomes complex and Gram-negative anaerobic cocci can be detected
- *After 3 days:* Gram-negative cocci and rods assume greater prominence. The anaerobes increase in numbers and fusobacteria and filaments can be detected
- *After 7 days:* The final phase of plaque maturation is marked with continued decrease of Gram-positive cocci and rods. The complex flora contains spirochetes, fusiform bacilli and vibrios as well as large numbers of Gram-negative cocci, bacilli and filamentous organisms. Sublingual plaque usually develops from supragingival plaque deposits and the conditions in pocket influence the type of colonizing organism. The environment is anaerobic and nutrients are supplied from the crevicular fluid. Out of the total, 90% of culturable organisms are anaerobic including *Bacteroides melaninogenicus, Fusobacterium nucleatum, Actinomyces* and *Spirochaetes.*

Non-bacterial microorganisms in plaque include *Mycoplasma* species, yeasts, protozoa and viruses.

The microorganism exists within an intercellular matrix that also contains a few host cells such as epithelial cells, macrophages and leukocytes.

- *Intercellular matrix:* 20–30% of the plaque
- *Organic constituents:* Polysaccharides, proteins, glycoproteins and lipids
- *Inorganic constituents:* Calcium, phosphorous with trace amounts of sodium, potassium and fluoride.

The inorganic constituents of subgingival plaque are derived from crevicular fluid, which is a *serum transudate.*

Formation of plaque: Dental plaque may be readily visualized on teeth within 2 days with no oral hygiene measures.

Areas: Gingival third of tooth, cracks, pits and fissures on occlusal surface, over hanging restorations and around malaligned teeth.

Determining Factors

Oral hygiene, diet, salivary composition and flow rate modify plaque formation. Formation of dental pellicle on the tooth surface constitutes the initial phase of plaque formation. Pellicle is derived from food debris and oral microorganism. Pellicle on the hard surfaces provides a substrate on which bacteria progressively accumulate to form dental plaque.

Clinical Examination

Thin plaque may be translucent and, therefore, not visible.

Stained plaque may be acquired, e.g. tobacco stained.

Thick plaque tooth may appear dull and dirty.

For identification of plaque, disclosing agents are used which stains plaque or by running explorer around the tooth surface mesial to distal surface.

Plaque Control

Technique for plaque removal and prevention of new plaque formation is called plaque control.

This includes:

- Mechanical plaque control
  - Toothbrushing
  - Dental floss
  - Interdental brushes
  - Oral irrigation devices.
- Chemical plaque control
  - Mouthwashes
  - Toothpastes.

Methods of plaque control include:

- Toothbrushes
- Dentifrices
- Interdental cleaning aids
  - Dental floss

  - Tapered wooden toothpicks
  - Small conical or cylindrical brushes
  - Single-tufted brushes
  - Miniature bottle brush.
- Gingival massage
- *Oral irrigation devices:* These work by directing a high pressure, steady or pulsating stream of water through a nozzle to the tooth surface or gingival sulcus
- Chemical plaque control
  - Chlorhexidine
  - Essential oil mouthwash (Phenol mouthwash): Listerine
  - Other products
    - ◊ Stannous fluoride
    - ◊ Cetylpyridinium chloride
    - ◊ Sanguinarine.

Correction of Other Causes of Plaque Accumulation

Such treatments are usually the responsibility of the dentist, but it may be that a reason for plaque accumulation is discovered by the hygienist in the course of scaling. This should be brought to the attention of the dentist in a tactful way, without discussing the problem with the patient first. Some of these having already been mentioned include:

- Overhanging restorations
- Carious cavities
- Poor contours on crowns
- Poor contacts between teeth
- Poor gingival contour (after ANUG)
- High frenal insertions
- Crowding and malaligned teeth
- Poor prosthetic or orthodontic appliances
- Lip-apart posture.

It is worth making special mention of the problem of the lip-apart posture. One should be cautious of subjecting the patient to gadgets, such as oral screens, and such uncomfortable procedures as taping the lips together at night. The real remedy lies in regularly and effectively removing all plaque from the teeth.

Plaque Control Instructions

- *Motivation:*
  - Receptiveness is required to understand the concepts of the pathogenesis, treatment and prevention of periodontal disease
  - Behavioral changes are required to adjust one's beliefs, practices and values to accommodate the required new oral hygiene habits
  - Change of habits is required to adopt a successful, self-administered daily plaque control regimen.
- *Education:*
  - To tell the patients that self-administered plaque control currently is the most important preventive and therapeutic procedure in periodontal therapy.
- *Repeated instruction:*
  - Plaque if not removed gets mineralized and forms calculus.
- *Frequency of plaque removal:* Cleaning once a day with all necessary aids is sufficient if it is performed meticulously. If plaque control is not adequate, a second brushing will help. In most patients, average cleaning lasts for 2 minutes every day and removes only 40% of plaque. So, emphasis must be placed on the efficiency of complete plaque removal at least once daily rather than on the frequency of brushing alone.

DENTAL CALCULUS

Dental calculus is the calcified plaque, or tartar, which cannot be removed by brushing but with the help of a dental scaler during regular dentist visits. It is similar to concrete, and consists of millions of bacterial cells calcified together with calcium phosphate derived from the saliva.

Classification

They are of two types; supragingival calculus and subgingival calculus.

Supragingival Calculus

Location: On the clinical crown coronal to the margin of the gingival and visible in the oral cavity.

Distribution: Most frequent sites are on the lingual surfaces of the mandibular anterior teeth opposite Wharton's duct and on the buccal surfaces of the maxillary molars opposite Stenson's duct. Crowns of teeth out of occlusion—nonfunctional or teeth that are neglected during daily plaque removal. Surfaces of dentures and dental prosthesis (Fig. 48.13).

Subgingival Calculus

On the clinical crown apical to the margin of the gingival usually in periodontal pockets, not visible upon oral examination.

Extents to bottom of the pocket and follows contour of soft tissue attachment (Fig. 48.14).

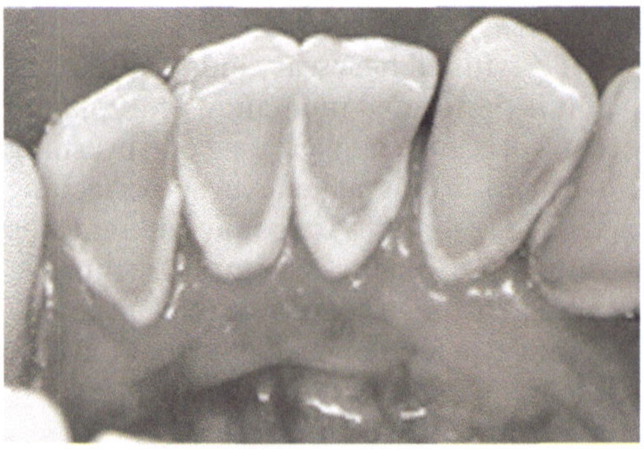

Fig. 48.13: Supragingival calculus
(For color version, see Plate 14)

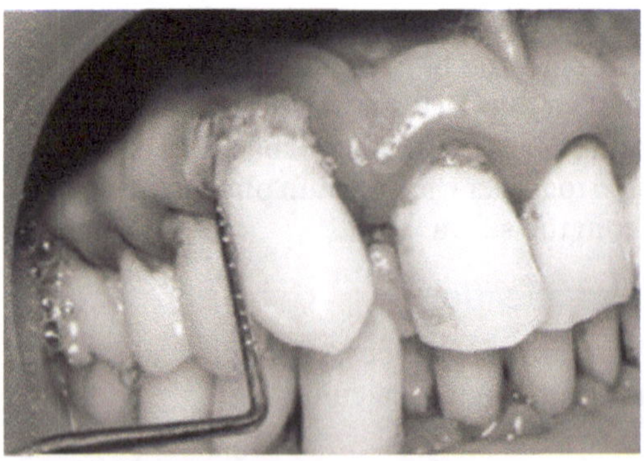

Fig. 48.14: Subgingival calculus
(For color version, see Plate 14)

Composition

Supragingival calculus consists of:

- Inorganic components:

Components	*Dry weight (in %)*
Inorganic	70–90
Calcium	27–29
Phosphorus	16–18
Carbonate	2–3
Sodium	1.5–2.5
Magnesium	0.6–0.8
Fluoride	0.003–0.04
Crystal forms	
Hydroxyapatite	58
Magnesium whitlockite	21
Octacalcium phosphate	12
Brushite	9

- Organic components:

Components	*Dry weight (in %)*
Mixture of protein-polysaccharide complexes, desquamated epithelial cells, leukocytes and various microorganisms	1.9–9.1
Carbohydrate (consists of glucose, galactose, rhamnose, mannose)	
Proteins	5.9–8.2
Lipids	0.2.

The four main crystal forms are:

1. Hydroxyapatite.
2. Magnesium whitlockite.
3. Octacalcium phosphate.
4. Brushite.

The composition of subgingival calculus is similar to that of supragingival calculus, except that it has:

- More magnesium whitlockite, less brushite and octacalcium phosphate
- Proteins present in supragingival calculus are salivary which are not present in subgingival calculus.

Attachment of calculus to tooth surface takes place by four ways:

1. Attachment by means of an organic pellicle.
2. Penetration of calculus bacteria into cementum.

3. Mechanical locking into surface irregularities.
4. Close apposition of calculus under surface depressions to the gently sloping mounds of the unaltered cementum surface.

Formation

Calculus is attached to dental plaque that has undergone mineralization. The plaque which is soft becomes harden due to precipitation of mineral salts between the 1st day and 14th day of plaque formation.

Saliva is the mineral source for supragingival calculus and gingival fluid for the subgingival calculus. Calcifications begin along the inner surface of the supragingival plaque and attached component of subgingival plaque adjacent to the tooth in separate foci, which increase in size and coalesce to form solid masses of calculus.

Rate of Formation

Calculus formation continues until it reaches a maximum after which it may be reduced in amount. The time required to reach the maximal level is 20 weeks.

Theories Regarding Mineralization

- Rise in the saturation levels of calcium and phosphate ions leads to precipitation of these minerals in the form of calculus
  - This can be caused due to rise in the pH of saliva
  - Colloidal proteins in saliva bind calcium and phosphate ions
  - Phosphate liberated from dental plaque desquamated epithelial cells and bacteria precipitate calcium phosphate by hydrolyzing organic phosphates in saliva.
- Seeding agent induce small foci of calcification that enlarge and coalesce to form a calcified mass.

Role of Microorganisms in the Mineralization

Mineralization of plaque starts extracellularly around the organisms. Filamentous organisms, diptheroids, and *Bacteroides* and *Veillonella* species have the ability to form intracellular apatite crystals.

Etiologic Significance

Calculus does not irritate the gingiva directly, but it provides a fixed nidus for the accumulation of plaque over it and holds plaque against gingiva.

Plaque initiates the gingival inflammation causing gingivitis. It leads to pocket formation. So, calculus in this way plays a significant role both for initiation and for progression of periodontal disease.

DENTAL STAINS

Dental stains are pigmented deposits on or in the tooth surface. Stains on the teeth can be either extrinsic or intrinsic.

- *Extrinsic:* Occurring on the external surface of the tooth, can usually be removed by prophylaxis
- *Intrinsic:* Stains which occur within the tooth substance and cannot be removed by normal prophylactic measures, e.g. hypoplastic enamel, tetracycline stain, fluorosis, dental caries, etc.

Attempts can be made to "bleach" intrinsic stain by the use of bleaching solution and exposure to the ultraviolet light. Alternatively and more commonly, the stained teeth are crowned or replaced in rare cases.

Extrinsic Stains

This is the province of the dental hygienist. This type of stain can be broadly divided into those of:

- Metallic origin
- Nonmetallic origin.

Metallic Stain

Various metals can stain the teeth either intrinsically or by extrinsically staining plaque. Contact with metals can come from:

- Occupational exposure among metal workers, etc.
- Drug therapy
- Metals used in dentistry.

Clinical Appearance

Metal	*Discoloration*
• Copper and brass	Green or bluish-green discoloration
• Nickel	Green
• Silver and gold	Black and pink
• Manganese	Black
• Mercury	Dirty green.

Etiology

Metal can be either inhaled and the dust directly deposited on the teeth, or alternatively, metallic dust or drug can be ingested and the stain deposited via saliva. In the former case, this is most common in metal workers, but as working condition in industry are now subject to stringent health regulations, this type of stain is now seen rarely.

Nonmetallic Stain

- *Green stain*
  - Etiology is by chromogenic bacteria staining plaque and chromogenic bacteria staining the remains of the primary cuticle.
- *Black stain*
  - Black or dark brown, continuous fine line of no appreciable thickness, follows the contour of the gingiva, about 1 mm away from soft tissue
  - More common in children and females
  - Etiology is not known, though some consider it stained remnants of primary enamel cuticle.

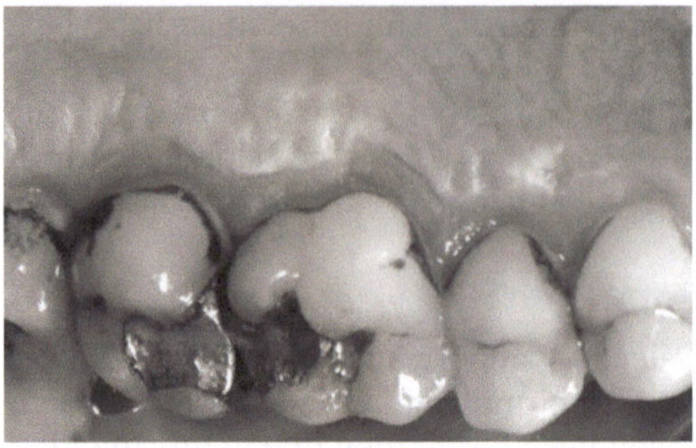

Fig. 48.15: Tobacco stains *(For color version, see Plate 14)*

- *Yellow stain*:
  - Dull yellowish discoloration of plaque by food pigments seen most commonly with poor oral hygiene.
- *Orange and red stain*:
  - Chromogenic bacteria staining plaque.
- *Tobacco stain*:
  - Light brown to black
  - Tar products from combustion of pipe, cigar and cigarettes can stain both plaque and calculus
  - Deposition varies with oral hygiene, and only to a lesser extent with tobacco consumption (Fig. 48.15).
- *Chlorhexidine stain*:
  - Brown to black stain occurs.

Intrinsic Stains

Blood-borne Pigmentations

Pigments from decomposed hemoglobin carried in the blood can be deposited in the teeth substance if the pulp is damaged in any way.

A wide range of colors include:

- Orange
- Brown
- Green
- Gray
- Black.

Drugs and metals used in dentistry are:

- Restorative materials
  - Copper amalgam: Bluish-green
  - Silver amalgam: Grey to black.

- Endodontic therapy
  - Silver nitrate: Bluish-black
  - Aureomycin: Yellowish
  - Certain chemicals in root canal sealers.

TRAUMA FROM OCCLUSION

Trauma from occlusion (TFO) can be defined as periodontal tissue injury caused by excessive occlusal forces, beyond the adaptive capacity of the periodontium. The occlusion that produces such injury is called traumatic occlusion. This traumatic occlusion may also cause painful spasms, injure the temporomandibular joint and produce excessive tooth wear.

Periodontal ligament and the alveolar bone require mechanical stimulus from occlusal forces in order to remain structurally sound. When occlusal forces are insufficient then periodontal tissues show atrophy but when occlusal forces exceed the physiologic limit, the injury is produced in periodontal tissues and is known as trauma from occlusion.

It must be understood that malocclusion does not necessarily produce trauma. On the other hand, anatomically and aesthetically acceptable dentition may produce injury to the periodontium.

The occlusion that produces periodontal injury is called traumatic occlusion or occlusal disharmony or functional imbalance or occlusal dystrophy. An increased occlusal force is not traumatic if the periodontal tissue can accommodate it.

Types

Trauma from occlusion may be of following types:

- *Acute trauma from occlusion:* A sudden change in occlusal forces caused by restorations or prosthetic appliances may alter the direction of occlusal forces on teeth. This causes tooth pain, increased mobility and sensitivity to percussion. If forces are removed by finishing restoration/appliance, then it may subside. Sometimes the tooth/teeth shift from the forces, causing self-correction of forces. Otherwise, periodontal abscess, necrosis or cemental tear may be produced. In few cases, symptom-free chronic condition may persist
- *Chronic trauma from occlusion:* It is more common than the acute one and is caused by gradual changes in the occlusion produced by tooth wear, drifting and extrusion of teeth combined with parafunctional habits such as bruxism and clenching. There is loosening of teeth, widening of periodontal ligament and angular defects in alveolar bone without pocket. In the initial phase of tooth mobility, there is alveolar bone resorption, reduction of periodontal ligament with increase in the width of periodontal ligament. In the second phase of tooth mobility, traumatic lesions heal with permanent widening of the periodontal ligament space along with adaptation to the increased forces
- *Primary trauma from occlusion:* In previously healthy periodontium, if there is alteration in the occlusal forces, it may cause primary trauma from occlusion. The alteration in the occlusal forces may be due to:
  - Insertion of a high filling
  - A prosthesis creating excessive force on abutment and antagonist teeth
  - The drifting of teeth or extrusion into the space of missing teeth
  - Orthodontic movement of teeth into functionally unacceptable positions.

  The forces do not initiate pocket formation because supragingival crestal fibers are not affected and so there is no apical migration of the junctional epithelium
- *Secondary trauma from occlusion*: When there is reduced capacity of the periodontium to withstand occlusal forces, then the previously well-tolerated occlusal force become traumatic. This type of tissue injury due to impairment of adaptive capacity of periodontium is known as secondary trauma from occlusion.

Clinical Features

Bone loss due to marginal inflammation reduces the periodontal attachment area resulting in increased burden on remaining tissue. Moreover, systemic disorders may inhibit anabolic activity or induce degenerative changes in the periodontium.

- *Changes produced by trauma from occlusion alone:* In the absence of local factors, i.e. plaque, calculus, etc. the trauma from occlusion may cause the following:
  - Widening of periodontal ligament
  - Angular defects in the alveolar bone without pocket formation
  - Loosening of teeth.
- *Other changes:* Based upon clinical impression rather than substantial evidence, the following clinical changes may be associated with trauma from occlusion:
  - Food impaction
  - Abnormal habits
  - Recession
  - Gingival bleeding, hyperplasia of gingiva
  - Cheek biting
  - Obscure facial pain
  - Pulpal hyperemia resulting in hypersensitivity to cold, pulpitis, pulp necrosis and pulp stone
  - Pericementitis
  - Limited excursion of mandible
  - Unlimited excursion of mandible
  - Blanching of gingiva on application of occlusal forces.

Box and Stillman considered trauma to be causative factor for the following signs of incipient periodontal diseases.

- *Traumatic crescent:* A crescent-shaped, bluish-red zone of gingiva confined to about one-sixth of the circumference of the root
- Congestion ischemia or hyperemia of the marginal gingival
- Recession of the gingiva, which may be asymmetrical, associated with resorption of the alveolar crest
- *McCall's festoon:* Discrete, semilunar enlargement of the marginal gingiva
- *Stillman's cleft:* Indentation in the gingival margin, generally on one side of the tooth. Two clefts frequently occur on the same tooth. Intermittent compression of the periodontal ligament followed by abnormal flushing of the gingival capillaries and enlargement and engorging of gingival vessels were considered to be responsible for clefting
- *Absence of stippling:* Interpreted as evidence of edema secondary to trauma
- Distended veins in the oral mucosa
- Sharply demarcated linear depressions in the alveolar mucosa, parallel to long axis of root and overlying the septal bone.

Pathological Migration of Teeth

Figure 48.16 shows clinical pathological migration of teeth, clinically.

Radiographic Signs

- Widening of the periodontal space often with thickening of the lamina dura along the lateral aspect of the root in the apical region and in bifurcation areas
- Vertical rather than horizontal destruction of interdental septum with formation of intrabony defects
- Root resorption
- Radiolucence and condensation of alveolar bone.

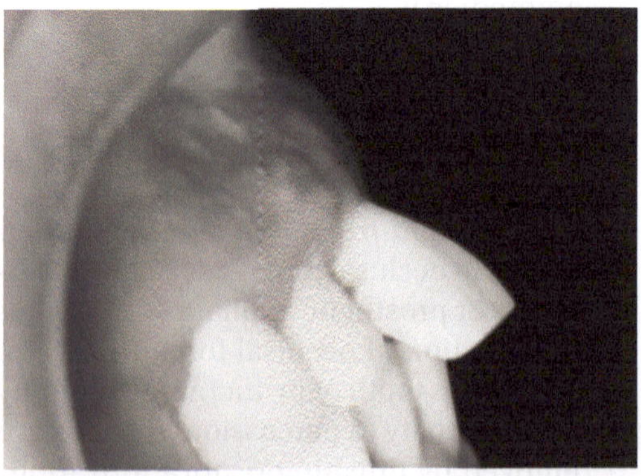

Fig. 48.16: Pathological migration of teeth due to trauma from occlusion

Physiological Adaptive Capacity of the Periodontium to Occlusal Forces

Periodontal tissue can adapt to increased occlusal forces by thickening and strengthening of the periodontal ligament and increase in the density of alveolar bone. When adaptive capacity is exceeded, destructive changes follow in the periodontal ligament, alveolar bone and in the tooth surface. The adaptive capacity varies in different persons and in the same person at different times. The effect of occlusal forces upon the periodontium is influenced by:

- Direction of occlusal forces
- Duration of occlusal forces
- Magnitude of occlusal forces
- Frequency of occlusal forces.

The principal fibers of periodontal ligament are so arranged that they can best accommodate occlusal forces directed in the long axis of the tooth. Constant pressure on the bone causes resorption, whereas intermittent force favors bone formation. Lateral or horizontal forces are accommodated by bone resorption in area of pressure and bone forming in area of tension. Torques or rotational forces cause both tension and pressure and usually injure the periodontium.

Effects of Insufficient Occlusal Forces

- Degeneration of periodontium
- Atrophy of periodontal fibers
- Osteoporosis of alveolar bone
- Reduction of bone height.

Hypofunction results from an open bite relationship, absence of junctional antagonists or unilateral chewing habits that neglect one side of the mouth.

Trauma from occlusion is a reversible change. There is repair once the offending forces are eliminated. Excessive forces should be corrected by the clinician. If this is not possible, then damage to the supporting tissues will continue. An increased occlusal force is not traumatic if the periodontium can accommodate it. A physiologic force may become traumatic if the adaptive capacity of the periodontal tissue is impaired.

Effects of Trauma from Occlusion on the Progression of the Marginal Periodontitis

The local irritants which initiate gingivitis and periodontal pockets affect the marginal gingiva, but trauma from occlusion occurs in the supporting tissues and does not affect the gingiva. Trauma from occlusion does not alter the inflammatory process but changes the tissue environment and the architecture of the area around the inflamed site. In the presence of inflammation, the change in the shape of the alveolar crest may be conducive to angular bone loss and infrabony pockets in some cases.

HALITOSIS

Halitosis or feter oris is defined as foul, offensive or bad breath. Bad breath is due to some physiological changes and some pathological causes. Pathologically, it may be due to local causes or systemic causes.

Physiologically, the change in breath is due to the following conditions:

- *Change with age:* In young children, odor is sweet and pleasant. As the age advances, it becomes disagreeable. This is due to local changes in mouth and also changes in metabolism
- *Changes during the day:* Usually, morning breath in all persons after getting from sleep is pungent and unpleasant. It is due to putrification of epithelial cells and food debris and saliva, which lay accumulated during sleep.

The odor is unpleasant due to pathological conditions; it may be local or systemic.

Local Causes

- *Retention of food around the teeth:* Food particles retained in cervical areas, interdental spaces, deep pockets and on the tongue may get decomposed by bacteria causing halitosis

- *Putrification of saliva:* Saliva due to stagnation and putrification by bacteria causes halitosis
- *Gingivitis and periodontitis:* Blood and pus formation due to bacterial action in these diseases produce halitosis
- *Dental caries:* Multiple caries are a common cause of halitosis. The food particles and saliva sustained in large cavities and the necrosed dentin and pulp cause halitosis
- *Coated tongue:* Accumulated food particle and desquamated epithelial cells on the rough surface of tongue cause halitosis. This is seen in gastrointestinal disturbances
- *Mouth breathing:* Unpleasant breath is due to reduced salivary flow, gingivitis of anterior teeth and change in bacterial flora
- *Dehydration:* Salivary secretion is reduced encouraging greater bacterial activity and causing foul breath
- *Artificial dentures:* Deposits of plaque, food and debris accumulate on denture surfaces. Putrification of food debris and stagnation of saliva deposits cause halitosis
- *Smokers' breath:* It is due to nicotine deposits in the mouth.

Systemic Causes

- *Halitosis from nasopharynx:* Chronic sinusitis, tonsillar infections, laryngitis, and pharyngitis are the common causes of halitosis
- *Aromatic food consumption:* For example, Onion, garlic; after absorption in the blood, the lungs exhale the aroma of the foodstuff
- Impaired digestion of fats
- *Metabolic diseases:* For example, diabetes causes typical foul breath of acetone. Leukemia results in ammoniacal odor
- *Lung disease:* Chronic bronchitis and lung gangrene produce foul odors. Pulmonary tuberculosis, empyema, and other infected conditions are associated with halitosis
- *Menstrual breath:* It appears with onset of periods.

Management

- Oral prophylaxis
- Restorations or extractions of carious teeth
- Periodontal surgery to eliminate pockets
- Proper brushing and mouthwash after meals. Mouth breathing can also be corrected by oral screens
- Dentures should be kept clean. They should not be worn at night
- Smoking should be reduced and stopped
- All pathological conditions should be treated
- Avoid aromatic food substances.

ORAL SEPSIS AND ITS EFFECTS ON GENERAL HEALTH

Theory of focal infection related to the ill effects of oral sepsis on the general health of an individual has been evaluated over the past few years. It is vital that dental professionals no longer view gingivitis simply as a precursor to periodontitis, but understand it as one of the underlying cause of oral inflammation and its potentially adverse impact on overall health. This theory of late has produced sufficient epidemiological and clinical evidence to prove its credentials.

Focus of infection was referred to a "circumscribed area of tissue, infected with exogenous pathogenic microorganisms, and usually located below the tooth in the surrounding gingival/periodontal membrane, mucous or cutaneous surface" of the oral cavity.

Mechanism of Focal Infection

Mechanism of focal infection causing periodontal disease has been illustrated in Figure 48.17.

Bacteria and soluble bacterial products can enter the bloodstream and can reach distance sites, e.g. the endothelium of blood vessels, where it can initiate a local inflammatory response and disease.

The two known mechanisms to explain the focal infection are:

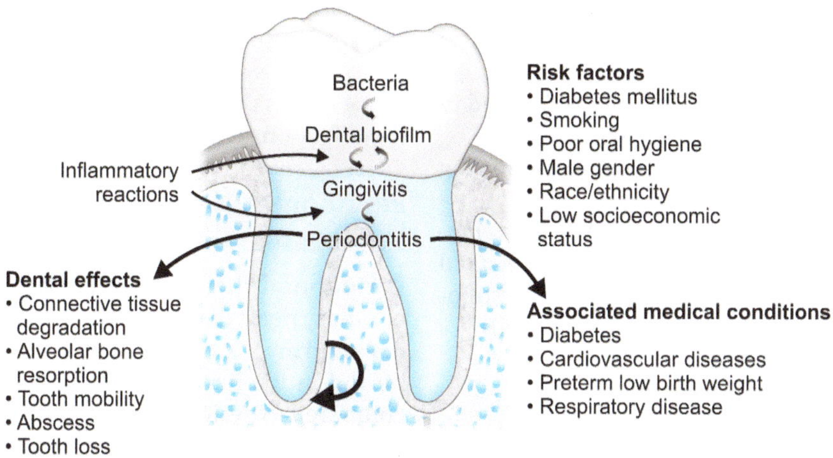

Fig. 48.17: Mechanism of focal infection originating from the tooth and periodontal diseases

- Hematogenous or lymphogenous metastasis of microorganisms from an infected focus to distant tissues
- Hematogenous or lymphogenous spread of toxins or other microorganism related products from an infected focus to distant tissues, causing hypersensitive reactions in the targeted tissues.

This localization and spread of microorganisms to distant body tissues is observed to be a function of environmental preference of the particular microorganism, rather than an inherent or developmental feature.

Oral Foci of Infection and its Spread

A variety of situations exist in the oral cavity, which are source of infection and which may set up distant metastasis. These include:

- Infected periapical lesions such as periapical granuloma, cyst and abscess
- Teeth with infected root canal
- Periodontal diseases with special reference to tooth extraction or manipulation.

Subgingival Environment as a Reservoir of Bacteria

The subgingival microbiota in patients with periodontitis provides a significant and persistent Gram-negative bacterial challenge to the host. These organisms and their products such as lipopolysaccharides have ready access to circulation through sulcular epithelium, which is ulcerated. Hence, bacteremia is common with mechanical trauma while eating, brushing, flossing, and scaling. This leads to an immunoinflammatory response by host producing variety of systemic disorders.

Significance of Oral Foci of Infection

There have been a vast number of reports based chiefly on clinical evidence to show that oral foci of infection either cause or aggravate many systemic conditions like:

Arthritis

Arthritis of the rheumatoid type is a disease of unknown etiology and the patient has a high antibody titer to a group of hemolytic streptococci. Because of the occurrence of streptococcal infection in the mouth, it may precede the initial or recurrent attacks.

Subacute Bacterial Endocarditis

Strong evidence has come in favor of oral infection, and its relation to subacute bacterial endocarditis (SABE) as:

- Similar bacterial microflora exists in the disease and oral cavity, dental pulp and in periapical lesions
- Disease symptoms have been observed in certain cases post tooth extraction
- Evidence of transient bacteremia following tooth extraction.

The causative organism of SABE is *Streptococcal viridans*. Numerous studies indicated that tooth extraction is often followed by streptococcal bacteremia that may cause SABE.

Gastrointestinal Diseases

These diseases have been periodically related to oral foci of infection. Gastric and duodenal ulcers have reportedly been produced experimentally by the injection of streptococci. But the low pH of the gastric secretion is an adequate defence against such infection.

Ocular Diseases

Ocular diseases have been attributed in the ophthalmologic literature to primary foci of infection such as those associated with the teeth, tonsils, sinuses, etc.

Skin Diseases

Skin diseases such as acne, tinea, eczema, scabies, urticaria, psoriasis, etc. may be related to oral foci or infection.

Renal Diseases

Streptococcus haemolyticus may be the causative organism but the chance of renal diseases due to oral foci of infection is very less.

Distant Spread of Odontogenic Infection

The spread of odontogenic infection through some potential space may lead to mediastinitis, mediastinal abscess, pleural effusion, empyema, pericarditis, cellulitis of face and Ludwig's angina.

Sometimes, a number of neurological complications may accompany odontogenic infections. These complications may be fatal. They include cavernous sinus thrombosis, brain abscess and meningitis. The mask area of the face is the dangerous area from which the infections can enter the brain.

Periodontal Disease and Coronary Heart Disease

Periodontal disease has been related to coronary heart disease (CHD) or atherosclerosis and myocardial infarction. Patients with periodontitis have 25% more risk for CHD compared to periodontally healthy individuals. Since CHD is a major cause of death, so it is important to identify this relationship amongst our patients in day-to-day practice. The level of oral hygiene is also associated with CHD. Patients with poor oral hygiene have two-fold increased risk for CHD.

Periodontal Disease and Diabetes Mellitus

The relationship between diabetes mellitus (DM) and periodontal disease has been extensively examined and found that DM increases risk of periodontitis. Periodontitis has been labeled as sixth complication of DM apart from retinopathy, nephropathy, neuropathy, etc. and control of periodontitis has beneficial effect on glycemic control of diabetic patient. Mechanical therapy with systemic antibiotics (Doxycycline) has been found to be effective in such cases.

Periodontal Disease and Pregnancy Outcome

Low birth weight infant (less than 2,500 g) and premature delivery (before 37 weeks) has been related to periodontitis in mother. Research has examined a relationship between preterm labor and maternal periodontal infection, which can be prevented by motivating potential mothers and pregnant women for good oral hygiene maintenance and carrying out prophylaxis at an early stage.

Periodontal Instrumentation and Oral Hygiene Aids

CHAPTER 49

INTRODUCTION

Periodontal instruments are designed for treating all types of gingival and periodontal diseases, such as scaling and root planing, curetting the gingiva or diseased tissue.

CLASSIFICATION OF PERIODONTAL INSTRUMENTS

Periodontal instruments are classified according to the purpose they serve.

- Periodontal probe
  - Functions
    - ◊ To locate the presence of periodontal pockets
    - ◊ To measure depth of periodontal pockets
    - ◊ To determine the course of pockets on individual teeth.
- Explorers
  - Functions
    - ◊ To locate presence of caries
    - ◊ To locate calculus deposits supragingivally/subgingivally.
- Scaling, root planing and curettage instruments
  - Functions
    - ◊ To remove calcified deposits on crown and root of teeth
    - ◊ To remove necrotic debris on tooth surface
    - ◊ To remove altered cementum from subgingival surfaces of root
    - ◊ Debridement of soft tissue lining the periodontal pockets.
  - *Hoe, chisel, file scalers:* Used to remove tenacious subgingival calculus
  - *Ultrasonic and sonic instruments:* Used for scaling and cleaning tooth surface and curetting soft tissue lining of pocket.
- Cleansing and polishing instruments
  Stainless steel instruments are commonly used. High carbon and tungsten carbide instruments are also available.

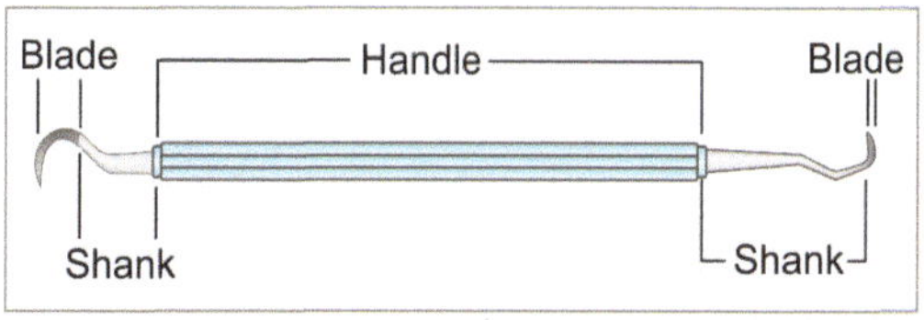

Fig. 49.1: Parts of a periodontal instrument

Each instrument can be divided into three parts (Fig. 49.1):

1. Working end blade or nib.
2. Shank.
3. Handle.

Periodontal Probes

These are tapered rod-like instruments calibrated in millimeters with a blunt, rounded tip. Shank is angled to allow easy insertion when measuring pocket depth.

Probe should be inserted with firm, gentle pressure to the bottom, aligning the shank parallel to long axis of tooth, e.g. William

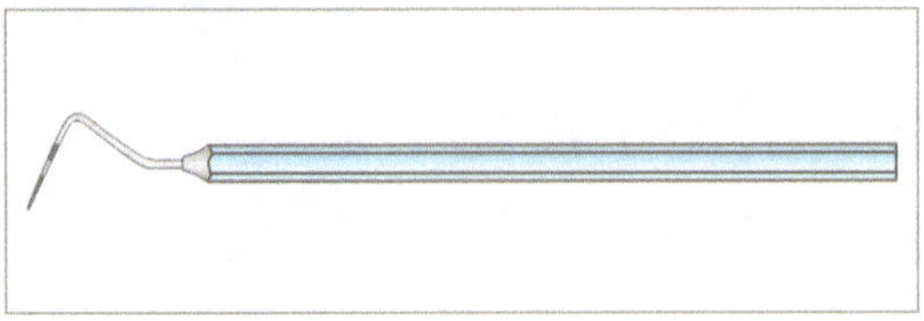

Fig. 49.2: Periodontal probe consists of handle, shank and calibrated working end

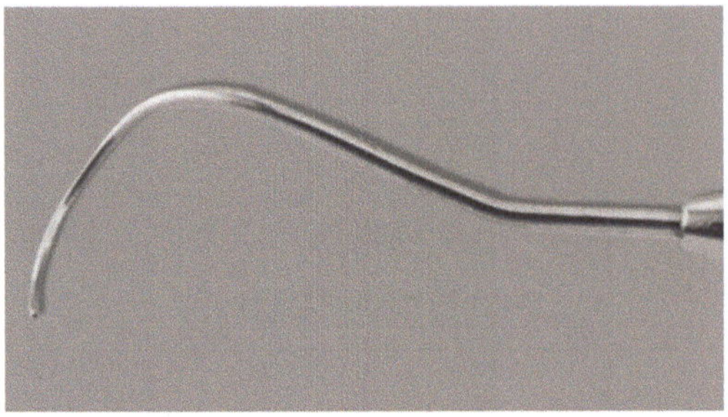

Fig. 49.3: Curved Naber's probe for detection of furcation areas

probe which has markings at 1,2,3,5,7,8,9,10 mm (Fig. 49.2) Color-coded probes are also available like World Health Organization (WHO) probe. Naber's probe is used to detect furcations (Fig. 49.3). New advancements in the field of probes have led to development of pressure-sensitive computerized electronic probes, e.g. Florida probe.

Sickle Scaler (Supragingival Scalers)

In these scalers, the working end is triangular in section with two straight cutting edges formed by the lateral surfaces and base of the triangle.

Sickle scalers may be straight or contra-angled (i.e. with a cranked shank so that they can be used on posterior teeth). This type of scaler is used primarily for the removal of supramarginal calculus.

Examples of sickle scalers are the commonly used Jacquette scalers which are usually in sets of three. The scaler is used with a pull stroke and is placed on the surface of the tooth below, i.e. apical to the calculus so that the surface joining the cutting edges makes an angle of something less than 90° with the root surface.

There are many variations of sickle-type scalers and all are used for supramarginal scaling or for slightly into the crevice.

Different sickle scalers available are U15/30, Ball, Indiana University. Sickles are available in large, medium and small size blades. Nevi 2 posterior are thin scalers to be inserted sub-lingually.

Curette

This is a very sharp fine-cutting instrument that has not been in the hygienist's armamentarium very long. It is often regarded as a surgical instrument and may be used for the removal of the unwanted necrotic surface of the inner wall of the periodontal pocket. The curette blade is basically shaped like a narrow spoon with the sides of the spoon forming two cutting edges. The bowl of the spoon curves longitudinally as well as from side to side; therefore, the cutting edge has a continuous rounded shape and there are no sharp curves. Curved blades and rounded toe allow better adaptation. The fine curettes are used for root planing and minute scaling. The instruments are usually paired with the appropriate corresponding blades for the mesial and distal surfaces of a tooth.

Both single- and double-ended curettes are available. There are two basic types of curette—universal and area specific (Table 49.1).

Modifications of Gracey Curettes

Gracey curettes are available in a rigid or a finishing type shank. Gracey 1516 and 1718 are modifications of 1112 and 1314 with more acutely angled shank and with 3 mm elongation, respectively.

Extended Shank Curettes

Hu-Friedy After Five* curettes are available with 3-mm-long terminal shank for extension into deeper pockets (Fig. 49.4).

Table 49.1: Comparison of area specific (Gracey) and universal curettes

Features	*Universal curette*	*Area-specific (Gracey curette)*
Area of use	One curette designed for all areas and surfaces	Set of many curettes for specific areas and surfaces
Cutting edge use	Both cutting edges used	One (outer) cutting edge used
Curvature	Curved in one plane	Curved in two planes up and to the side
Blade angle	No offset blade, beveled at 90° to shank, e.g. Barnhart curettes 12 and 56, Columbia curettes 1314, 2R2L, 4R4L	Offset blade, face beveled at 60°, e.g. Gracey #12 and 34: Anterior teeth, Gracey #56: Anterior and premolar teeth, Gracey # 78 and 910: Posterior teeth—buccal and lingual surfaces, Gracey #1112: Posterior mesial surface, Gracey 1914: Posterior distal surface

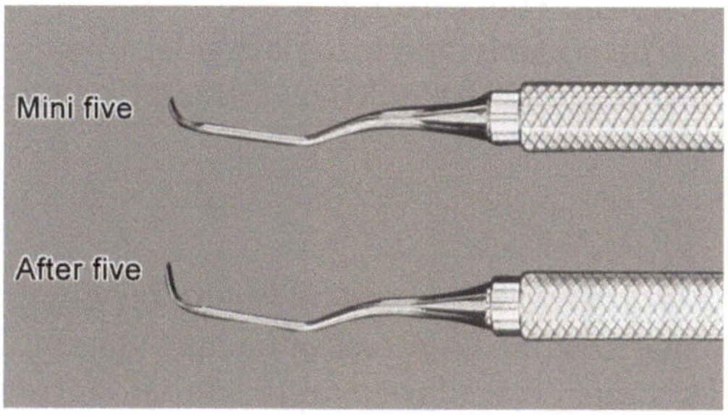

Fig. 49.4: Comparison of Mini Five® and After Five® curettes

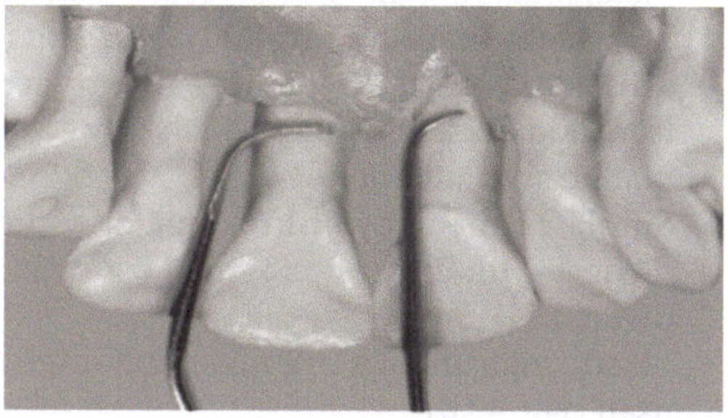

Fig. 49.5: Comparison between standard Gracey #56 (right) with a rigid Mini #56 (left) curettes

Mini-bladed Curettes

- This is also modification of the standard Gracey curette
- The working end is thinner. This has the advantage of easy access in narrow areas such as the furcation and the concavities on the roots
- The working length is half the length of the Gracey curette. This provides good access on the midline region on the anterior tooth roots. Also, it allows good access on the tight pockets, developmental grooves, etc.
- The lower shank is 3 mm longer than a standard Gracey curette
- As the working end is thinner, there are chances of instrument breakage due to inappropriate force while attempting to remove large pieces of calculus (Fig. 49.5).

Gracey Curettes

- This is also a modification of Gracey curette
- The working end is 50% shorter than a Gracey curette
- The curvature of the working end is more. It curves more upwards. This enables good adaptation on the root surfaces and curvatures
- The lower shank is longer. The shank is marked with bands at the 5 mm mark and the 10 mm mark. This marking provides the clinician an approximate depth of the working end within the periodontal pocket
- There are identification marks placed on the cutting end and the handles of these instruments. This makes it easier for the clinician to identify the cutting edge as well as the mesial or distal curettes
- This is a set of four curettes.

Langer and Mini-Langer Curettes

- This design is a combination of a standard Gracey curette and a universal curette
- The shank design is similar to a Gracey curette, but the blade is designed 90° like that of universal curette
- This makes it a much more versatile instrument
- It is available as an extended shank (After Five®) or mini blade (Mini Five®) designs.

Plastic Instruments for Implants

- Metallic instruments are not recommended for use on titanium implant abutments. This is because it may remove the surface layer and cause scratches which may favor plaque accumulation
- Similarly, the use of ultrasonic or sonic devices with metal tips is also contraindicated
- Plastic instruments are most commonly used (Fig. 49.6)
- Instrumentation is usually done only around the supragingival region
- The working ends of these plastic instruments are basically of four designs:
    1. Wrench-shaped.
    2. Crescent-shaped.
    3. Hoe-like.
    4. Working ends similar to metal periodontal instruments such as a sickle, probe or curette.

Hoe Scalers

- Single or double-ended instrument with a thin blade
- The blade is designed at a 99° angulation which ends in a flat terminal surface
- The junction of this flattened terminal surface and the inner aspect of the blade forms the cutting edge which is beveled at 45°
- The blade has a gradual curvature providing the required 2-point contact on the tooth during scaling
- The outer surface of the blade is convex
- The hoe scaler is of two types: Mesial/distal hoe and buccal/lingual hoe
- This scaler is used to remove gross amounts of supragingival calculus and some subgingival calculus.

File Scalers

Files scalers have series of blades on a base. Their function is to crush or fracture tenacious calculus. Nowadays, curettes are preferred since files tend to gouge and roughen root surface (Fig. 49.7A).

Chisel Scalers

Chisel scalers are designed for proximal surfaces of closely placed teeth usually in anterior part of mouth where other scalers cannot be used. They are double-ended instruments with straight shank at one end and curved at another (Fig. 49.7B).

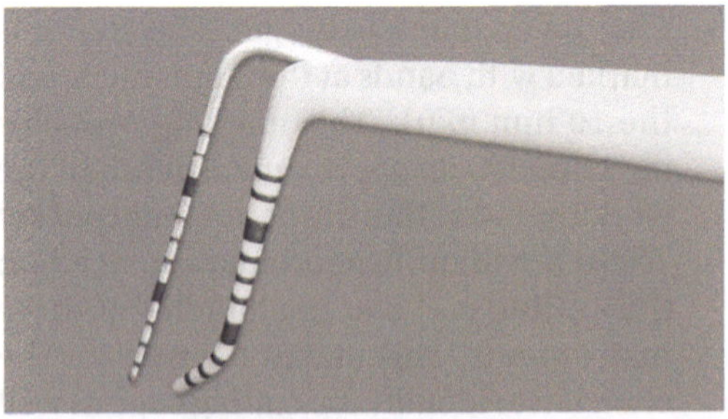

Fig. 49.6: Plastic probes

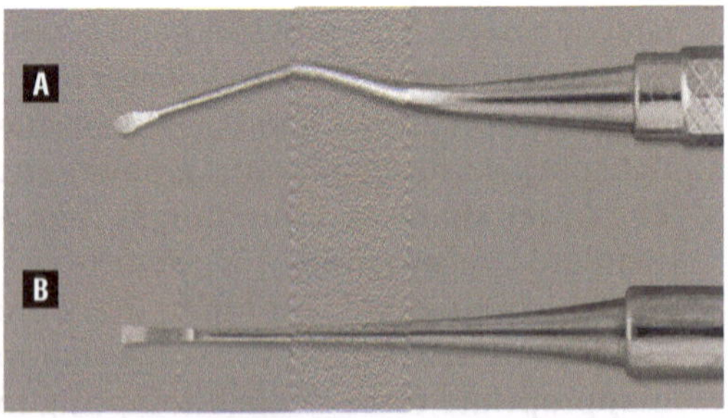

Figs 49.7A and B: (A) File scaler and (B) Chisel scaler

Sonic Scalers

Handpieces designed for high and low speed use compressed air and water delivered through hose. Sonic handpiece uses a variety of specially designed tips that vibrate in the elliptical pattern at a frequency of about 2,500–6,000 cycles per second. This is well-suited to remove soft deposits.

Ultrasonic Scalers

The ultrasonic scaler has gained a very large acceptance as a useful tool since its first introduction about 20 years ago. The earliest unit developed for scaling was the Cavitron 30 and this has over the years been succeeded by improved versions until we reach the unit in common use today (Fig. 49.8). The unit basically converts the usual mains electricity current to a frequency of about 25,000 Hz. This is converted at the handpiece from electromagnetic to mechanical vibrations of the same frequency and these vibrations are transmitted to the working tip of the instrument, which has a movement range (amplitude) of 0.001 in 1/1000.

A great deal of heat is evolved in the energy conversion and a water spray is incorporated in the handpiece both for its cooling effect and for its role in the "cavitational" effect which takes place, i.e. the fluid under the 25,000 times per second vibrational effect "cold boils" and is vaporized into an accelerated spray which plays a great part in the cleansing effect.

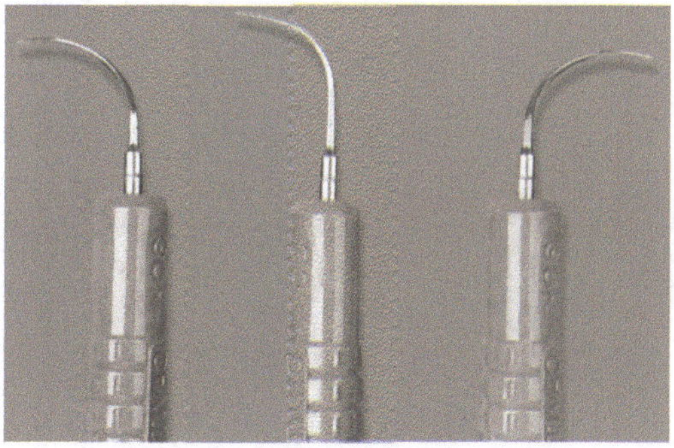

Fig. 49.8: Cavitron ultrasonic tips

There are now many types of ultrasonic scaler, and the inserts vary considerably. Most present day ultrasonic units are self-tuning, i.e. they automatically adjust the frequency for each insert used depending on its size and weight. The amount of amplitude of the scaler tips is regulated by the "power" control. The smallest power setting consistent with a good result for each patient should be selected.

It has been found that usually the ultrasonic scaling is about 20–25% quicker than manual scaling. However, it is not a replacement to hand scaling and this must follow the initial ultrasonic treatment.

Types

These are of two types; magnetostrictive and piezoelectric.

1. *Magnetostrictive:* It consists of a 16-coil special handpiece which magnetically changes dimension of a metal stack when electrical energy is applied, creating elliptical movement of the tip. The frequency range of the tip is about 25,000–30,000 cycles per second. All the sides of the tips are active and will work when adapted to the tooth. Significant generation of heat necessitates water spray for cooling to dissipate the heat generated.
2. *Piezoelectric:* In these systems, electric energy is applied to a crystal which emits vibrations in a linear pattern at frequency of about 25,000–40,000 cycles per second. In piezoelectric units, only the two sides of the tip are active and will work when adapted to the tooth, since the motion of the tip is linear. There is minimal heat generation and water is for lavage only.

Advantages

- Patients on the whole prefer the ultrasonic scaling
- Heavy supragingival deposits and heavy stains are easily removed, and calculus and debris are flushed away from the area and

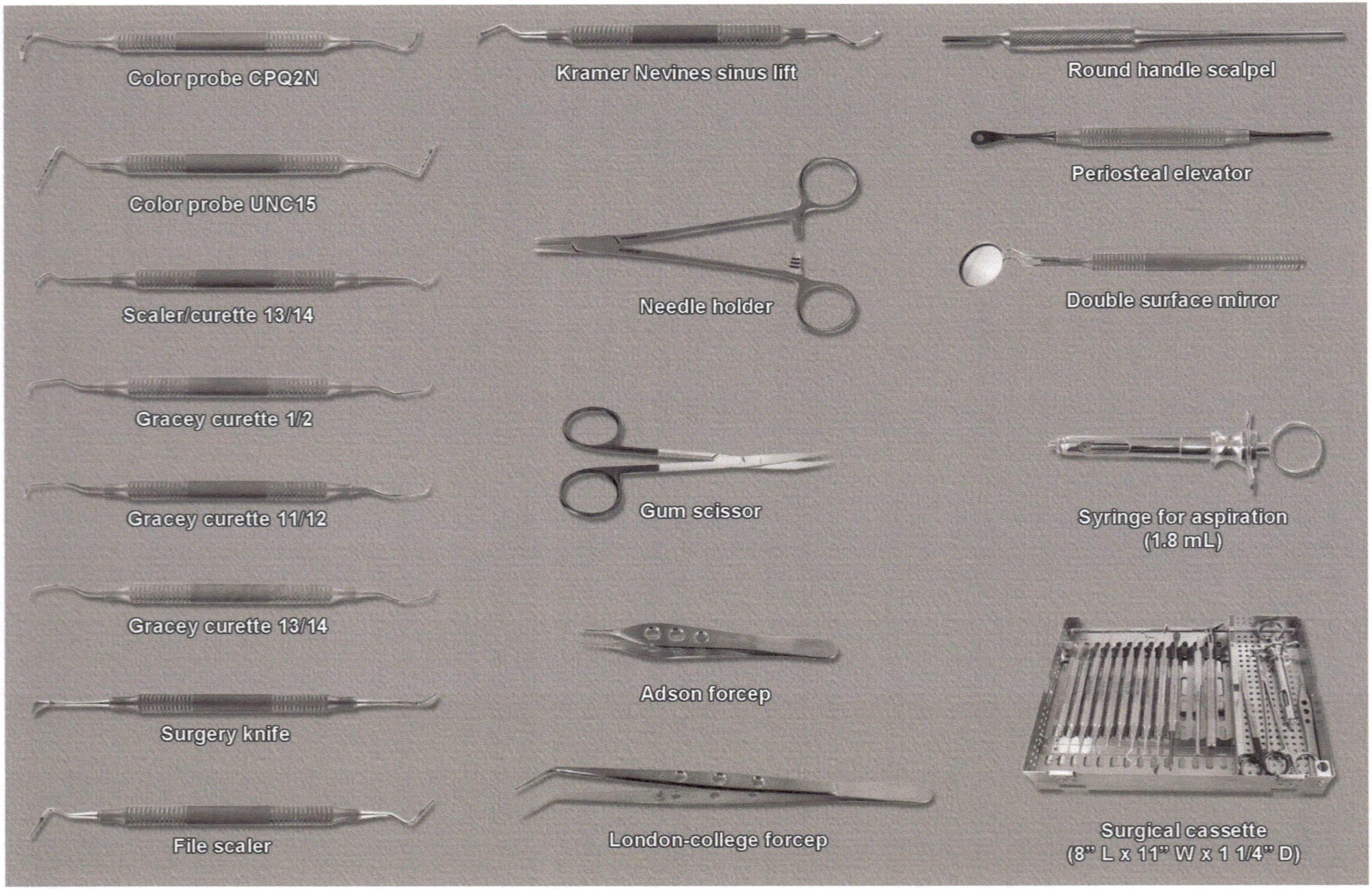

Fig. 49.9: Periodontal surgical kit (Color probe CPQ2N, Color probe UNC15, Scaler/curette 13/14, Gracey curette 1/2, Gracey curette 1/12, Gracey curette 13/14, Surgery knife, File scaler, Kramer Nevines sinus lift, Needle holder, Gum scissor, Adson forcep, London-college forcep, Round handle scalpel, Periosteal elevator, Double surface mirror, Syringe for aspiration, Surgical casette)

from the gingival crevice and pocket. It is, thus, much easier to clean up the really "dirty" mouth
- There is less fatigue for the operator.

Disadvantages

- False sense of security, depending on a gadget rather than on one's own critical judgment
- Certain loss of fine tactile sense
- Danger of spreading infection through aerosol effect
- Sometimes difficult to control large water flow
- Servicing of unit can be a problem.

Suprasson P-Max provides both non-autoclavable and autoclavable handpieces and various instrument tips, which apart from scaling, can do the functions of root planing, amalgam plugging, prosthesis loosening, root canal preparation and gutta-percha condensation. It can also work with an antiseptic irrigating solution.

PERIODONTAL SURGICAL KIT

Instruments used for periodontal surgeries are illustrated in Figure 49.9.

GENERAL PRINCIPLES OF INSTRUMENTATION

Effective instrumentation is governed by a number of general principles that are mutual to all instruments:

Accessibility (Positioning of Patient and Operator)

The patient should be in supine position and placed so that the mouth is close to resting elbow of clinician. The clinician should be comfortably seated with flat flap on the floor and thighs parallel to floor. For maxillary arch, the patient should be asked to raise the chair and for mandibular arch, to lower it for proper visibility.

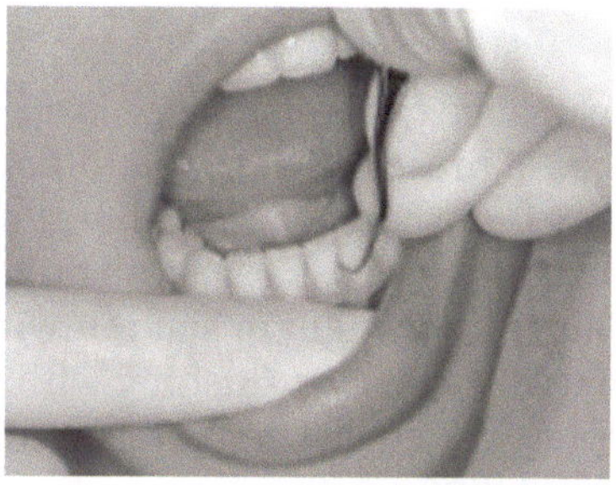

Fig. 49.10: Retracting lips with index finger of nonoperating hand

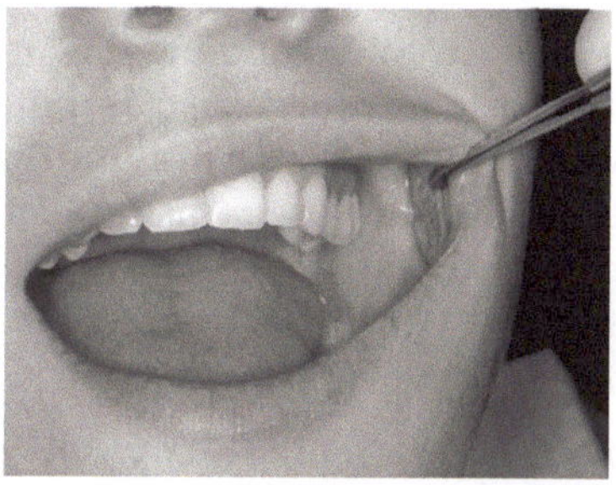

Fig. 49.11: Retracting cheek with mirror

Visibility, Illumination and Retraction

Whenever possible, direct vision with direct illumination from dental light is most desirable. If this is not possible then indirect vision may be obtained with the help of a mouth mirror. Retraction can be carried out with the help of:

- Use mirror to deflect cheek and fingers of nonoperating hand to deflect lips
- Use mirror to retract tongue and cheek (Fig. 49.10)
- Use mirror alone or fingers of nonoperating hand for cheek and lip (Fig. 49.11)
- Combinations of preceding methods.

While retracting, avoid irritating the angles of mouth and use petroleum jelly for cracking lips before any procedure.

Condition of Instruments (Sharpness)

The instruments before use should be checked for sharpness as it enhances tactile sensation for more precision. Also, instruments should be sterile and clean.

Maintaining a Clean Field

Instrumentation can be hampered in operative field by the presence of saliva, blood and debris as it obscures visibility and makes tooth surfaces slippery to establish firm finger rest. Therefore, adequate suction with the help of a saliva ejector, flushing with water and wiping with square gauze is essential for proper visibility.

Instrument Handling

Stability of instrument and hand is primary requisite for controlled instrumentation. The two major methods in handling the periodontal instruments are instrument grasp and finger rest.

Instrument Grasp

A proper grasp is essential for precise control of movements made during periodontal instrumentation. Standard pen grasp has been shown in Figure 49.12.

Modified pen grasp is most stable and effective for periodontal instruments and provides greatest control. The thumb, index finger and middle finger are used to hold instruments as a pen, but the middle finger is positioned so that the side of the pad next to the finger nail is resting on the instrument shank (Fig. 49.13). The index finger is bent at second joint and positioned well above the middle finger on same side of handle.

This leads to the formation of a triangle of forces, or tripod effect that increases control as it counteracts the tendency of the instrument to turn uncontrollably between fingers when scaling force is applied. This increases the tactile sensitivity. Other grasps used are palm and thumb grasp during sharpening and manipulation of air and water syringes (Fig. 49.14).

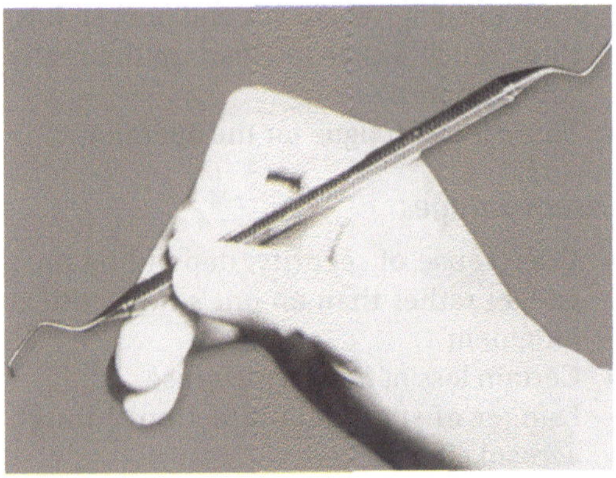

Fig. 49.12: Standard pen grasp. The side of the middle finger rests on the shank

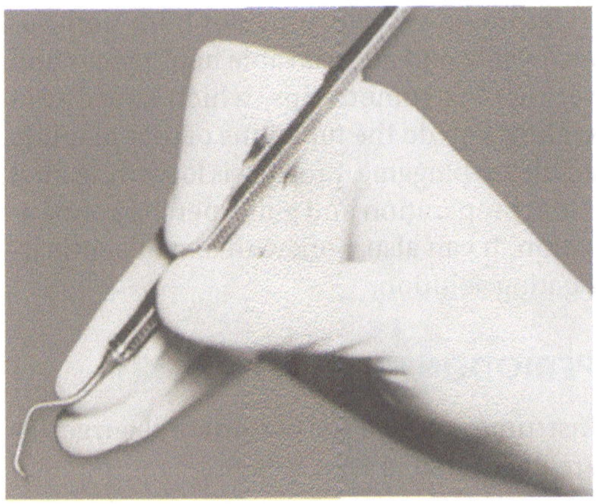

Fig. 49.13: Modified pen grasp. The pad of the middle finger rests on the shank

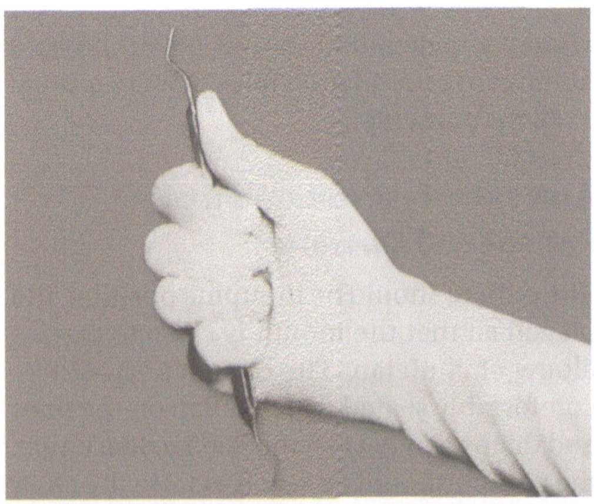

Fig. 49.14: Palm and thumb grasp used to stabilize instruments during sharpening

Finger Rest

It aids to stabilize the hand and the instrument by providing a firm fulcrum as the movements are made to activate the instrument. The fourth (ring) finger is preferred for finger rest though third (middle) can also be used but it restricts the arc of movement. Maximal control is achieved by keeping middle finger between the ring finger and shank of instrument. This built up fulcrum plays an important role in wrist forearm action which further activates powerful working strokes for calculus removal. These two fingers should be kept as one unit fulcrum during scaling and root planing, whenever possible. Finger rests may be classified as intraoral and extraoral.

Variations in intraoral finger rests are:

- *Conventional:* The finger rest is established on tooth surfaces immediately adjacent to working area
- *Cross arch:* The finger rest is established on tooth surface on other side of same arch
- *Opposite arch:* The finger rest is established on tooth surfaces on the opposite arch
- *Finger on finger:* The finger rest is established on the index finger or thumb of the nonoperating hand.

Extraoral fulcrums are essential for effective instrumentation of some aspects of the maxillary posterior teeth.

The two most commonly used intraoral rests are as follows:

- *Palm up:* Backs of the middle and fourth fingers are rested on the skin overlying the lateral aspect of the mandibles on the right side of face
- *Palm down*: Front surfaces of the middle and fourth fingers are rested on the skin overlying lateral aspect of mandible on the left side of face.

Intraoral finger rests and extraoral fulcrums reinforcement: Index finger or thumb of the nonoperating hand is applied to the handle or shank of the instrument for added control and pressure against the tooth.

Instrument Adaptation

Adaptation

Adaptation refers to the manner in which the working end of a periodontal instrument is placed against the surface of a tooth. Its objective is to make working end of instrument conform to the contour of the tooth.

Angulation

Angulation refers to the angle between the face of a bladed instrument and the tooth surface. Appropriate angulation is required for removal of calculus. During scaling and root planing, correct angulation is between 45° and 90°. For gingival curettage, angulation greater than 90° is established to engage and remove pocket lining.

Lateral Pressure

Lateral pressure refers to the pressure created when force is applied against surface of a tooth with cutting edge of a bladed instrument. Lateral pressure may be firm, moderate or light.

Strokes

The basic strokes used during instrumentation are:

- The exploratory stroke is light, "feeling" stroke that is used with probes and explorers
- The scaling stroke is a short, powerful pull stroke used with bladed instruments for removal of supra- and subgingival calculus
- The root planing stroke is a moderate to light pull stroke that is used for final smoothing and planing of root surface.

Principles of Use

1. Determine the correct cutting edge.
2. Make sure that lower shanks are parallel to the surface to be instrumented.
3. When using intraoral finger rests, keep fourth and middle fingers together in a built up fulcrum for maximum control and wrist-arm action.
4. Use extraoral fulcrums or mandibular finger rests for optimal angulation when working on maxillary posterior teeth.

5. Concentrate on using lower third of the cutting edge for calculus removal, especially on line angles.
6. Allow the wrist and forearm to carry the burden of the strokes rather than flexing the finger.
7. Roll the handle slightly between thumb and fingers to keep the blade adapted.
8. Modulate lateral pressure from firm to moderate to light depending upon the nature of calculus.

Root planing (smoothening the cemental surface) can be performed with sharp curettes. At the same time, fine calculus is removed.

In use, the correct curette (of a set) is chosen so that one working edge lies against the root surface to be planned (or against the epithelium of the pocket wall). The instrument is placed in this way below the calculus or at the bottom of the crevice with the blade making something less than 90° with the root surface. It is used with a pull stroke in a vertical (but sometimes in a horizontal or diagonal) direction.

PRINCIPLES OF SHARPENING

1. Choose a stone suitable for the instrument to be sharpened, one that is of an appropriate shape and abrasiveness.
2. Use a sterilized sharpening stone if the instrument to be sharpened will not be resterilized before it is used on a patient.
3. Establish the proper angle between the sharpening stone and the surface of the instrument on the basis of an understanding of its design.
4. Maintain a stable, firm grasp of both the instrument and the sharpening stone. This ensures that the proper angulation is maintained throughout the controlled sharpening stroke. In this manner, the entire surface of the instrument can be reduced evenly, and the cutting edge will not be improperly beveled.
5. Avoid excessive pressure as it will quicken the speed of the stone to grind the surface of the instrument and may soften the instrument's life unnecessarily.
6. Avoid the formation of a "wire edge" with minute filamentous projections of metal extending as a roughened ledge from the sharpening cutting edge. When the instrument is used on root surfaces, these projections will produce a grooved rather than a smooth surface. A wire edge occurs when the direction of the sharpening stroke is away from, rather than into or toward, the cutting edge. When back and forth or up and down sharpening strokes are used, formation of a wire edge can be avoided by finishing with a down stroke toward the cutting edge.
7. Lubricate the stone during sharpening. This minimizes clogging of the abrasive surface of the sharpening stone with metal particles removed from the instrument. It also reduces heat produced by friction. Use oil for natural stones and water for synthetic stones.
8. Sharpen instruments at the first sign of dullness. A grossly dull instrument is very insufficient and requires more pressure when used, which hinders control. Furthermore, sharpening such an instrument requires the removal of a great deal of metal to produce a sharp cutting edge. This shortens the effective life of the instrument.

TOOTH POLISHING

Tooth polishing is the act of smoothing the tooth surface so as to prevent the accumulation of plaque on the tooth surface area. The most commonly used instrument is prophy cup, a small motorized rubber cup, which is used along with an abrasive polishing compound.

Rubber Cup

Rubber cups are used with polishing paste or prophylactic paste. These pastes usually contain fluoride as an anti-cavity agent. Rubber cups should never be used over the cementum area as it may lead to cemental erosion.

Bristle Brush

These should be used with caution only in the crown areas covered by enamel, as they might injure cementum and gingival tissues. They are used in conjugation with the prophylaxis pastes.

Dental Tape

Indicated for polishing the proximal surfaces and inaccessible areas where other polishing instruments are hard to reach. It is used in conjugation with polishing paste. Care should be taken to avoid injury to the gingiva.

Air-powder Polishing

This system delivers an air-powder slurry of warm water and sodium bicarbonate for polishing. It is very effective for the removal of external stains and soft deposits on the tooth surface. It should not be used in patients with respiratory illness, hypertension and hemodialysis.

One of the most important aspects of prevention is the provision of smooth well-polished surfaces which become plaque coated and stain less easily than rough or unpolished surfaces. The polishing is also necessary to remove any stains left after scaling.

Some Basic Principles to be used for Polishing of Teeth

It is almost always necessary to use techniques and materials which avoid the production of heat. Both tooth substance and restorative materials will be adversely affected by overheating. Therefore, where possible, slow speeds should be used and the composition of rubber wheels, pastes, etc. should be checked to confirm that there are no ingredients which may be harmful to tooth surface or to filling materials (e.g. amalgams may be seriously affected by sulfur, which is contained in some rubber polishing discs).

Harsh polishing pastes such as pumice should not, in normal circumstances, be used on enamel surfaces, unless the severe scratching, whose results may be somewhat desirable as in etching techniques used in the currently developing methods of incisal tip rebuilding with materials such as Novafil, or in fissure sealing.

POLISHING METHODS

Natural Tooth Surfaces

Since well-polished smooth enamel surfaces retain plaque less well than rough surfaces, it is necessary to polish all tooth surfaces after the removal of plaque and calculus which has been carried out as a routine prophylaxis or as a part of a periodontal treatment. Many of the commercially available prophylaxis and polishing pastes are too abrasive, even flour of pumice will remove the more acid-resistant surface layer or scratch. It has been shown that more enamel abrasion may result from dentists' polishing than from toothbrush and dentifrice usage. This would support those patients who complained, "My teeth seem to get dirtier much quicker since I had them cleaned by the dentist." It is also some sort of basis for another belief that scaling and polishing "takes the enamel off". Of course, all these complaints were and still are hotly denied as "old wives tales" but occasionally there is an element of truth, perhaps wrongly interpreted, in these beliefs.

For safety, therefore, one hesitates to use the conventional pumice containing polishing pastes. Additionally, motor driven polishing brushes should rarely be used on enamel, the finishing polish being carried out with small webbed cups (of the crescent type) held in a special angle polishing head or an old contra-angle handpiece kept solely for this purpose.

Therefore, "safe" polishing materials such as zirconium silicate (e.g. Zircate), tin oxide or even zinc oxide should be used. In the case of a scaling procedure which is prolonged over three or four visits, and where, say, a quadrant is completed at each visit, neglect of polishing at the termination of each visit will allow plaque to accumulate as early as before. In addition, the feel of well-polished teeth gives the patient a greater incentive to carry out home care procedures in order to keep the present smooth, clean feeling for as long as possible.

Procedure for Polishing the Teeth

The procedure for polishing the teeth, therefore, follows a pattern:

1. Very careful scaling, and if an ultrasonic unit is used, much stain may be removed by judicious use of the tip. It should be remembered that deeply pitted stains are unlikely to be removed by a mechanical polishing method such as the motor-driven brush and paste without reducing the surface of the surrounding enamel markedly where possible. The proximal surfaces of the teeth and gingivae to the contact points are polished with strips.
2. A disclosing solution is then applied to the teeth to be polished and the patient asked to rinse this away after a few seconds. Any obvious gross stains may be removed by hand instrumentation. The teeth are then polished by using a rubber cup loaded with zirconium silicate paste (or powder, made up to a paste with water) running at a fairly low speed. All surfaces are polished and the edges of the cup introduced into the embrasures to polish the proximal surfaces as well as possible. The occlusal surfaces should not be forgotten.
3. A final polish (e.g. at termination of treatment in the adult) should include the use of a fluoride containing polishing paste (such as zirconium silicate treatment paste). A disclosing solution is again used and any residual stains are repolished. The patient is asked to see the result of using a disclosing solution on clean teeth and then to run his tongue over the surface. "This is your target from now on", he is told.

ORAL HYGIENE AIDS

The aim of oral hygiene, as carried out by the individual, is to remove all particles of food from the mouth after eating and drinking. In addition, the action of toothbrushing gives tone to the gums and keeps them firm and healthy.

Since bacteria can begin to act on food particles within 2 minutes of eating, for any oral hygiene practice to be effective, it must be undertaken at once. As a minimum precaution, the teeth should be brushed after breakfast, after lunch and most important of all, after the last food or drink at night.

Toothbrush and Toothbrushing

There is multitude of different shapes, textures, sizes and patterns of toothbrushes available in market. Dentists recommended most of these brushes, according to each buyer. There are brushes available with long head, short head, and all grades of hardness of natural bristle and similarly with plastic fibers. Some brushes seem to be quite inappropriate for tooth cleaning; others would appear to be not only ineffective but also harmful, though all these have claims to dentists' recommendation.

- Toothbrush design and construction has changed over the years, but, in spite of this, many dentists have remained faithful on their original concepts
- Our attitude to cleaning has changed. We consider attention to plaque and gingivae more important than removal of food debris, and enamel polishing or "whitening".

Many dentists still believe and staunchly defend their long-held view that nylon bristle is harmful and that the use of natural bristle is essential.

When nylon-bristled brushes were developed initially, the manufacturers, of course, followed the same hardness formula as was apparently desired by the masses. But man-made fiber was much less moisture absorbent and therefore when wetted as usual by the user, it did not soften but remained hard or extra hard. The gingivae (and even enamel) were often damaged and at that time nylon bristles acquired some disrepute.

Eventually, fine gauge plastic filaments like Tynex® were introduced and these are superior to natural bristles for the following reasons:

- Plastic bristles can be quality and size controlled to very fine limits
- The plastic bristles are potentially cleaner than natural bristles, as they do not absorb fluids and organisms as readily as natural bristles
- Natural bristles take longer to dry than the plastic. Thus, if a dry brush is required, a twice daily brushing need at least two brushes.

Faulty Brushing

- Most people wet the brush under a running cold tap before loading with dentifrice
- Brushing goes on until the toothpaste has foamed so much in the mouth that it then becomes necessary to spit and rinse. At this point, however, much or little has been achieved in brushing around all the teeth, most people do not continue brushing after this initial rinsing of the mouth. Few reload the brush and start again. The effect of the initial and/or continuous brush wetting action is to make natural bristles soft and soggy. For this reason, the majority of toothbrushes sold in this country were of the 'hard' or 'extra hard' type
- If the patient's gums bleed when brushing, the one should find out if the reason is gingivitis associated with plaque (as it usually is) then careful training in brushing is necessary with the appropriate brush and the patient told to brush in spite of the bleeding.

Choice of Toothbrush

The bristled toothbrush appeared in the year 1600 in China was first patented in America in 1857. They are available in various sizes, shapes, hardness and arrangement of bristles (Fig. 49.15). The American Dental Association has described the range of dimensions of acceptable brushes. Brushing surface 1-1.25 inches long (25.4–31.8 mm), 5/16 to 3/8 inch (7.9-9.5 mm) wide, with 2-4 rows of bristles and 5-12 tufts per row.

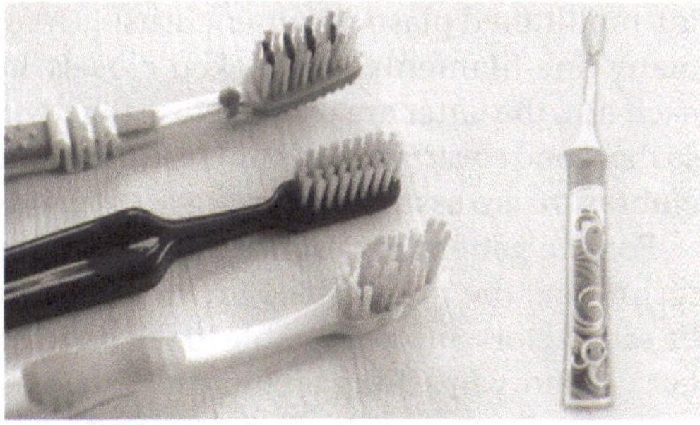

Fig. 49.15: Different types of toothbrushes

Bristle hardness is directly proportional to square of diameter and inversely proportional to square of length diameters of commonly used bristles range from 0.007 inch (0.2 mm) for soft brushes to 0.012 inch (0.3 mm) for medium and 0.014 inch (0.4 mm) for hard brushes. For most patients, short-headed brushes with straight cut, round ended, soft to medium nylon bristles arranged in three to four rows of tufts are recommended.

Desirable Qualities

- Manmade (controllable) filaments: Generally, 0.007–0.011 mm in width with "rounded" filament ends
- Soft to medium in hardness
- Short head (about 1 inch) with straight handle of 6 inch length
- Straight trim
- Multitufted.

As the condition of the gingivae and the brushing requirements vary with each patient, it is probable that no one type of brush may be adequate for every individual. The choice of brush must be made to suit the individual. In general, the type found to be most satisfactory is a multitufted plastic filament brush. Here, many fine filaments are packed closely in each tuft, the latter are placed close together so that good coverage of the tooth surface and embrasure are assessed.

For the generally taught "roll" brushing technique, the multitufted brush seems to be satisfactory and acceptable to the patient. For vibratory brushing techniques (such as is recommended in the Bass method), the brushes with 0.007 inch filaments are more satisfactory.

Automatic toothbrushes: All the powered brushes which are recommended have quite small heads with multitufted filament bristles (Fig. 49.16). The potential for damage to the tooth substance or gingiva by powered brushes, a point frequently brought up by dentists, is limited by the fact that no powered brush can exert the same pressure which can be demonstrated by the healthy limbed manual individual. The automatic brush would stall before the excessive pressure can be exerted. Users of automatic brushes must be carefully taught how to use them effectively. There is no easy way even with these brushes. The advantage of powered brush is that it is easier for the less manually dexterous to achieve some sort of result, and once a reasonable skill is acquired, there is a saving in time over manual brushing. The potential disadvantage of this appliance is that the patient can be lulled into believing that all it has to do is to purchase one of these and everything will be done for him. There would appear to be little difference in effect between automatic brushes, which have arc oscillations, reciprocal, horizontal movement or a combination of both.

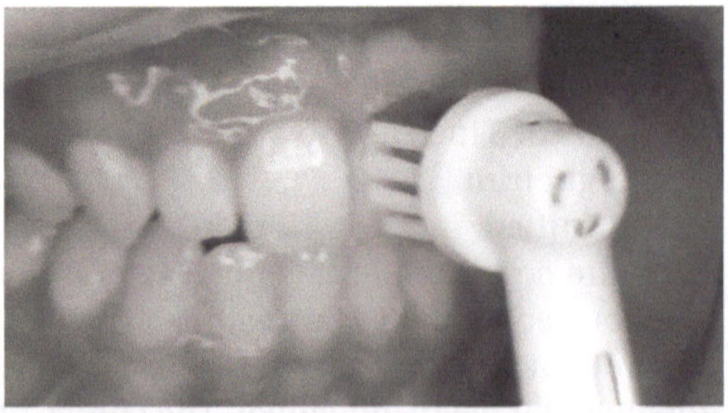

Fig. 49.16: Use of automatic toothbrush

Experience with these brushes from the earliest days of their development leads to the conclusion that only continuously powered, i.e. rechargeable brushes, are readily acceptable. Brushes with conventional replaceable batteries suffer from the disadvantage of an immediate lessening of torque from the first day of use. Another problem with automatic brushes is their high cost, repair and servicing. It is often difficult to restore the brush to satisfactory use if water enters the switch mechanism.

Manual versus automatic brushing: All patients, where possible, should be taught initially an effective plaque removal technique with the manual brush. If the patient is manually incapable (or incapacitated) or even too lazy to spend enough time, then an automatic brush may be recommended and demonstrated. Some of those who are unable to brush may want to use an automatic toothbrush. It is just as important in these cases to go over again the patient's technique of using the new brush. The correct brushing technique has been explained in Figures 49.17 to 49.20.

TOOTHBRUSHING TECHNIQUES

Although, it would be a desirable goal, it is not possible to achieve 100% plaque removal in any but the exceptional patient. We may try very hard to teach various techniques and follow this up with floss instruction and the use of interdental cleaners. Nevertheless, many (if not most) of our patients will fall short of our aims for them. And, it is important to emphasize here that most of our patients will have a greatly improved gingival condition, some even demonstrating complete resolution of the inflammation. It thus appears obvious that

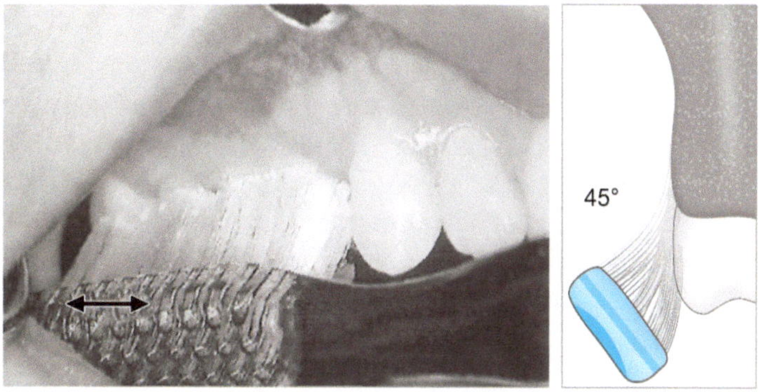

Fig. 49.17: Brushing the outer surfaces of the upper posterior teeth at an angle of 45° *(For color version, see Plate 14)*

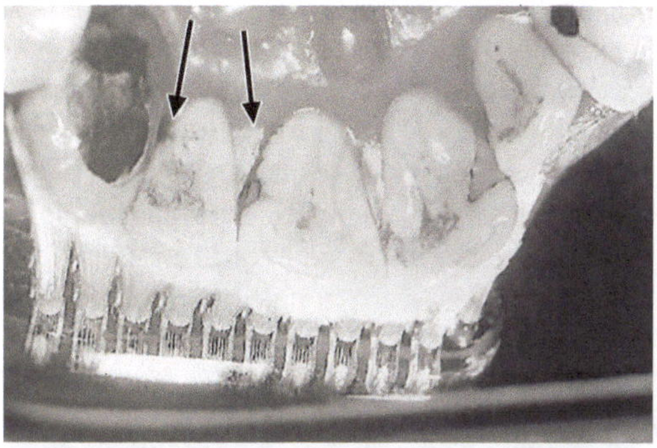

Fig. 49.18: Brushing the outer surfaces of the upper anterior teeth *(For color version, see Plate 15)*

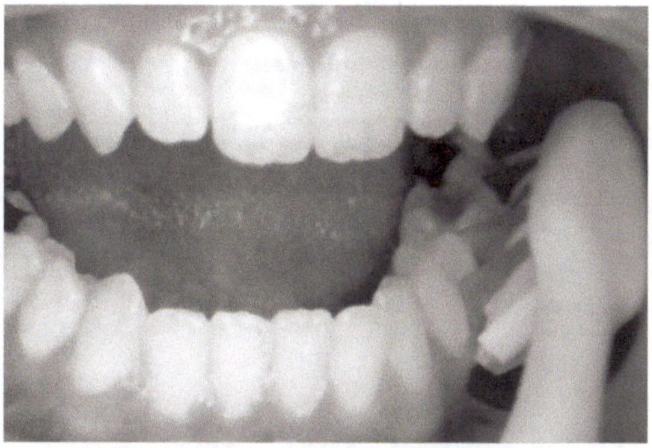

Fig. 49.19: Brushing the outer surfaces of the lower posterior teeth *(For color version, see Plate 15)*

the tissue resistance of most of our patients can cope with a certain amount of residual plaque and this would indicate that the dentist or hygienist should not make a spot judgment on the first visit as to how much training in oral hygiene methods a patient requires (Fig. 49.21). It will be necessary to assess the patient's response over a few visits, and perhaps even after a visit or two, as to how much effort or thoroughness of plaque removal is required for each patient (Fig. 49.22A and B). There are some who will have little gingival inflammation and perhaps no caries, but a notable amount of plaque around the teeth, others will have a minimal amount of adherent microorganisms and yet may demonstrate acute inflammation. We must, therefore, modify our approach to each patient depending on the reaction observed.

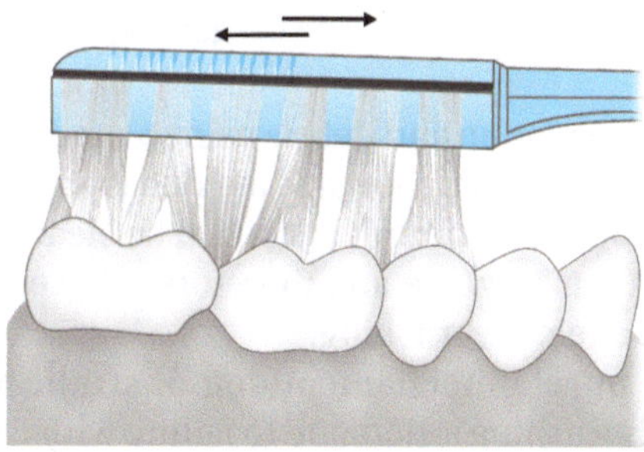

Fig. 49.20: Brushing the chewing surfaces of all teeth

It must be stressed by the teacher of oral hygiene that terms such as correct (or incorrect) brushing should not be used. There is no right or wrong way to brush teeth. The result is more important than the method. Therefore, if the patient declares that he can

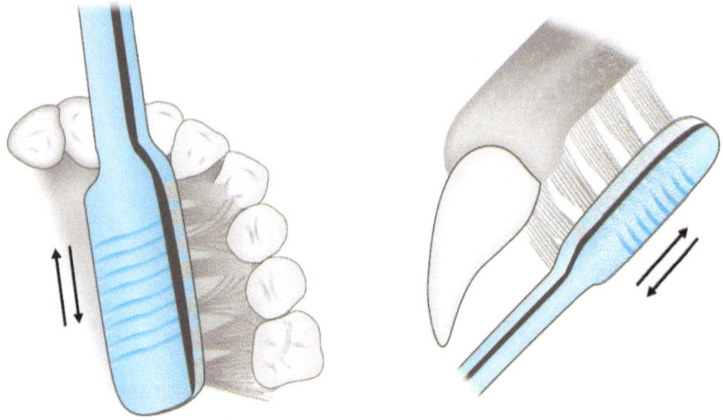

Fig. 49.21: Strokes used for the palatal surfaces of maxillary teeth

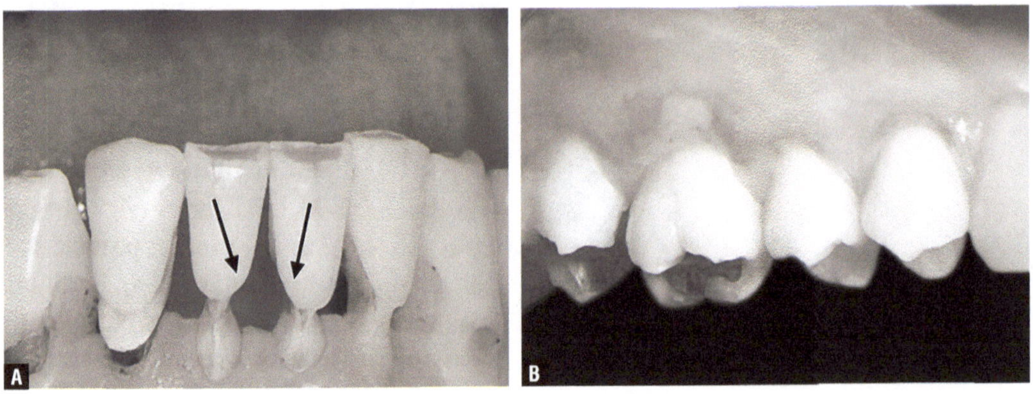

Figs 49.22A and B: (A) Damage to teeth and (B) adjacent soft tissue due to excessive scrubbing technique *(For color version, see Plate 15)*

remove plaque and debris using a method of his own, and can show this method is effective, we would be wrong to insist that he cleans his teeth our way. We are, therefore, concerned with effective brushing.

A purely mechanical demonstration of toothbrushing is doomed to failure with most patients. It is necessary to explain to the patient just why he or she is being asked to carry out procedures, which are sometimes quite difficult and also time consuming. The explanation should not just be a general one, but should relate to the patient's problems and be an actual part of the presentation.

Motivation

The nature of plaque and its adhesion to the tooth is carefully explained. The role played by plaque in production of caries and periodontal disease is outlined with emphasis on preventive role of toothbrushing.

Education

The fact that there is not one single "right" way to brush is emphasized. The right way is anyone of a number of different methods which will suit the particular patient (Some oral hygiene teachers give their patients instructions on brushing and insist that these are carried out before any scaling is performed. The reason given is that any gingival improvement is then convincingly proved to the patient to have been achieved by his own effort with the brush. On the other hand, it may be unfair to the patient to jeopardize early healing just to prove a point. Gingival inflammation will resolve much quicker if the calculus is removed).

At this stage, the teeth are painted with a disclosing solution and the plaque adhering to the teeth are pointed out to the patient. This indicates the areas, which have been missed during home brushing (Figs 49.23A and B). The plaque is gently scraped off a tooth with the side of a probe to demonstrate how easy it is to remove mechanically. A suitable brush is selected for the patient and he is told that this is his brush, which will be sealed up and kept for training at every visit. Therefore, it is advisable to purchase brushes, which are supplied in container, which can be closed.

Demonstration

The patient is asked to bring the brush that he has been using at home, but not to buy a new one. It is examined for suitability and the patient is then asked to demonstrate completely how the usual brushing is carried out. It helps to set a stopwatch at the commencement. After observing the patient's routine, the time to completion is announced. This is usually of the order of 20-30 seconds, although the brusher often insists that he has taken 2 minutes).

Errors in brushing, areas omitted and lack of organized method are pointed out. An almost constant error is that patients wet the toothbrush before commencing. They should be told that this is an incorrect thing to do, and the much worst procedure—the use of hot water—will damage the bristles. Life-size models are used for individual toothbrush demonstrations.

Each quadrant of the mouth is divided into three areas, posterior, middle, anterior, and for the brushing purposes, these are further subdivided into buccal/labial side and lingual or palatal side. The patient is recommended to brush each of these 6 areas with 8 strokes of the brush, thus making a total of 48 strokes for each quadrant or approximately 200 strokes for complete mouth. It has been found that as noted above, the patient has little concept of time taken for brushing but can readily count 200 strokes. Furthermore, the strokes relate to specific areas of the mouth while even if say a timer is provided, there is no guarantee that the patient will brush any more methodically. There are many brushing methods. The dentist or hygienist should not complicate by using too many different techniques, but should be able to demonstrate at least two methods.

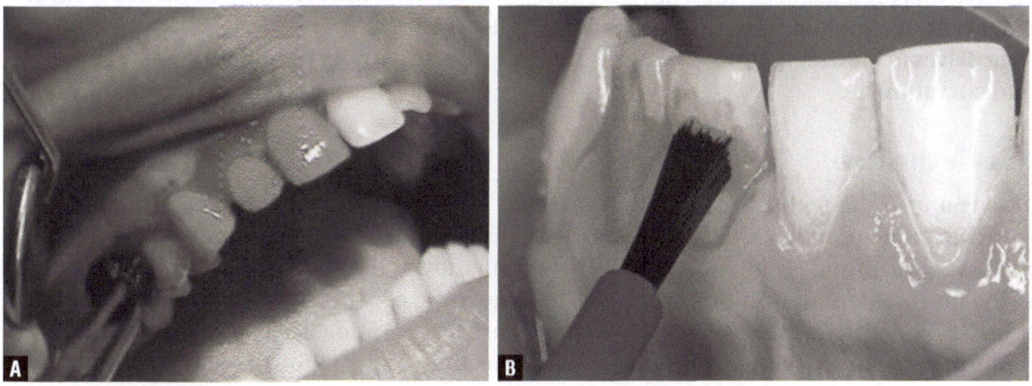

Figs 49.23A and B: Disclosing solution used to identify plaque for patient education

(For color version, see Plate 15)

Roll Technique

The average patients do not easily acquire effective toothbrushing techniques. Therefore, exotic and overcomplicated methods should be avoided. Perhaps, most widely taught (routinely) is the "roll" method, although this still offers difficulties to those who lack manual dexterity, or who have limited wrist movement. The brush is placed on the first of our 12 designated sectors of the jaw with the bristles on the alveolar mucosa pointing away from the occlusal surface. The sides of the bristles press against the attached gingiva and sulcus area. The bristles are rolled across the gingival toward the occlusal keeping the sides of the bristles pressed firmly against the tissues (they should appear to blanch) and with many of the bristles sweeping through the embrasures. This stroke is repeated eight times in each region. Assuring that the buccal area was brushed, this is followed by the lingual and repeated around the whole arch. The occlusal surfaces are then brushed with the tips of the bristles from lingual and buccal and back. The emphasis in all the brushing is that the brush should be used as a broom—to sweep—not as a scrubbing brush to scour. The brush is often held vertically for the lingual surfaces of the upper and lower incisor teeth. Finally, the occlusal surfaces are scrubbed.

The toothbrush should be applied to the teeth so that the sides of bristles, not the ends, contact the teeth. In this way, the bristles adapt themselves to the irregularities in embrasures, and curvatures.

Bass Technique

This is one of the techniques which has recently become popular, although described many years ago, and is dependent on the use of the fine filament multitufted brushes. The brush is applied in the same section by section pattern as previously but the bristles direction at an angle of 45° to the long axis of the teeth and pointing toward the gingival sulcus

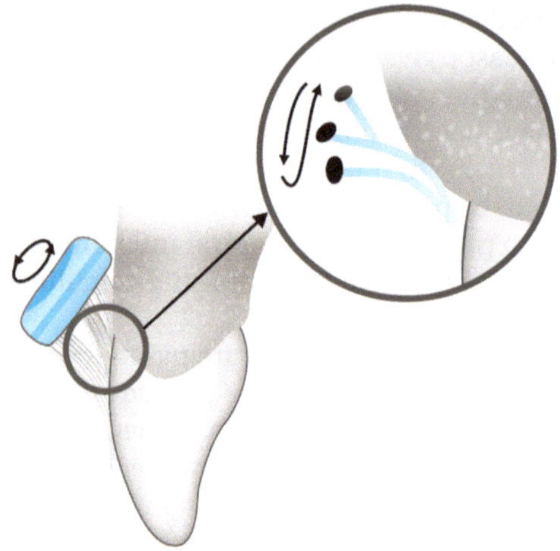

Fig. 49.24: Bristle angulation in Bass technique

(Fig. 49.24). The bristles in fact are made to enter the sulcus and the brush rotated and vibrated firmly in a small circle without moving the bristles ends from the crevice. In this way, the gingival areas of the tooth and the "pockets" are cleaned. The action is repeated in adjacent areas following the previously described pattern. Some dentists advocate a to-and-fro motion of the bristles in the sulcus area instead of the circular motion. There would appear to be little to choose between the two actions. The lingual area of the anterior teeth is brushed using the same action but holding the brush head vertically. In our experience, the average patient has great difficulty in:

- Identifying 45° angulation
- Finding the gingival sulcus with the bristle tips.

Charters Technique

This is nowadays not used so often as the Bass method and consists of a substantially similar action except that the brush is placed with the bristles pointing occlusally at an angle of 45°, i.e. there is no action of bristle in the gingival sulcus but the vibrating motion concentration on cleaning the proximal embrasures

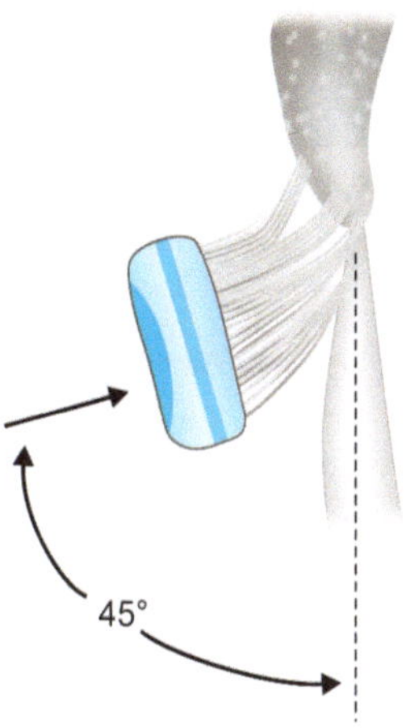

Fig. 49.25: Bristle angulation in Charters technique

(Fig. 49.25). This technique is used only where there is already loss of soft tissues interdentally. It is also used in areas of wound healing after periodontal surgery.

These various methods should not be taught to patients indiscriminately but the patient's ability to achieve successful plaque removal with the simplest methods should first be evaluated and here differences in tooth alignment, arch form and size, inclination and manual ability may bring about modification in teaching methods. This emphasizes the need for personal "one to one" training and the disadvantages of group "teaching". The brushing technique should befit the patient, not vice versa.

Assessment

After each demonstration, the patient is asked to brush his own teeth similarly, and the dentist or hygienist may help by placing the patient's brush in the correct position and helping to guide the wrist or hand action.

Following this, disclosing agents are used and the amount of residual plaque is demonstrated. A similar procedure is adopted on the following visit approximately one week later, with the disclosed plaque indicating areas that have been overlooked. Further training is given and complete training requires 3–4 visits.

Clinical Comments on Oral Hygiene Aids

Toothbrushing remains the most important single method of plaque control, but there are two possible dangers involved in it.

1. *Omissions:* Adequate brushing is not simple and often the gingival margins or interdental spaces are missed, thus leaving plaque in the most dangerous areas.
2. *Excesses:* With the hard brush and very abrasive paste or powder, gingival recession can be caused, leaving areas of exposed cementum, which might be very sensitive. Excessive brushing may wear deep crescent-shaped areas in the dentin of the exposed root, which is not protected by enamel. This is more usually seen in older patients but may occur in younger patients where a tooth is prominently placed because of crowding. Nevertheless, toothbrush trauma, as this is often termed, should not be over emphasized during oral hygiene instruction, unless signs of damage are appearing. It is more important to stress the value of brushing than the dangers and the hygienist should bear in mind that there is much more damage done by a lack of brushing than by excessive brushing.

METHODS OF PERFORMING ORAL HYGIENE AND REMOVING DEBRIS

Dentifrices

These are aids to the cleansing and polishing action of the brush due to its content of an abrasive, detergent and an antiseptic agent.

Instrumental

The toothpick is a useful mechanical agent for removal of food impacted between teeth. Similarly floss, silk thread may be pulled between teeth. These should be burnt or discarded after use.

Datun has been used as a mechanical aid for cleaning teeth since a long time and is an accepted custom in towns and villages. These are useful except that all surfaces and especially molar teeth cannot be reached and cleaned easily with it.

Toothbrushes are accepted as a useful aid in cleaning teeth when moved correctly on all surfaces of teeth except the interdental spaces. Choice should be made with regard to shape and size of the mouth. Carelessly kept toothbrushes are sources of gum infection.

Mouthwashes

Simple rinsing of the mouth mechanically removes easily detachable or soluble debris. Adding alkali, salts, or soap or hydrogen peroxide increases the detergent power for insoluble debris. Mouthwashes are frequently used to remove bacteria and their byproducts by irrigation. Better results are obtained if used with compressed air.

DENTIFRICES

Toothpastes have two principal functions:

1. Their abrasiveness helps in the removal of plaque and stains.
2. They leave a feeling of freshness in the mouth.

A large number of different toothpastes are available and many of them have special ingredients added in an attempt to prevent dental disease. Some examples of these additives are:

- Antibacterial agents, such as chlorhexidine
- Calculus inhibitors, such as urea, pyrophosphate
- Emulsifying agents
- Fluorides.

Composition

The composition of toothpaste been is given in Table 49.2.

Types

Different types of toothpastes are discussed in Table 49.3.

Table 49.2: Composition of a toothpaste

Ingredient	*Percent by weight*
Calcium pyrophosphate	40.00
Sorbitol (70% aqueous solution)	20.40
Glycerine	10.20
Sodium coconut monoglyceride sulfonate	0.82
Sodium lauryl sulfate	0.80
Sodium carboxymethyl cellulose	1.00
Magnesium aluminum silicate	0.40
Stannous fluoride	0.40
Flavor (spearmint)	0.90
Color	0.05
Sweetener (potassium salt of 6-methyloxathiazinone dioxide)	0.05
Water and minors	balance

Table 49.3: Types of toothpastes

Type of toothpaste	*Composition*	*Characteristic features*
Anti-caries/ cavity protection toothpastes	Sodium fluoride and sodium monofluoro-phosphate	Contain fluoride to stop tooth enamel decalcification and protect teeth from tooth decay and cavities
Plaque and gingivitis prevention toothpastes	Sodium lauryl Sulfate, triclosane, zinc and stannous ions	Antibacterial and prevent the formation of dental plaque
Tooth whitening toothpastes	Papain, Dimethicone	Have either higher abrasion value than normal toothpastes to mechanically remove food, smoking and other stains from teeth

The abrasiveness of toothpaste should be adequate to aid plaque removal, but not enough to cause abrasion of the teeth. In general, none of the toothpastes available are more abrasive than the tooth powders that are not recommended.

Novelty toothpastes are specifically for children and may well encourage them to clean their teeth. They are available in different flavors and colors.

Although the removal of debris and plaque from the tooth surfaces and gingivae is almost entirely a mechanical one, the importance of a good dentifrice should not be minimized. A report (1974) on dentifrices by an independent nondental organization was widely publicized as proclaiming that toothpastes were unnecessary as it was "the brush that did the cleaning".

It is sensible to recommend two or three brands, which we believe to have a constantly maintained formulation. One of the dangers of recommending "supermarket toothpastes" is that they are often products made by unknown manufacturers and sometimes sold on a temporary basis while they are profitable or popular.

The dentifrices that are usually recommended should be purely on therapeutic basis, which contain fluoride compounds, and have been developed and marketed after research and testing.

Special Purpose Dentifrices

Some patients who have sensitive cervical areas on their teeth may benefit from the use of desensitizing pastes such as Sensodyne, Emoform, Thermodent, etc. Although many patients state that they have been advised to use pastes to treat gingivitis or periodontitis, there is no justification for such a recommendation. The only possible value of such dentifrices is in the symptomatic treatment of sensitivity of dentin. Before prescribing these toothpastes, a thorough investigation into more definite causes should be carried out.

When these pastes are used, the patient should be instructed to brush with a small amount on a toothbrush as they would with a normal paste followed by rubbing the paste with a finger into the sensitive areas.

INTERDENTAL CLEANING AIDS

The toothbrush can clean the labial, lingual and occlusal surfaces of the teeth reasonably well except for the proximal surfaces. What must be emphasized, however, is that toothbrushing, when carefully practiced, should suffice to give the diligent patient a simple method of achieving a high degree of protection from various oral diseases. Anything other than brushing is looked upon as special skill and hence seldom persevered with. An illustration of this is that patients will often, as they sit themselves in the dental chair, apologize for not brushing that day or after the last meal. No patient ever arrives apologizing for not using floss or wood sticks. Therefore, every effort should be made with the patient's brushing technique. However, for the well-motivated

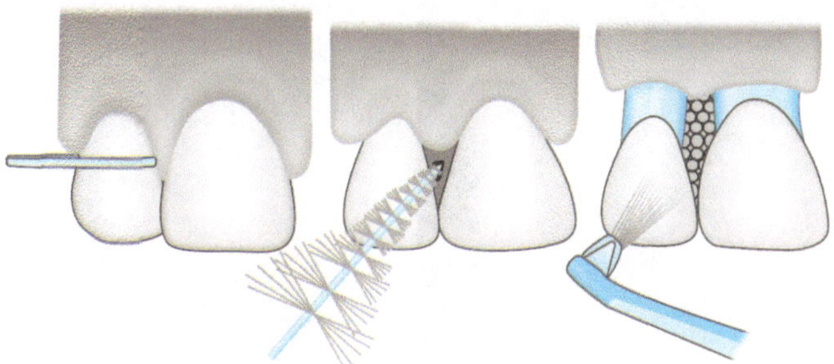

Fig. 49.26: Various interdental aids

patients, there are various aids that might be used to improve interdental cleaning (Fig. 49.26).

Dental Floss (Waxed and Unwaxed)

The waxed floss has been used for generations with satisfactory results whereas the average patient accepts the use of a toothbrush as part of the daily routine, flossing is not so naturally accepted and considerable difficulty is experienced in handling it.

Technique of Flossing

Even if the technique is apparently mastered, patients subsequently give up after use over a short period of time. Therefore, careful demonstration is always necessary. Written instructions are useful only after there has been practical training and practice in handling. It has been found easier to cut off a 6-inch length of floss and tie the ends together to form a loop. This is then held as in the illustration between left thumb and right index finger in order to clean the upper left quadrant (Figs 49.27A and B). The fingers are reversed for the right quadrant. The loop is held between both index fingers for the lower teeth. The floss is held taut between the fingers and is gently worked from the occlusal through the contact point down to the gingival crevice where, if possible, it is slid along, the tooth surface just under the crevice and the two hands are brought as near together as possible, thus wrapping the floss around half the circumference of the tooth. In this position, the floss is gently drawn occlusally while being kept firmly against the tooth surface. The action is repeated and then the surface of the neighboring tooth across the embrasure is similarly treated. The patient is instructed to clean all the proximal surfaces changing grip as indicated. Where it is not possible to introduce the floss through a contact point (e.g. soldered contacts of bridge pontics or splints), the material is passed under the contact using a floss threader.

The patients usually have more difficulty handling unwaxed floss and it is very doubtful whether any supposed advantage will outweigh the difficulties encountered, or will bring measurable benefits. Hill Lew and Glickman demonstrated that there was no significant difference in results achieved by toothbrushing and toothbrushing followed by the use of floss, either waxed or unwaxed. There are many flossing devices on the market but none is recommended because they are no easier to handle than the floss itself.

Wood Sticks

Many patients will fairly readily take to the use of wood sticks (stimudents, interdents). These, together with other interdental cleaners of measurable dimensions, should

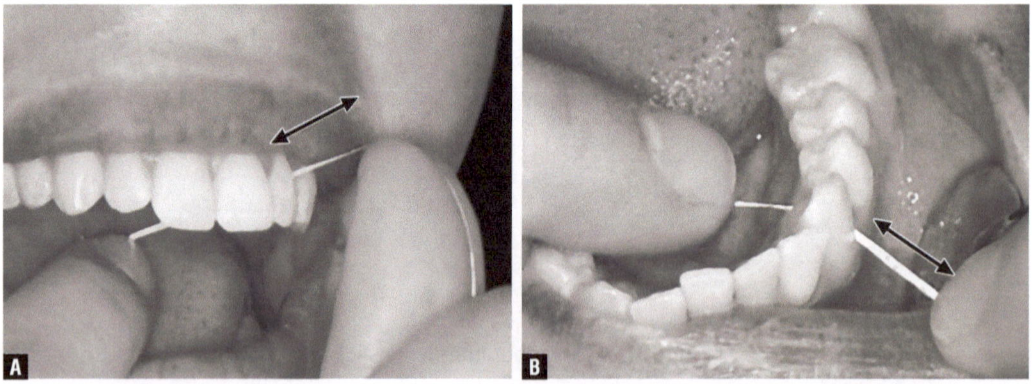

Figs 49.27A and B: Use of floss to clean interdental areas *(For color version, see Plate 16)*

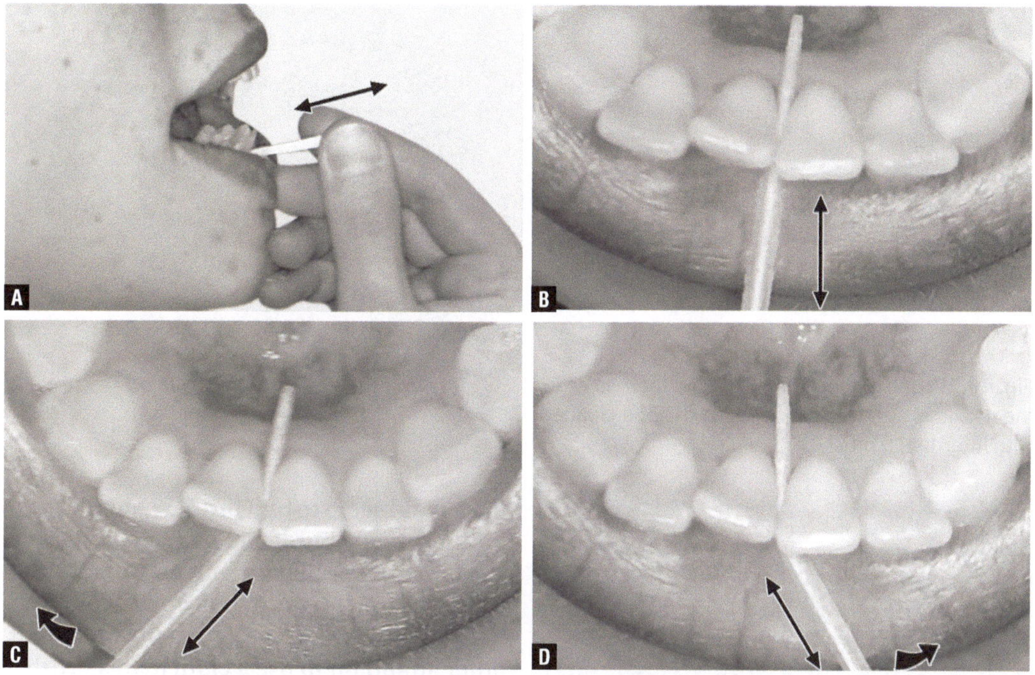

Figs 49.28A to D: Note the angulation and method of applying a wood stick *(For color version, see Plate 16)*

be recommended only where there is sufficient interdental space not filled by gingival tissue. Care is necessary in teaching the use of wood sticks. They should not be used as tooth picks, which is what the patient will tend to do, but the stick should be inserted into the embrasure, pointed end first, with the stick at the angle of 45° to the long axis of the tooth, and the sharp edge away from the gingiva. The stick is rubbed about 12 times in each space with the tip pointing coronally. A methodical approach should be emphasized, that is, the patient should start from a fixed point in the mouth and work round the mouth back to the same point.

There should be some order in using the sticks so that no space is missed out. There may be some difficulty in reaching spaces in the posterior part of the mouth, and other devices or techniques may have to be employed. The wood sticks, based on the original idea of toothpicks, are quite inexpensive and may be sufficient for some patients because they are made of hardwood and do not compress when in use. Surprisingly, they require a little more space than the more compressible stimudents (Fig. 49.28A to D).

Rubber points: Some toothbrushes have a rubber point in the handle which patients find reasonably easy to use as an extension of normal toothbrushing. Other rubber tips may be fitted to special handles.

Interdental Brushes

Interdental brush has the advantage that they will reach the posterior areas easily and patients do not often have difficulty in their use.

They have the advantage of being reasonably inexpensive. It is also possible to clean the embrasures from both lingual and labial aspects of the jaws (Fig. 49.29). Other small brushes may be disposable and attached to metal handles by a screw ring (Perio aid). Different types of interdental brushes are show in Figures 49.30A and B.

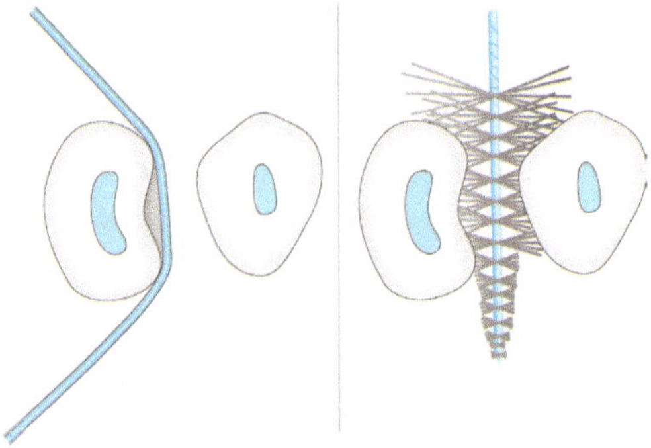

Fig. 49.29: If the space between the teeth is wide, the proximal surfaces of the teeth may be cleaned with interdental brushes

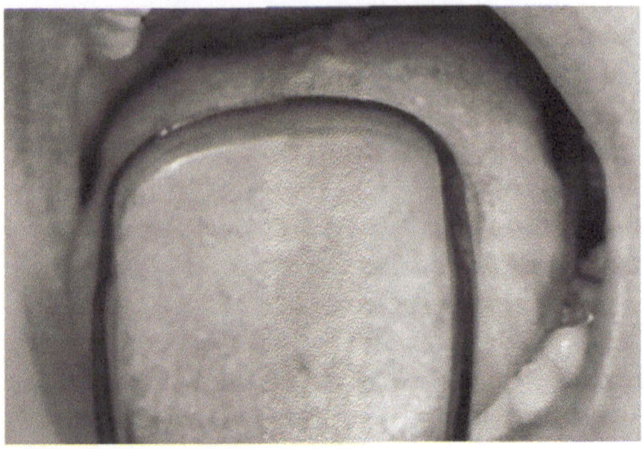

Fig. 49.31: Tongue scraper

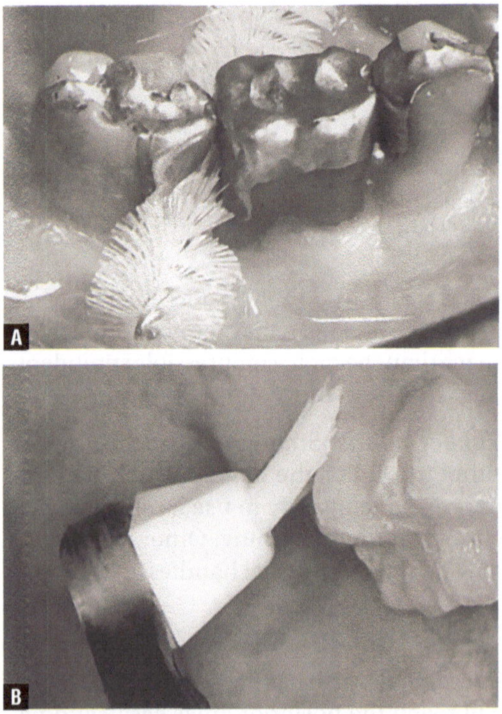

Figs 49.30A and B: (A) Bottlebrush type of interdental cleaner; (B) Unitufted brush for inaccessible areas *(For color version, see Plate 16)*

Polishing Cloth

These may be used (thin toweling cut to the shape of the fingers and sometimes sewn to an average shape by dental staff) to polish the surfaces of all teeth before brushing. However, this would seem to be a further complication for the already burdened patient but may be treated as a special armamentarium for the difficult case, e.g. the handicapped child and here it may be much easier for the mother or other attendant to use a cloth than a brush.

Tongue Scraper

Tongue scrapers facilitate the removal of bacterial accumulation and debris from the dorsum of tongue that are a major cause of halitosis (Fig. 49.31).

Water Irrigation Outfits

Powered dental irrigation devices are designed to eliminate plaque and debris through mechanical action of a jet of stream of water. Use of water or antimicrobial agents with pulsating irrigation devices has been used as an adjunct to mechanical plaque control in dental practice. These appliances, which are expensive with limited effect on plaque control, have very little justification in oral hygiene training.

ORAL PROPHYLAXIS IN GINGIVAL AND PERIODONTAL DISEASES

Oral hygiene indicates the state of cleanliness of the oral cavity. These are the measures, which the patient takes care at home to ensure that his dental health is maintained at its optimum level and thus he ensures strong and healthy teeth and gums, which are free from disease. It is also designated as home care or oral physiotherapy and are, in other words, preventive measures taken by the individual himself.

Poor oral hygiene is the important cause of dental diseases. The food debris and bacteria get accumulated round the teeth and give rise to bacterial plaque, dental caries, formation and deposition of calculus, halitosis and periodontal diseases. Poor oral hygiene predisposes to herpetic and Vincent's stomatitis and even throat infections.

If a person is blessed with perfect dentition and he takes appropriate diet containing roughage like fruits and vegetables which require chewing and mastication with its associated movements of the tongue and lips, then it can be presumed that these will produce satisfactory cleansing of teeth and gums. But the frequency of abnormal dentition and malocclusion and the defective mastication of food result in lodgment of food particles between the teeth. These food residues become mechanical irritants and source of bacterial infection that may spread to the gums and teeth.

ORAL PROPHYLAXIS

Oral prophylaxis is the measure taken by the dental surgeon and his staff to prevent dental diseases. It is carried out as a preparation of the mouth for oral surgical procedures and placement of prosthodontic restorations. The objectives are to have a disease-free mouth.

- Removal of soft and hard deposits, e.g. dental plaque and calculus. This prevents caries and periodontal diseases
- The roughened tooth surfaces are polished and smoothened
- Pinpoint carious cavities are polished to prevent further spread
- The dentures and restorations are checked and polished
- Overhanging contours of restorations are finished and polished to prevent trauma to oral tissues and lodgment of food
- Sharp cusps and ragged edges are rounded off
- Prophylactic odontotomy is carried out
- Pits and fissures are sealed off with sealing agents
- Correct brushing technique is taught at chairside
- Application of fluorides for prevention of caries is carried out in children (2% sodium fluoride)
- Abnormal habits are corrected, e.g. lip biting, thumb sucking, etc.
- Complete dental checkup is done to detect diseases early
- Application of disclosing solution to demonstrate dental plaque
- X-rays are taken if necessary to locate proximal caries.

It is an established fact that dental plaque is the primary cause for the initiation and progression of periodontal diseases. As the plaque matures its bacterial flora changes from normal commensal organism to more pathogenic flora. Moreover, the deposition of calcium salts from saliva into the soft plaque results in the mineralization and formation of dental calculus. Dental calculus being highly irregular in structure results in the attachment of abundant quantities of dental plaque having very high number of pathogenic bacteria. Calculus keeps the pathogenic dental plaque in continuous touch with the gingival tissues resulting in the gingival and periodontal disease.

In order to control the initiation and further progression of gingival and periodontal diseases, it is necessary to check the growth of dental plaque as well as calculus. Therefore, oral prophylaxis becomes one of the most important aspects of the treatment and control of gingival and periodontal diseases.

Goals of Oral Prophylaxis

Since the oral prophylaxis removes the hard and soft deposits from the teeth, it helps the oral tissues in the following manner:

- *Prevention of onset of disease:* Gingival and periodontal disease starts with the local deposits like food debris, materia alba, plaque and calculus. They affect the tissues in the following manner:
  - *Mechanical*: They cause irritation to gingival tissues, thus leading to inflammation
  - *Bacterial*: Microorganisms grow over the deposits. They liberate toxic substances and enzymes, which are poisonous in nature and cause degeneration of connective tissue.

  Therefore, oral prophylaxis by removing these deposits prevents gingival and periodontal diseases.

  It is an important phase to educate the patient for proper toothbrushing, and use of gum stimulation, which helps in proper keratinization of gingiva and protection against bacteria and their enzymatic effects.
- *Prevention from spread of disease:* Once the disease starts, it tends to spread into deeper tissues of periodontal ligament, cementum and alveolar bone. If the oral prophylaxis is done in the initial phase, then the degeneration of periodontal ligament and resorption of alveolar bone can be checked.

  It is very important in systemic diseases, which are aggravated if oral prophylaxis is not performed, or oral hygiene is not maintained.
- *Prevention of recurrence of disease:* Recurrence of periodontal disease is very common among the noncooperative patients. Since they do not take care of oral hygiene, the disease process restarts and sometimes complicates the situation. Therefore, oral prophylaxis instructions for proper brushing and gum massage are essential to prevent recurrence of treated cases
- Oral prophylaxis improves the aesthetics by removing tartar and other mucinous sticky material from teeth
- It provides a feeling of freshness in mouth
- It checks the bad oral breath (Feter oris)
- It prepares the mouth for further surgical procedures
- It is a good start for apprehensive children who are scared of dental treatment
- It prepares the teeth for topical application of fluoride, or other chemical applicants
- It motivates the individual to develop adequate habits of personal oral care.

Oral prophylaxis does not only include simple scaling and polishing of teeth but it also includes other corrective measures such as:

- *Prophylactic fillings:* The susceptible areas on the occlusal surface of teeth like deep fissures and grooves are either beveled to eliminate the catch points or filled with restorative materials
- *Preventive orthodontic:* In this, maloccluded teeth are corrected so that areas, which are not approachable by brushes, are corrected as well as space maintainers are given to children to prevent any tilting of teeth, thus preserving the space of the permanent teeth
- *Correction of defective fillings:* All-over extended fillings particularly the class II restorations should be corrected. The overextension of filling results in the collection of large quantities of plaque underneath, leading to periodontal disease
- *Filling of all carious lesions:* All cavities should be properly filled and contoured so as to reduce the chances of plaque accumulation
- *Correction of food impaction:* All plunger cusps are corrected with the help of diamond stones so as to remove the areas of food impaction, which can act as secondary factor leading to gingival and periodontal diseases
- *Extraction and immediate prosthesis:* All hopeless teeth should be extracted immediately which cannot be maintained by any therapy. Spaces should be then filled by appropriate prosthesis so that mesial and occlusal drifting of the teeth can be checked.

Working Protocol of a Dental Hygienist

CHAPTER 50

INTRODUCTION

The dental hygienist is a key figure in the prevention of periodontal disease and in the maintenance of health in treated patients. Although, the progress made in the prevention of caries may seem all too little, the progress made in the prevention of periodontal disease is unfortunately much less.

The hygienist's duty is to teach effective brushing technique to remove plaque. All patients accept the act of brushing as a natural part of their daily routine. It is just the learning of a new brushing technique that is difficult. But very few patients, however willing and keen they seem at the time of training, will not permanently accept flossing programs or the use of other gadgets, except possibly interdental wood sticks.

SCALING AND POLISHING

Calculus, whether supramarginal or submarginal, is the supreme plaque holder. If calculus is not removed, the success of any brushing instruction is prejudiced. It is also unfair to expect the patient to carry out home care procedures which are always quite difficult for some if the teeth are left in a roughened state either through lack of polishing or because calculus still remains. This is not to say that we should not commence brushing instruction from the first oral hygiene visit. But we should also, at the same time, help the patient in our way by beginning to clean and polish the surfaces of all teeth. Thus, careful scaling is the most important factor in the prevention of periodontal disease. It is also a factor in the maintenance of the treated case. No matter how well we teach our patients to carry out plaque elimination procedures, most will still form calculus in some regions and will require regular thorough scaling.

Student hygienist needs to be shown in the preclinical period and subsequently on patients, the grasp and correct positioning of instruments for each area of the dental arches to be scaled. Therefore, although the general principles in relation to scaling, root planing and instrument care will be discussed here, the student's main learning must be via repeated practice. The early methods of training vary considerably between dental institutions. It used to be the practice for the student to use scaling instruments to remove paint carefully from door knobs without scratching the metal underneath or some form of glue were baked onto the roots of ivory or real teeth for the same purpose. It must be the responsibility of the staff of the dental hygiene institutions to devise their own early training methods. Apart from the scaling procedure, the hygienist may be required to carry out root planing also.

Scaling: It is the removal of adherent calcified deposit (calculus) from the surfaces of the teeth. If the deposits are coronal to the gum margin, the procedure is said to be supramarginal, and conversely, if the deposits are "hidden" below the gum, the scaling is termed submarginal.

Root planing: The root surfaces may be covered by fine spots or rings of hard calculus, some of which may be so firmly attached that finger of calculus project into defects in the cementum. With suitable fine instruments (hoes and curette), the calculus is planned away together with any damaged or nonvital cementum. During root planning, a certain amount of gingival curettage takes place as an incidental—this is the removal of diseased epithelial lining of the inside wall of the crevice or pocket.

Before commencing scaling, a great deal must be known about the patient who must have been examined first by the dentist, who after having taken a complete history and thus formulated a treatment plan, will ask the dental hygienist to carry out the scaling and to give instruction in home care. There are those patients who will require special premedication before scaling.

Patients with a history of rheumatic fever, organic heart murmurs, valvular lesions, pre- and post-cardiac surgery patients, all require not only gentle care, but also an antibiotic cover against temporary bacteremia which may occur during or immediately after scaling.

At the first visit, this pretreatment care is easy, because the dentist has probably arranged cover. It is at subsequent visit for the continuation of scaling that the dental hygienist can make omissions unless a routine practice of noting on the patient's chart boldly for the special care, which is necessary, is emphasized.

All the instruments necessary for the session should be sharp, clean and sterilized. The operation area should be immaculate with no stains on the spittoon bowl and a clean rinsing cup is placed in position and is filled with warm water after the patient has been seated.

The relevant radiographs and other information should be available for study during the time the patient is being treated. The information given in the X-rays should be followed as much as possible.

The patient is seated comfortably in the chair—any denture being removed and placed in a covered bowl of water, a box of tissue is handed to a female patient if she is wearing lipstick for its removal, and the chair adjusted to a good working position. It is advisable for the hygienist to be seated whenever possible while working.

The dental hygienist tutor should make sure that the seated scaling posture adopted by the student is a correct and unstrained one, with the feet planted firmly on the floor and the thigh supported by the stool. Before commencing work, the patient's teeth should be examined carefully and the presence of gross calculus (supramarginal and subgingival) should be noted. Although the calculus on the crown surfaces is usually easily visualized, it is not enough to do this alone.

Calculus can mimic enamel and can be missed. The use of an air blower (chip syringe, or a gentle puff of air from the unit syringe) will dry the tooth surface and any calculus will readily show up. Subgingival calculus will also frequently be disclosed by the use of the air syringe which opens up the crevice and reveals the dark (seruminal) calculus—it may also show by direct vision as a purple or dark discoloration of the marginal gingiva, often associated with inflammation and swelling of these areas.

The calculus must be palpated or felt with an explorer. The crevice or sulcus may be probed gently using a cross calculus probe. The student should practice repeatedly the tactile recognition of the presence of submarginal calculus. Once the touch and feeling have been acquired, a marked improvement in scaling skill results. This probing will also detect (in conjunction with the X-ray appearances) the presence of restorative (filling) overhangs and also some hidden carious cavities.

The hygienist may be called upon to carry out scaling as part of the initial preparation of a periodontally involved case, and a number of visits may be devoted to thorough scaling, and also training the patient in homecare methods. The result of this is often a marked improvement that reduces the requirement of periodontal surgery subsequently. The patient's ability to cooperate by maintenance methods following treatment can be evaluated and this stage enables the causative factors to be ascertained and probably eliminated. The purely prophylactic scaling where there is no gingival inflammation or abnormal crevicular depth can be completed in one visit, otherwise where there is any gingival inflammation present, it must be stressed that it is not necessary to dismiss the patient in one visit.

There must be a follow up, at least a week after the scaling and oral cavity checked for resolution of the gingival inflammation or for any remaining calculus. Any such areas with calculus, however, firmly deposited, will retain the inflammation and will stand out from the healthier pink gingiva.

For more extensive calculus deposits, both supra- and submarginal, the scaling is usually carried out on a quadrant basis separately, at different visits, spaced a week apart. In the subsequent visit before another quadrant is treated, the previously scaled one is carefully examined for any missed deposits and removed. At the termination of each visit, the areas treated should be polished to achieve as smooth surface as possible in order to lessen further plaque deposition and recalcification. It is not absolutely essential to carry out such treatment always on a quadrant basis and some workers prefer to scale all-round the mouth (or one arch) to the limits of all reachable calculus, and then at a subsequent visit, remove deeper deposits which have become more accessible through gum shrinkage.

It should be stressed that all too commonly taught division of scaling into "gross scaling" and "fine scaling" as two separate operations is to be depreciated and the dental hygienist should try to achieve the maximum removal of deposits consistent with the patient's tolerance and the technical facility of the operation. Haphazard "digs" in different areas of the mouth will be inefficient, leave areas untreated, and will waste time. Furthermore, scaling strokes should overlap so that no areas are missed (as in mowing a lawn).

After completion of oral prophylaxis, dental hygienist must summarize the brushing technique as discussed in the section below.

Points to Consider While Toothbrushing

The purpose of toothbrushing is to remove the particles of food from between the teeth and the pits and fissures on the occlusal surfaces. This will help to prevent bacterial and plaque accumulation. It must be stressed that, except for the occlusal surfaces, the teeth should never be brushed across, as this will eventually damage the enamel.

There are certain important points that should be taken care of while brushing.

- With the bristles resting on the gums, always use a sweeping movement from the gums toward the biting surface of the teeth. The gum margins and tooth surfaces on the tongue side of the teeth must be cleaned as well as those which face the cheek and lips
- Brush the upper teeth with a downward motion
- Brush the lower teeth with an upward motion
- Brush the chewing surfaces of the upper and lower teeth using a rotary motion
- Brush the teeth in a definite order
- Brush the tongue if it is coated
- Vigorously rinse the mouth.

Vigorous mouth rinsing can remove much of the food particles. It is not as efficient as toothbrushing but is useful when the latter is occasionally not possible. The fluid must be forced between the teeth to cleanse the areas where dental caries so easily starts.

Control of Pain Sensations During Oral Prophylaxis

Although, it may be possible to scale many patients without the use of anesthetics, either topical or injectable, it is frequently necessary and advisable to use a topical anesthetic. This should be discussed with the patient first, and the numb sensations that will ensue are described. The usual method is to apply the liquid, by the use of cotton bud or tiny pellet of cotton soaked in topical anesthetic, by painting over the area to be scaled (e.g. topical xylocaine). The patient should be told not to swallow, but may spit out, whenever necessary. Aerosol sprays of topical anesthetic should not be used, as the flow of this to the back of the mouth cannot be controlled very easily. Furthermore, patients should be advised that great care should be exercised particularly with children when food is taken in within 60 minutes following the use of topical anesthetics, because of the danger of lip/cheek/tongue biting due to anesthetization of oral tissues and pharynx.

Antibiotic Prophylaxis

Oral hygiene prophylaxis (scaling) involves manipulation of gingival and periodontal tissues. Patients seeking oral prophylaxis having a medical history, like insulin-dependent diabetes, hemophilia, subacute bacterial endocarditis, chronic obstructive pulmonary disease, compromised immunity, cases of cardiac, hepatic, renal diseases, and patient who have undergone joint replacement surgery in the last 2 years require prophylactic antibiotic cover before undergoing dental and periodontal treatment.

All such patients should be treated under the supervision of a registered dental surgeon who is competent to prescribe suitable antibiotic before the start of the treatment to avoid any future systemic complications.

RESPONSIBILITIES OF A HYGIENIST

The responsibilities of the dental hygienist in patient education are:

- To build confidence in the patient that the dental services he receives are the best for his individual needs
- Dental care is the continuous process. Regular dental appointments are to be expected and the patient will be informed for periodic dental prophylaxis, X-rays, and examination by the dentist at specific intervals
- The patient is motivated to carry out his part of the dental care schedule by assuming responsibility for his own mouth cleanliness through toothbrushing, gum massage and flossing
- The dental hygienist is capable in preparing comprehensive dental histories, thus saving much time for the dentist and the patient. His understanding of total health, in relation to dental health, provides a background for obtaining facts that otherwise may be overlooked
- The dental hygienist can allay fears, misapprehensions and misunderstanding in reference to the dental services to be undertaken
- Most important is his ability to teach scientific accuracy, dental health, personal nutrition needs and recommended procedures.

Public Health Aspect of Dentistry

CHAPTER 51

INTRODUCTION

Public health aspect of dentistry deals with dental health education of the public in order to achieve the following goals:

- Prevention of onset of dental diseases
- Prevention of mutilating effects of dental diseases by:
  - Early detection
  - Early treatment of diseases.
- Prevention of recurrence of the diseases by recall visits after thorough treatment.

PREVENTIVE DENTISTRY

The main aim of public health dentistry is to reduce the diseases of the hard and soft tissues of the oral cavity and reduce the time required to treat these diseases. This is carried through the following methods:

- Dental health education gives emphasis on the importance of oral hygiene lectures and annual dental inspections. Dental health education is carried out through:
  - Lectures with audio-visual aids
  - Posters used as a motivating force
  - Dental health education with models and charts
  - Films and slides
  - Radio and television programs.
- Periodic check-up by annual dental inspection. This is done every 6 months to observe following things:
  - Oral hygiene status
  - Condition of teeth and surrounding investing tissues.
- Oral physiotherapy and home care with the help of following means:
  - Proper toothbrushing and gingival massage
  - Interdental cleaning and massage
  - Dental floss and dental tape
  - Oral rinsing with water
  - Fibrous diet for better cleaning aids.
- Preventive treatment or oral prophylaxis to remove the following:
  - Materia alba is soft deposit on the gingival third of crowns consisting of mucous, soft food debris, epithelial cells, and bacterial masses
  - Mucinous films and plaque commonly seen on the interproximal surfaces, consisting of colloidal materials and bacteria
  - Calculus deposit.

Oral Prophylaxis

Oral prophylaxis consists of:

- *Scaling*: By hand instruments or ultrasonic scalers
- *Polishing and removal of stains*: By using pumice and hydrogen peroxide
- Removal of occlusal irregularities
- *Prophylactic restoration:* Restoration of pits and fissures of posterior teeth by prophylactic odontomy/sealants
- Prophylactic orthodontic treatment

- *Elimination of abnormal habits:* Thumb sucking, mouth breathing, lip biting, bruxism
- Fluoridation for dental caries prevention.

Fluorides

Fluoride ions reach the enamel matrix and form calcium fluorapatite crystals in place of hydroxyapatite, which is more caries resistant. Fluorides can be administered:

- During enamel development: By systemic administration through fluoride in the table salt or adding fluoride into water to make the concentration of fluoride 1 ppm
- After the development of teeth is completed, topical fluoride administration by
  - Use of fluoride toothpaste
  - Topical fluoride application in the form of
    - ◊ 2% sodium fluoride
    - ◊ Stannous fluoride
    - ◊ Acidulated fluoride gel.
- Diet and nutrition
  - During pregnancy, balance diet is to be taken along with fluorides
  - Nonsticky food containing proteins to be given
  - Infant breastfeeding emphasized up to 6 months of age.
- Dental health surveys
  - Dental surgeons for educating the children and their parents about dental health
  - Dental clinics in public sector
  - Dental clinics along with all the hospitals.
- The common causes of gingivitis and periodontitis have been stated and it is necessary that preventive measures should be directed against these predisposing factors. The methods to be adopted are as follows:
  - *The use of fibrous food:* Part of the diet should include food that requires thorough chewing, as mastication has a stimulating effect on the tissues supporting the teeth in the normal mouth
  - *Brushing the gums and the care of dentures or removable appliances:* Oral hygiene as described previously is essential in the prevention of gingival diseases. It is important to use a brush with not too hard bristles and to be careful that every part of the gum margin of all the teeth is brushed systematically. The gentle friction on the gum hardens its epithelium or outer covering. In fact in order to emphasize the value of this procedure, a toothbrush is sometimes called a mouth brush
  - *Interdental cleaning aids:* A space may develop between the teeth, which may be due to periodontitis or to recession of the gums. This is difficult to clean even with a correctly designed brush. To keep the gums in the spaces in a healthy condition, the use of a narrow stimulators made of wood or plastic are required, but these should only be used under expert guidance as incorrect use may cause injury to gums and particularly if they are softened and damaged by the disease. If stimulators are prescribed, it is essential that they should be used regularly and in the correct manner
  - *Removal of calculus/deposits*: The amount of calculus deposited and the rate of deposition vary considerably in different persons and even in the same individual at different times. The teeth should be scaled at frequent intervals as indicated by a dentist
  - *Habitually open mouth:* This habit can be overcome with the cooperation of the teacher and parent with the dentist. In some cases, there is nasal obstruction and the opinion of an ear, nose and throat specialist should be obtained
  - *Prevention of malocclusion due to irregular oral habits*: Various habits are a

frequent cause of malocclusion and these should be corrected. Sometimes the habit may indicate an abnormal feeling of insecurity which itself requires investigation and treatment.

Fluoridation of Domestic Water Supplies

It has been discovered that many natural water supplies throughout the world, including some in Great Britain and India, contain very small quantities of fluoride. After many exhaustive studies involving the dental examination of large groups of people, the amount of fluoride in the water has been shown to have an effect on the teeth.

Communities whose water supply is deficient in fluoride have more dental caries than those with a water supply containing sufficient fluoride. The actual amount of fluoride is important and in temperate climates, the consumption of water is such that the optimum concentration is 1.0–1.2 parts of fluoride per million parts of water (ppm).

Investigations were originally started in 1945 in the United States of America and Canada to judge the effect of adding just the right amount of fluoride to the water supplies so making good the deficiency. On the other hand, in some districts there is too much fluoride occurring naturally in the water supply and this may cause mottled enamel in the inhabitants. In some of these places, the amount of fluoride has been reduced to the optimum level so avoiding this effect on the enamel. The restoration of fluoride to the optimum level does not in any way affect the color, taste or smell of the water.

The benefit of fluoride is greatest when the teeth are being formed and it is, therefore, important that the correct amount of fluoride should be taken by the expectant mother, for the deciduous teeth are partly mineralized before birth as well as after the birth at least until adult life is reached.

AIMS AND OBJECTIVES OF DENTAL HEALTH EDUCATION

Health is defined as a state of complete physical, mental and social well-being, not merely the absence of disease or infirmity—World Health Organization.

Dental health is defined as the adoption and maintenance of sound oral health practices and the use of oral health services judiciously, which result in improvement of the oral health status of both the individual and the community.

Public health is concerned with and is directed towards the improvement and protection of the health of a group, community, state or of a population in aggregate.

Concept of public health: Public health is the planning, carrying out and evaluation of health measures and system services so that both maintain and improve the health of a population group, and prevent and control diseases within that population group.

Oral hygiene may be defined as the science that deals with the preservation of health of oral tissues. It includes the measures carried out by patients for the prevention of diseases of the oral tissues. The practice of good oral hygiene includes the following:

- The maintenance of teeth free of plaque and calcified deposits and to prevent dental caries and gingival irritation
- The removal of hard and soft deposits and the teaching of methods to keep the mouth free of them
- Procedures must be carried out by the patient to keep the mouth free of plaque, stains and calculus.

For the prevention of plaque accumulation or its regular removal, the most important preventive measure is the effective use of the toothbrush. Till date only the mechanical action of the brush has been regularly shown to remove the bacterial and other deposits. Once gingivitis does occur, it becomes easier to motivate the patient because then the ill effects of bacterial accumulation on the teeth can be demonstrated by the use of disclosing solution. This will convince the patient to maintain good oral hygiene.

The Primary Objectives of Health Education (World Health Organization, 1969)

- To persuade people
  - To adopt and sustain health practice
  - To use judiciously and wisely health services available to them
  - To take their own decisions both individually and collectively to improve their health status and environment.

For the prevention and control of dental ill health, patient must understand that:

- Dental disease can be controlled if individuals would adopt and sustain the healthy life practices of controlling sugar intake and effective plaque removal
- The correct use of the available dental services can aid in the early diagnosis and treatment of disease
- The health of the mouth can be improved by the community taking steps to alter the environment by implementing fluoridation of public water supplies
- Dental ill health is greatly influenced by individual behavior; therefore, health education by modifying habits detrimental to dental wellbeing should be an important preventive health measure.

DENTAL HEALTH AND CHILDREN

The three most important factors related to health of children are:

- Adequate diet
- Good oral hygiene
- Regular and adequate dental care.

One of the most important factors is a balanced diet, low in easily fermentable carbohydrates. In addition to diet control, one of the parents should be educated in brushing the primary teeth regularly as soon as they erupt. The brushing should be continued until the child is old enough to be instructed in the proper and systematic use of the toothbrush. Periodic and continuous visits beginning at 2 years of age should be made to dentist. Carious teeth should be restored as soon as the lesions become evident clinically or radiographically. Topical applications of fluoride should be made at least once a year. Every effort should be made to preserve the primary teeth, until the time of their normal exfoliation and the eruption of the permanent teeth.

In addition to the importance of diet control, the parents should be stressed upon the significance of the child's first permanent molar. These teeth are most frequently neglected in comparison to teeth, since many parents mistake them for the primary teeth.

Thumb sucking is considered by many to be normal in a child 2.5–3 years of age. If the habit persists beyond this age, it is desirable to discourage the habit at an early age, before it becomes deep seated.

The teaching profession is in a favorable position to help the prevention of dental diseases. School teaching staff, caring for school children over long intervals of time, can to a marked degree control the standard of oral hygiene and dental instruction, and observe habits that are harmful. Moreover, they can also influence parents, who frequently seek advice of teachers. Together they can do much to lessen dental diseases.

Both parents and teachers are in a position to set a personal example in this respect. It is of great importance that there should be a continuous emphasis laid on maintenance of oral hygiene both at home and at school. This objective is aided by adopting the following regime.

- Meals should be taken at regular times. Aerated drinks like Pepsi, Cola, etc. should be limited
- Sticky snacks such as bread, sweet confectionery products should not be taken in between meals
- Fibrous food such as a slice of apple should be taken at the end of a meal.

ROLE OF DENTAL HYGIENIST IN TOBACCO CESSATION

Tobacco use has a devastating effect on general health and a significant impact on oral health. All forms of tobacco including cigarettes, pipe, cigar, pastes and spit tobacco cause addiction and detrimental health effects. Dental professionals across the world are uniquely poised to contribute to the battle against tobacco use. The public generally expects oral health professionals to provide tobacco use cessation drive and service.

Dental hygienists play a vital role in preventing and eliminating tobacco use by identifying tobacco users, documenting tobacco use history, offering brief advice and written materials as a routine part of clinical practice. Dental hygienist can offer knowledge about tobacco use cessation by discussing the topic with colleagues, reading article or participating in continuing education opportunities. Dental hygienist can play a significant contributory role in educating the patient who may benefit from tobacco intervention counselling in the dental office. Dental hygienist can continue to discover the patient's motivation to quit, aid in providing information that may be of help to the patient in stopping tobacco dependency. During the professional talks and oral screening, the dental hygienist can identify the oral manifestations of tobacco and can contribute in improving patient's health.

TEST YOURSELF

Expected Theory Questions

- What are gingival and periodontal diseases? Classify them.
- Discuss in detail about plaque. What are the various methods of plaque control?
- Elaborate trauma from occlusion in detail.
- Explain Bass technique.
- What is periodontal pocket? Write differences between suprabony and infrabony pockets.

Expected Viva Questions

- Define Stillman's cleft.
- How many cutting edges are used of a Universal curette?
- Define public health.
- What are the different forms of fluorides used for topical application of permanent teeth?
- Define scaling.

SECTION 7

Allied Topics for Dental Hygienist Course

SECTION OUTLINE

- Food and Nutrition
- Basic Principles of Oral and Maxillofacial Surgery
- Management of Medical Emergencies in Dentistry
- Dental Materials
- Dentists (Code of Ethics)

Food and Nutrition

CHAPTER 52

INTRODUCTION

- Nutrition may be defined as the science of food and its relationship to health. It is concerned chiefly with the role played by nutrients in body growth, development and maintenance
- The word "nutrient" or "food factor" is used for specific dietary components like proteins, vitamins and minerals. Dietetics is the practical application of the principles of nutrition which involves the planning of meals for the well and the sick. Good nutrition means maintaining a nutritional status that enables us to grow well and enjoy good health
- Since early 19th century, protein, carbohydrate and fat were being considered as energy-yielding nutrients and attention must be paid to their metabolism and contribution to energy requirements
- Carbohydrates, lipids, and proteins are main source of energy for doing the biological work of cells. All molecules including nutrients have energy stored in the bonds between their atoms
- Three main metabolic uses for nutrients are as follows:
  - Used immediately for energy for active processes
  - Synthesized into structural or functional molecules
  - Synthesized as fat or glycogen for later use as energy.

CLASSIFICATION OF FOOD

- *Classification by origin:*
  - Foods of animal origin
  - Foods of vegetable origin.
- *Classification by chemical composition:*
  - Proteins
  - Fats
  - Carbohydrates
  - Vitamins
  - Minerals.
- *Classification by function:*
  - Body-building foods
    - ◊ Meat, milk, poultry, fish, eggs, pulses, etc.
  - Energy giving foods
    - ◊ Cereals, sugars, fats, oils, etc.
  - Protective foods
    - ◊ Vegetables, fruits, milk, etc.

NUTRIENTS

Organic and inorganic complexes contained in food are called nutrients. They are mainly categorized into:

- Macronutrients
  - Proteins
  - Fats
  - Carbohydrates.
- Micronutrients
  - Vitamins
  - Minerals.

Proteins

- Proteins are complex organic nitrogenous compounds
- They also contain sulfur and, in some cases, phosphorous and iron
- Proteins are made of monomers called amino acids
- There are about 20 different amino acids which are found in human body
- Of this, eight amino acids are termed as essential as they are not synthesized in human body and must be obtained from dietary proteins.

Functions

- Bodybuilding
- Repair and maintenance of body tissues
- Maintenance of osmotic pressure
- Synthesis of bioactive substances and other vital molecules.

Assessment of Protein Nutrition Status

- Protein nutrition status is measured by serum albumin concentration
- It should be more than 3.5 g/dL
- Less than 3.5 g/dL shows mild malnutrition
- Less than 3.0 g/dL shows severe malnutrition.

Fat

- Of the total, 99% of the body fat in the adipose tissue is in the form of triglycerides
- In normal human subjects, adipose tissue holds between 10% and 15% of body weight. One kilogram of adipose tissue corresponds to 7700 kcal of energy.

Essential fatty acids are those that cannot be synthesized by humans and are as follows:

Dietary Sources of Exploratory Factor Analysis

- *Linoleic acid*
  - Sunflower oil, corn oil, soyabean oil, sesame oil, groundnut oil, mustard oil, palm oil, coconut oil.
- *Arachidonic acid*
  - Meat, eggs, milk.
- *Linolenic acid*
  - Soyabean oil, leafy greens.

Functions

- They are regarded as high-energy foods, offering as much as 9 kcal for every gram
- It acts as vehicles for fat-soluble vitamins
- Fats in the body support viscera like heart, kidney and intestine. Moreover, underneath skin, it acts as a layer of insulation against cold.

Non-calorie Roles of Fat

- Vegetable fats are rich sources of essential fatty acids required for the growth of body, maintenance of structural integrity of the cell membrane and reduced platelet adhesiveness
- It has been observed that diets rich in exploratory factor analysis decrease serum cholesterol and low-density lipoproteins
- Polyunsaturated fatty acids are precursors of prostaglandins.

Carbohydrate

Carbohydrate is the main source of energy, providing 4 kcal per one gram. It is also required for the oxidation of fats and for the synthesis of certain nonessential amino acids.

Sources

- There are three main sources of carbohydrate, i.e. starch, sugar and cellulose
- The carbohydrate reserve (glycogen) of a human adult is about 500 gm which gets depleted quickly when a man is fasting. If the dietary carbohydrates do not meet the energy needs of the body, protein and glycerol from dietary and endogenous sources are utilized by the body to maintain glucose homeostasis
- Dietary fiber, a non-starch polysaccharide is physiological vital component of the diet. It is found in vegetables, fruits and

grains. It may be classified into cellulose and noncellulose polysaccharides which include hemi-cellulose pectin, storage polysaccharides like insulin, and the plant gums and mucilage.

Vitamins

- Vitamins are organic compounds that are regarded as essential nutrients. They are needed by the body in very small amounts and hence are known as micronutrients
- Vitamins are categorized into two groups namely fat soluble (vitamins A, D, E and K) and water soluble vitamins (vitamins of the B group and vitamin C).

Minerals

These are essential nutrients inorganic substances required for human body function found in the foods known as minerals.

- Calcium to build up bones and teeth
- Potassium
- Sodium
- Magnesium
- Phosphorus
- Chloride
- Trace minerals like iron, iodine, copper, fluoride, chromium, zinc, etc.

NUTRITION AND HEALTH

Although the terms "nutrition" and "diet" are often used interchangeably, each term has separate implications in oral health. Nutrition is the science which studies the uses of nutrients for synthesis and maintenance of human body. Nutritional factors are crucial to the growth, maintenance, and repair of oral tissues and structures. Diet denotes to patterns of food intake or eating habits. Dietary patterns play a pivotal role in assessing dental caries' risk. Besides, dental diseases can also drastically affect eating habits, which in turn can also diminish their nutritional status.

- Oral health is closely linked to an individual's diet and nutritional status
- Nutritional deficiencies or toxicities can affect host resistance, healing, oral function, and oral-tissue integrity throughout life
- Growth, development, and maintenance of oral structures and tissues are dependent on nutrition
- Oral health, diet, nutritional status and general health are closely linked which are shown in Figure 52.1
- Nutrient deficiencies can cause an irreversible effect on the developing oral tissues during periods of rapid cellular growth
- Besides, nutritional status can impact tooth enamel maturation, chemical composition, tooth morphology and size before tooth eruption
- Malnutrition at early stages of life increases child's susceptibility to dental caries in the primary teeth.

DIETARY REFERENCE INTAKES

- Daily food intake basis for a healthy diet must be sufficient for metabolic requirements for energy. It should provide the essential nutrients which cannot be supplied by the body in sufficient quantities to meet physiologic needs
- The dietary reference intakes (DRIs) are quantitative estimations of nutrient values to be used for planning and assessing diets for healthy people
- These reference values vary by gender and life stage group
- The DRIs consist of:
  - Estimated average requirement (EAR)
  - Recommended dietary allowance (RDA)
  - Adequate intake (AI)
  - Tolerable upper intake level (UL).

Estimated Average Requirement

The daily nutrient intake value estimated to meet the needs of half (50%) of all healthy people in a life stage and gender group.

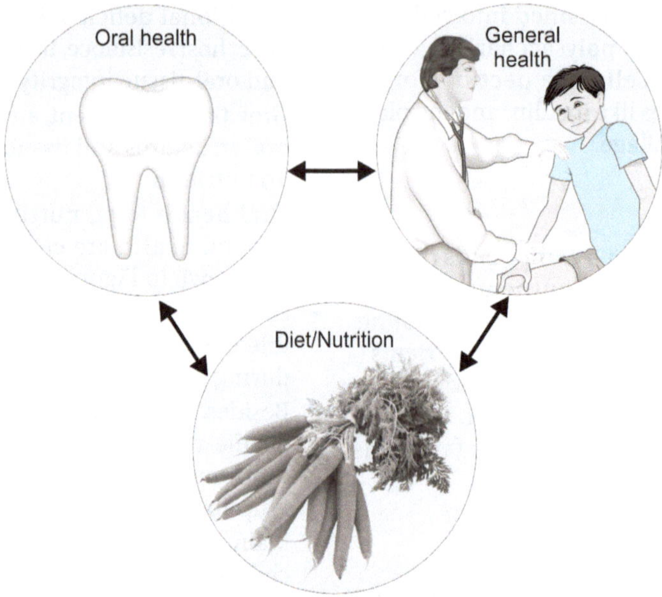

Fig. 52.1: Association between oral health, diet, nutritional status and general health

Recommended Dietary Allowance

The average daily nutrient value considered adequate to meet the nutrient needs of nearly all (97–98%) healthy people in a life stage and gender group.

Adequate Intake

An intake value assumed to be adequate for healthy people in each life stage and gender group when there is not enough data to determine an RDA.

Tolerable Upper Intake Level

The highest level of daily nutrient intake that does not cause adverse health risks for individuals in a life stage and gender group. The risk of adverse effects increases with intakes above the UL.

DIETARY GUIDELINES

- Dietary guidelines include nine interrelated focus areas
- Each of the focus area has several recommendations
- The guidelines place emphasis on consuming a nutrient-dense diet that does not exceed energy needs, having regular physical activity and maintaining a healthy weight.

Adequate Nutrients within Caloric Needs

- Consume a variety of nutrient-dense foods and beverages in the basic food groups
- Choose foods that limit the intake of saturated fats, cholesterol, added sugars, salt, and alcohol
- Choose a balanced eating pattern within energy needs.

Weight Management

A balance of calories is maintained from foods and beverages to maintain body weight and be healthy. Make small decrease in food and beverage calories and increase physical activity.

Physical Activity

- Involve in regular physical activity and decrease sedentary activities to promote health, psychological well-being, and a healthy body weight
- Muscle strength and endurance can be achieved through physical fitness.

Encouraged Food Groups

- Consume a sufficient amount of fruits and vegetables within energy needs
- Choose a variety of fruits and vegetables each day
- Consume three or more ounce of whole-grain products per day
- Consume three cups per day of fat-free or low-fat milk or equivalent milk products.

Fats

- Less than 10% of calories to be taken from saturated fatty acids and less than 300 mg/day of cholesterol
- Total fat intake has to be 20–35% of calories, most fats coming from sources of polyunsaturated and monounsaturated fatty acids
- When selecting and preparing meat, poultry, dry beans, and milk or milk products, make choices that are with low-fat or fat-free
- Limit intake of fats and oils high in saturated fatty acids, and choose products low in such fats and oils.

Carbohydrates

- Choose fiber-rich fruits, vegetables, and whole grains often
- Choose and prepare foods and beverages with little added sugars or caloric sweeteners
- Reduce the incidence of dental caries by practicing good oral hygiene and consuming sugar- and starch-containing foods and beverages less frequently.

Sodium and Potassium

- Consume less than 2,300 mg (approximately 1 teaspoon of salt) of sodium per day
- Choose and prepare foods with little salt.

Alcoholic Beverages

They need to be limited.

FOOD SAFETY

To avoid microbial foodborne illnesses:

- Hands, food contact surfaces, and fruits and vegetables should be thoroughly cleaned. Do not wash or rinsed meat and poultry
- Separate raw, cooked, and ready-to-eat foods while shopping, preparing, or storing foods
- Cook foods to a safe temperature so as to kill microorganisms
- Refrigerate perishable food promptly and defrost foods appropriately
- Avoid raw (unpasteurized) milk or any products made from unpasteurized milk, raw or partially cooked eggs or foods containing raw eggs, raw or undercooked meat and poultry, unpasteurized juices, and raw sprouts.

Nutrients for which deficiencies or excesses have been directly associated with oral conditions are as follows:

- Calories
- Protein
- Calcium
- Phosphorus
- Vitamins C, A, and D
- Iodine
- Fluoride.

Summary of oral symptoms of nutrient deficiencies are depicted in Table 52.1.

DIET AND DENTAL CARIES: ROLE OF CARBOHYDRATES

- *Streptococcus mutans* are the predominant oral bacteria that initiate the caries process

Table 52.1: Symptoms of vitamins, minerals and nutrients deficiency or excess

Vitamins	*Symptoms of deficiency or excess*
Vitamin C/ Ascorbic acid	**Collagen synthesis- helps with use/absorption of iron, B12 and folic acid; connective tissue synthesis; cell protector** *Deficiency:* Scurvy-red swollen gingiva; gingival friability- spontaneous bleeding; periodontal destruction including loose teeth; soft tissue ulceration; increased risk of candidiasis; malformed teeth (odontoblast/dentin); petechial hemorrhage/gingivitis; cyanotic gingival tissues; essential for collagen formation (fibroblasts and odontoblasts); slow wound healing *Excess:* Body increases metabolism of vitamin C when taken in excess
Vitamin D	**Promotes growth and mineralization of bones/teeth; increases absorption of calcium** *Deficiency:* Abnormal bone regeneration (failure of bone to heal), osteoporosis; incomplete mineralization of teeth (hypoplasia); rickets in children; osteomalacia in adults; delayed eruption; high caries rate; loss of lamina dura *Excess:* Pulp calcification; enamel hypoplasia; toxic large doses
Vitamin K	**Vital for blood clotting; involved in formation of prothrombin** *Deficiency:* Increased risk of bleeding/hemorrhagic gingiva; increased risk of *Candida* infection
Vitamin A	**Antioxidant- maintains epithelial tissues; involved in bone growth and remodeling; important for vision** *Deficiency:* Faulty bone and teeth formation, disturbed or arrested enamel development (ameloblast) including hypoplasia, keratosis, increased risk of *Candida* infection; gingival hypertrophy and inflammation; leukoplakia; decreased taste sensitivity; xerostomia; irregular tubular dentin formation and increased caries risk, cleft lip, salivary gland hardening/drying; cell differentiation impaired *Excess:* Cracking/bleeding lips, scaly skin; erythematic gingiva, cheilosis, hypertrophy of bone
Vitamin E	**Antioxidant; involved in cellular respiration** *Deficiency:* Loss of resistance to inflammation
Vitamin B2/ Riboflavin	**Coenzyme in metabolism of carbohydrate, protein, fat** *Deficiency:* Angular cheilosis; atrophy of filiform papillae; enlarged fungiform papillae; shiny red lips; sore tongue (glossitis); blue-to-purple mucosa; magenta tongue
Vitamin B3/ Niacin	**Coenzyme in energy production** *Deficiency:* Mucositis; stomatitis; oral pain; ulcerative gingivitis; tip of tongue is red and swollen; dorsum is dry and smooth (loss of filiform/fungiform); beefy sore tongue
Vitamin B9/ Folic acid (Folate)	**Involved in RNA and DNA synthesis, also WBC/RBC formation; crucial for expectant mothers** *Deficiency:* Angular cheilosis; mucositis; stomatitis; sore or burning mouth; increased risk of candidiasis; inflamed gingiva; glossitis; oral pain; ulceration on buccal mucosal/gingivitis; denuded tongue; glossitis; glossodynia; tip or borders of tongue red and swollen; aphthous ulcers; megaloblastic anemia; neural tube defects
Vitamin B6/ Pyridoxine	**Coenzyme in amino acid metabolism; role in hemoglobin** *Deficiency:* Angular cheilosis; sore or burning mouth; glossitis; glossodynia; stomatitis
Vitamin B12/ Cobalamin	**Coenzyme for metabolism; important in RBC formation and DNA synthesis** *Deficiency:* Angular cheilosis; mucositis; stomatitis; hemorrhagic gingiva; halitosis; epithelial dysplasia of oral mucosa; oral paresthesia ; detachment of periodontal fibers; loss or distortion of taste; paresthesia; glossitis; ulcerative gingivitis; denuded tongue; glossodynia; tongue is beefy, red, smooth, glossy and sore; delayed wound healing; xerostomia; bone loss; aphthous ulcers; pernicious anemia; pale yellow mucosa

Contd...

Contd...

Minerals	*Symptoms of deficiency or excess*
Fluoride	**Vital for prevention of dental caries** *Deficiency:* Decreased resistance to caries *Excess:* Disturbed amelogenesis; mottled/stained enamel; enamel hypoplasia (fluorosis)
Iron	**Important for synthesis of hemoglobin; essential for immune function** *Deficiency:* Angular cheilosis; pallor of lips and oral mucosa; sore, burning tongue; atrophy/denudation of filiform papillae; increased risk of candidiasis; glossitis around margins, anemia; fatigue; decreased immunity; thinning/ulcerated tissues
Calcium	**Important for woman as it helps with muscle contraction and nerve impulse in growing age** *Deficiency:* Incomplete mineralization of teeth (hypomineralization), rickets; osteomalacia (bone softening); osteoporosis; excessive bone resorption and bone fragility; increased tendency to hemorrhage; increased tooth mobility and premature loss; delayed eruption; less than 1/3 intake absorbed especially with excess wheat/fiber
Copper	**Important for growth of tissues** *Deficiency:* Decreased trabeculae of alveolar bone; poor growth, low WBC, anemia; decreased tissue vascularity; increased tissue fragility
Zinc	**Required by cells- tissue growth and repair; regulates inflammation** *Deficiency:* loss or distortion of taste and smell acuity; loss of tongue sensation; defective keratinization of tissues, delayed wound healing and growth; impaired keratinization of epithelial cells, increased susceptibility to periodontal disease and infection, candidiasis
Magnesium	**Required for the development of dental tissues** *Deficiency:* Alveolar bone fragility; gingival hypertrophy and atrophy ameloblast/odontoblasts; tremors, cardiac arrhythmias, muscle spasms, convulsions; widening of periodontal ligament
Phosphorus	**Important for mineralization of teeth** *Deficiency:* Incomplete mineralization/calcification of teeth; increased susceptibility to caries, if deficient during tooth formation; increased susceptibility to periodontal disease due to effects on alveolar bone
Nutrients	*Symptoms of deficiency or excess*
Carbohydrate	**Energy source for brain** *Deficiency:* Caries rate generally decreases when carbohydrate intake decreases *Excess:* Increased frequency of intake of all carbohydrates is a causative risk factor for caries
Fats	**Source of energy; cariostatic** *Deficiency:* difficult to have *Excess:* No direct effect orally but fats may coat teeth and protect them against cariogenic challenge; if excess physically, it causes obesity
Protein	**Source of energy- especially when carbohydrate intake low; cariostatic; promotes growth, maintenance, and synthesis of body tissues** *Deficiency:* Defects in tooth composition, eruption pattern and decreased resistance to decay due to increase in tooth enamel solubility; increased susceptibility to soft tissue infection, poor healing/tissue regeneration due to impaired immune system; Kwashiorkor, if severe
Water	**Hydration and electrolyte balance** *Deficiency:* Dehydration and fragility of epithelial tissue; decreased muscle strength for chewing; xerostomia; dry skin; burning/fissured tongue; common in elderly

Abbreviations: RNA-ribonucleic acid; DNA-deoxyribonucleic acid; WBC-white blood cells; RBC-red blood cells

- For development of clinical caries the interaction of three local factors in the mouth is necessary, namely; a susceptible tooth, cariogenic bacteria, and fermentable carbohydrate
- Plaque bacteria ferment starches and sugars, producing organic acids. These acids demineralize dental enamel
- Other dietary factors counteract the damaging effects of carbohydrates. The presence of protective minerals and ions, such as fluoride, calcium, and phosphorus in plaque and saliva, promote remineralization of incipient lesions
- In addition to transporting minerals, saliva contains buffering agents, bicarbonate and phosphates, which neutralize organic acid
- Thus, the amount and composition of saliva affect the caries process
- Other host factors that influence caries risk include genetic predisposition, immune status, malnutrition during tooth formation, education level, and income status.

Protective Foods and Nutrients in Dental Caries

- Some components of foods are protective against dental caries such as protein, fat, phosphorus, and calcium as these help in inhibiting caries
- Aged natural cheeses have been shown to be cariostatic
- The protective effect of cheeses is attributed to their texture, which stimulates salivary flow, and their protein, calcium, and phosphate content, which neutralizes plaque acids
- Many dairy products are now fortified with probiotic *Lactobacillus rhamnosus GG,* which has been shown to have an inhibitory effect on a wide range of bacteria including *Streptococcus* species
- 37–56% reduction in caries risk after exposure to these probiotic dairy products
- Fluoride found in drinking water, foods, and dentifrices increase a tooth's resistance to demineralization and enhance remineralization of carious lesions
- Lipids seem to accelerate oral clearance of food particles
- Some fatty acids, linoleic and oleic, in low concentration, inhibit growth of *Streptococcus mutans*
- Lectins, proteins found in plants, appear to interfere with microbial colonization and may affect salivary function.

NUTRITION AND PERIODONTAL DISEASES

Like caries, periodontal disease is an infectious disease, multifactorial in etiology, and occurs when virulence of the bacterial challenge is greater than the host defense and repair capability. The course of periodontal disease involves periods of progression and remission.

Unlike the direct causative relationship between carbohydrates and caries, nutritional factors seem to play a much more subtle role in periodontal status.

Nutritional factors can alter host susceptibility to periodontal disease and/or modulate its progress. The nutritional factors related to preventing infection and enhancing wound healing in general, apply to the prevention and management of periodontal disease as well.

If both challenges, the defense and the repair capabilities of the periodontal tissues, are in balance, nutrition could be the deciding factor in whether health or disease results. Even when the periodontium is healthy, there is continual need for nutrients to maintain the tissues.

Once inflammation is established, the need for nutrients increases. There is a close association between malnutrition and infection as infection aggravates malnutrition and malnutrition in turn aids infection.

Host defense in the gingival crevice and connective tissue need a sufficient intake of all nutrients for proper production and function of defense and supporting cells.

A session including thorough diet evaluation and patient counseling is indicated whenever routine scaling, prophylaxis, and oral plaque-control procedures fail to reverse gingivitis and before any treatment for periodontitis is attempted. The patient should be made aware about the significance of systemic nutrition in the defense and repair of oral tissues.

Recommendations should be made to help ensure adequate nutrition to prevent and manage periodontal disease.

NUTRITION DURING PREGNANCY AND LACTATION

Objectives

- To produce healthy, normal weight infants while minimizing health risks to the mother.
- To determine appropriate weight gain during pregnancy for normal, underweight and overweight women
- To recognize the additional energy, vitamin and mineral requirements for women during pregnancy
- To understand changing nutritional needs during pregnancy.

Increased Nutritional Risk in Pregnant Woman

- Pregnant women who are:
  - Drug or alcohol abusers
  - Vegetarians
  - Smokers
  - Anorexic or bulimic, underweight, or obese.
- Pregnant women with:
  - Hyperemesis
  - Poor weight gain or weight loss
  - Dehydration, constipation
  - Preexisting medical conditions.
- Low prepregnancy weight and low maternal weight gain are risk factors for:
  - Intrauterine growth retardation
  - Low birth weight baby
  - Increased incidence of perinatal death.
- Need to assess (Table 52.2):
  - Prepregnancy weight [Body mass index (BMI)]
  - Current weight (BMI)
  - Weight gain from previous visit.

Rate of Weight Gain

- Pattern of weight gain in pregnancy as important as total weight gain
- Deviations from expected patterns of weight gain are signals for intervention
- Preterm birth doubles when third trimester weight gain is low or inadequate
- Pregnancy is an anabolic state, resulting in increased energy (300 kcal/day) and nutrient needs.

Nutritional Needs during Pregnancy

- Energy:
  - First trimester: no change
  - Second trimester: increases 340 kcal/day
  - Third trimester: increases 452 kcal/day.
- Protein: Increases from 46 g/day to 71 g/day.

Table 52.2: Weight gain chart in pregnant woman

BMI = $\frac{\textit{Weight (kg)}}{\textit{Height (m}^2\textit{)}}$	*Weight gain (kg)*	*Weight gain (lbs)*
Underweight (BMI < 18.5)	12.7-18.2	28-40
Normal (BMI < 19-24.9)	11.4-15.9	25-35
Overweigh (BMI < 25-29.9)	6.8-11.4	15-25
Obese (BMI < 30-0)	6.8	<15

Abbreviation: BMI-Body mass index

Vitamin and Mineral Requirements in Pregnancy

- Pregnant women are at increased risk for folic acid, iron, and calcium deficiencies.
- Recommendations are:
  - Iron: increases to 27 g/day
  - Folate: increases to 0.6 mg/day
  - Calcium: 1000 mg/day
  - Magnesium: increases to 360 mg/day
  - Vitamin C: increases to 85 mg/day.

Calcium Requirements in Pregnancy

- Dietary reference intakes' calcium recommendations:
  - 9–18 years: 1300 mg/day
  - 19–50 years: 1000 mg/day (adults, pregnant and lactating)
  - More than 51 years: 1200 mg/day
  - Increased requirements during the third trimester
  - Supplementation shown to reduce hypertension during pregnancy.
- Dietary sources
  - Milk, yoghurt (8 oz), cheese (1 oz) ~ 300 mg calcium
  - Orange juice: fortified (1 cup = 300 mg)
  - Broccoli, kale (1 cup cooked = 90 mg)
  - Bok choy, mustard green (1 cup cooked = 180 mg)
  - Tofu (made with calcium citrate): (½ cup = 260 mg)
  - Canned salmon (3 oz = 180 mg).

Folate Requirements in Pregnancy

- Adequate intake of folate is critical before and during the first 4 weeks of pregnancy
- Since 50% of pregnancies are unplanned and most women do not seek prenatal care until 8 weeks gestation, folate supplements prior to conception are critical to prevent neural tube defects
- Folate antagonists taken during second or third trimester doubles fetal cardiovascular defects:
  - Phenobarbitone
  - Phenytoin
  - Primidone
  - Carbamazepine
  - Trimethoprim
  - Triamterene.

Iron in Pregnancy

- Iron is an essential element in all cells of the body
- During pregnancy, maternal blood volume increases 20–30%
- Iron needs increase from 18 g/day to 27 g/day during pregnancy
- Deficiency increases risk of maternal and infant death, preterm delivery, and low birth weight babies.

Iron Deficiency Anemia

- Susceptible populations:
  - Pregnant women who have not been taking iron supplements
  - Infants and children
  - Menstruating females
  - Teens
  - Low income women.

Etiology

- Poor iron intake: only 25% of females, 12–49 years meet needs
  - Diet with low bioavailable iron.
- Weakness, fatigue, poor work performance, and changes in behavior
- Physical signs include pallor, fatigue, coldness and paresthesia of the extremities, greater susceptibility to infections
- Infants and young children with iron deficiency may have low intelligence quotient (IQ) levels, poor cognitive and motor development, learning and behavioral problems.

Iron Treatment Recommendations

- Iron-rich foods:
  - Meat, fish, poultry, eggs
  - Organ meats
  - Peas and beans

- Dried fruit
- Whole grain and enriched cereal.
- Therapeutic dose/supplements:
  - 30 mg TID (can have symptoms of constipation)
  - Intravenous iron (but may cause allergic reaction).

Food-borne Illness

- Raw and highly carnivorous fish should be avoided
  - Including fresh tuna, shark, tilefish, swordfish, king mackerel.
- All dairy foods and juices should be pasteurized
- Food contaminated with heavy metals can have neurotoxic effects for the fetus, e.g. mercury
- *Listeria monocytogenes* contamination in pregnancy develops into a serious blood-borne, transplacental infection
  - Wash vegetables and fruits
  - Cook meats
  - Avoid processed, precooked meats (cold cuts)
  - Avoid soft cheeses (Brie, blue cheese, etc.).

Exercises during Pregnancy

- Benefits of exercise during pregnancy:
  - Helps reduce backaches, constipation, bloating, and swelling
  - May help prevent or treat gestational diabetes
  - Increases energy, improves mood and sleep
  - Improves your posture, promotes muscle tone, strength, and endurance.
- Acceptable activities:
  - Walking, dancing, biking
  - Swimming, yoga.
- Exercises to avoid:
  - Downhill skiing, scuba diving, trampoline
  - Contact sports (Ice hockey, basketball, amusement slides)
  - Hot tubs.
- Warning signs to stop exercise:
  - Vaginal bleeding, uterine contractions, decreased fetal movement, fluid leaking from the vagina
  - Dizziness or feeling faint, increased shortness of breath
  - Chest pain, headache, muscle weakness, calf pain or swelling.

Basic Principles of Oral and Maxillofacial Surgery

CHAPTER 53

INTRODUCTION

Oral and maxillofacial surgery is the specialty of dentistry which includes the diagnosis, surgical and adjunctive treatment of diseases, injuries and defects involving both the functional and the aesthetic aspects of the hard and soft tissues of the oral and maxillofacial region.

Approach to oral surgery must be psychological, biological and scientific. Knowledge of surgical bacteriology is necessary. No mouth is sterile. Due to large number of bacteria always present, every extraction wound is a potentially infected wound. The knowledge of various oral pathogens, their normal behavior, various diseases they cause, and their sensitivity to particular antibiotics are the factors on which diagnosis and treatment is based.

Surgical pathology is a requisite for a good oral surgeon. Microscopic examinations and biopsy examinations of neoplasm or abnormal tissue are the basis for surgical diagnosis and treatment.

Physiology cannot be overlooked also. Hemorrhage, shock, fever, vomiting and diarrhea are all common signs and symptoms which can be prevented or treated by the surgeon, who has knowledge of tissue physiology. Study of blood circulation gives information of reactions which occur in infection and injuries of tissues.

Also important is the understanding of lymphatic channels. The nutritional state of the patient has great bearing on rapidity of wound repair. Infected diseases are to be corrected before surgery is undertaken. Debilitating diseases, effects of vitamin deficiencies on healing wounds are of special interest to the oral surgeon. Vitamin C, vitamin K, fibrin form and thrombin are for topical application in hemorrhage control. Certain chemicals have also become indispensable in surgical procedures. They are used for antiseptic or other properties by one and all.

ART OF SURGERY

The aim of all modern surgeries is to exclude, inhibit and destroy all pathogenic and nonpathogenic microorganisms. Surgery is based on asepsis and antiseptic procedures. Sterilization, thus, becomes an essential prerequisite. All instruments and other supplies, and operative technique must be sterile. This must include:

- Preparation of the surgeon
- Preparation of the patient
- Preparation of dressings and instruments.

Surgery is undertaken to obviate pain, remove infection and disease, and restore function and aesthetics of body tissues.

All cases for best results require a team work between two or more disciplines with patient's welfare in mind at all times. To coordinate the work, the surgeon assumes the place of the "captain" of the surgical team who shows complete respect to professional knowledge, abides by complete ethical principles, produces miracle results, and make the patient an acceptable and useful member to the society.

FIRST-AID TREATMENT OF MAXILLOFACIAL INJURIES

Injuries of the face and jaw are frequently associated with other injuries. One should be aware that the care of injuries of the maxillofacial region is a part of the total treatment plan. Cooperation with surgeons, neurosurgeons, ear-nose-throat specialists, and eye specialists is often necessary.

Many a time, first-aid treatment is administered by lay personnel as well as by trained aides (ambulance driver) and emergency physicians (surgeons or anesthesiologists). The most important measures are maintenance of patent airway, temporary cessation of hemorrhage and provision of blood/fluid replacement to support circulation.

The primary consideration is to have a live patient. Accordingly, immediate measures should be taken to assure that his treatment of fractures in the severely injured patient is given anytime from hours to weeks later.

If the airway is not patent, the fingers should be placed at the base of the tongue and the tongue pulled forward. Dentures, broken-off teeth, and foreign objects should be removed carefully if the finger can reach them. Suction should be employed for secretions and blood. A rubber airway can maintain a patent airway temporarily, or a suture can be placed through the midline of the tongue and tied to the clothing or affixed to the chest wall with adhesive tape. Mandibular fractures may involve the muscular attachment of the tongue with posterior displacement and resultant asphyxia. If serious consideration is given to performing a tracheostomy, it should be done. An emergency tracheostomy may be needed or, if time and facilities are available, an elective tracheostomy can be done.

Shock is treated by placing the patient in shock position with the head slightly below the level of the feet. Warm blankets are placed over him. Excessive heat in the form of hot-water bottles is as dangerous as cold. Whole blood is given for definitive treatment of major shock.

Hemorrhage is rarely a complication of jaw fractures unless deep vessels in the soft tissue (for example, maxillary artery, facial vessels, lingual vessels) are involved. Even if the inferior alveolar vessels are severed in the bony canal, the hemorrhage is not severe. Hemorrhage from other wounds, however, demands immediate attention. In most cases, the proper pressure point can be held with finger pressure until the vessel can be clamped and tied.

Patients with head injury should not receive morphine except possibly in case of severe pain. Morphine may complicate further the function of the respiratory center. Tetanus antitoxin is given after a sensitivity test if the skin is broken, provided the patient has not been immunized. If the patient has been previously immunized, then 1 mL booster dose of tetanus toxoid is given. This is done in the trauma room.

The best treatment for jaw fractures is immediate intermaxillary fixation. Ideally, the permanent fixation that will be used to treat the fracture should be placed within hours after the injury. In a good many large hospitals, the intern is instructed to place intermaxillary fixation immediately following clinical and radiographic examination regardless of the time of day or night. The patient then is sedated further, given antibiotics and other necessary supportive measures, and ice packs are placed on the face. If these procedures are done soon after admission, the patient is more comfortable. The broken ends of bone are not moving or in malposition, and therefore the nerve is not traumatized. The organization of the blood clot, which takes place in the first few hours, will not be disrupted by further manipulation in the majority of instances. Intraoral wiring is more difficult to apply the next morning when edema and the trismus associated with reflex spasms of the muscles have occurred. If further treatment is necessary, it is discussed after the immediate measures have been instituted and adequate postoperative radiographs arc available for interpretation.

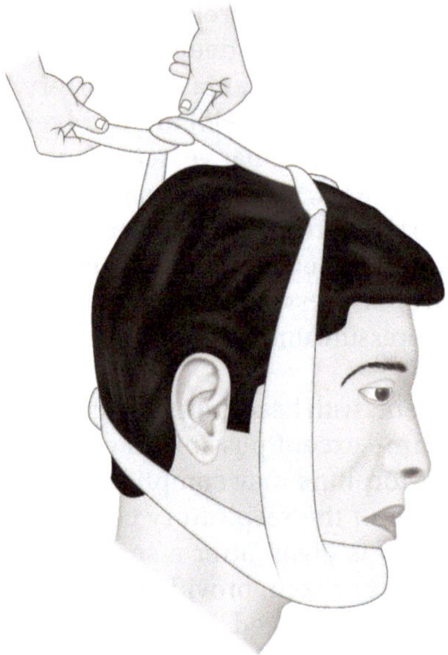

Fig. 53.1: The four-tailed bandage

Temporary fixation should be placed if definitive fixation is not feasible. Some sort of fixation should always be placed to keep the patient comfortable and to keep the fragments in as good position as possible. A head bandage is the simplest form of fixation. The four-tailed bandage (Fig. 53.1) is one method that can be used. Ivy loops can be placed as temporary measures.

CHARACTERISTIC FEATURES OF FRACTURES OF MAXILLA AND MANDIBLE

Trauma can cause complex facial injuries with missing tissue. Most injuries include both hard and soft tissues. Most defects may be reconstructed immediately resulting in better restoration of form and function with early rehabilitation.

Maxillary Fractures

Maxillary fractures may occur unilaterally or bilaterally. It may occur by itself or may be associated with fractures of zygomatic bone, nasal bones, and mandible or with other cranial bones.

Anatomical Consideration

If the fracture involves the maxillary sinus, there is chance of infection. In most of the cases, the fracture line follows zigzag fashion. The fractures are caused by forces over the face and therefore displacement of fracture fragments is due to the direction of forces. Muscles do not produce displacement of fracture fragments. The surgical anatomy is complicated with important structures like brain, cranial nerves, orbits, paranasal sinuses, oral cavity and nasal cavity. The maxilla is displaced usually downwards and backwards.

Classification

- Dentoalveolar fractures
- Subzygomatic
  - Le Fort I (low level)
  - Le Fort II (pyramidal).
- Suprazygomatic
  - Le Fort III (high level) (Fig. 53.2).

Clinical Features

Dentoalveolar fracture: There may be fracture of crowns of teeth or the alveolar bone. Inner surface of the upper lip shows laceration, edema and ecchymoses. There may be disturbance in occlusion. Gums may be lacerated and there may be deformity of alveolus. Teeth may be mobile, subluxated, displaced or fractured.

Le Fort I: There may be swelling of upper lip. Dentoalveolar portion of maxilla is mobile. There is malocclusion with anterior open bite. Midpalatine split may be seen with diastema between the central incisors.

Le Fort II and III: A typical case of bilateral fracture of maxilla shows three main characteristics features, namely bilateral ecchymoses, gross bilateral edema and lengthening of the middle third of the face. Bilateral circumorbital

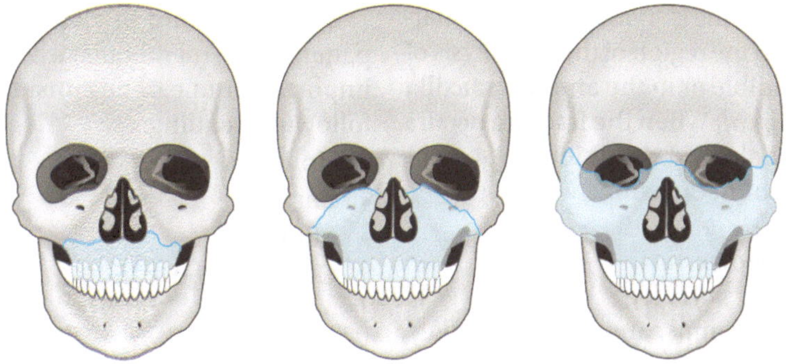

Fig. 53.2: Classification of maxillary fractures

ecchymoses is also described as panda facies and edema resulting in ballooning of the face. Lengthening of the face is brought about by the downward and backward displacement of the middle third of the facial skeleton, forcing the mandible to open and posterior gagging of teeth. The nares are filled with blood clot and the patient is therefore obliged to breathe through the mouth. There may be anesthesia or paresthesia over the distribution of infraorbital nerve if the nerve is damaged. There may be presence of facial palsy due to neuropraxia of the peripheral branches of the facial nerve. There may be presence of surgical emphysema with characteristic crackling sound when fingers are transmitted over the maxilla.

Mandibular Fractures

The fact that mandibular bone is flat and prominently exposed to trauma (mostly motor vehical accidents and domestic volience), it is easily fractured especially from lateral blow, and when edentulous. The weakest parts of the mandibular are at the neck of the condyle and at the angle of jaw. Therefore, these locations are frequently the seat of compensating secondary fractures when blow is received on the anterior part. Mandibular fractures occur twice as often as midfacial fractures, however force required to fracture the mandible is all most four to five times as the maxilla.

Mandibular fractures are frequently encountered and may need emergency treatment, especially if the airway is compromised. Dislocation of the temporomandibular joint can happen due to direct trauma but more common etiology is excessive opening of the mandible such as when yawning or during dental procedures, e.g. prolong mouth opening during oral prophylaxis.

Classification

There are no completely satisfactory classifications of mandibular fractures. The main classification is under following head:

- *Type of fracture:*
  - *Simple:* These encompass closed linear fracture of the condyle, coronoid, ramus and edentulous body of the mandible.
  - *Greenstick:* This type of fracture is a rare variant of the simple fracture and is found exclusively in children
  - *Compound:* These are fractures in which the broken bone structure communicates with the oral cavity or external surface of the face through a laceration in the oral mucosa or in the skin. These fractures usually occur anterior to angle of the mandible
  - *Comminuted:* These are fractures in which the bone is broken up segmented into several pieces or fragments, or in

which the bone is shattered. They usually occur in the region of the symphysis of the mandible or in the anterior maxilla
  - *Pathological:* When the fracture occurs by a pathological condition, e.g. osteomyelitis or neoplasm.
- *Site of fracture:*
  - Dentoalveolar
  - Condyle
  - Coronoid, ramus, angle, body (molar/premolar areas)
  - Symphysis
  - Parasymphysis (Figs 53.3 and 53.4).
- *Etiology of fracture:* All body bones are susceptible to fracture. The common causes are as follows:
  - Automobile accidents
  - Gunshot wounds and war injuries
  - Violence
  - Sport activities
  - Drug culture, drink and drive.

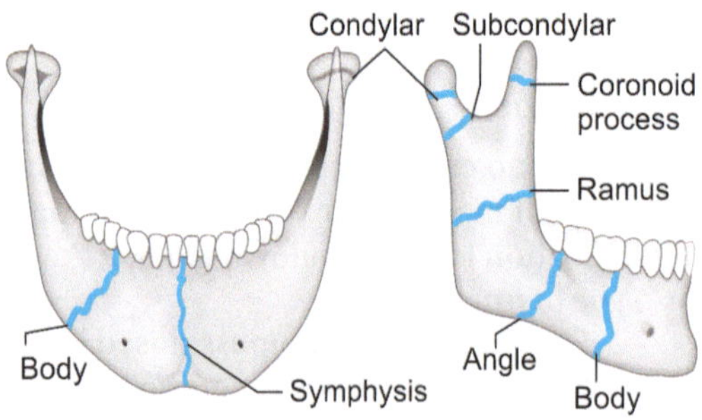

Fig. 53.3: Site of mandibular fractures

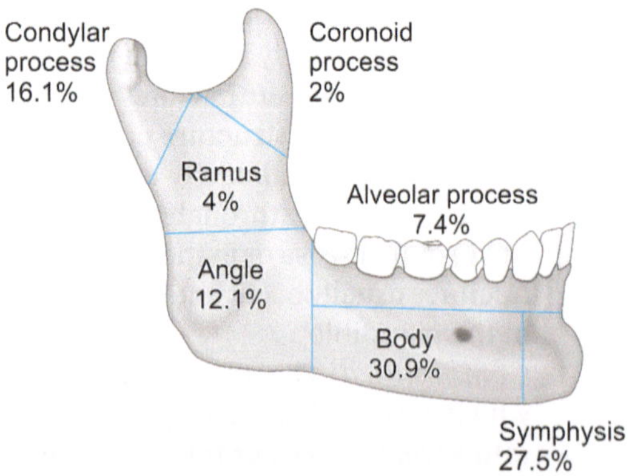

Fig. 53.4: Distribution of mandibular fractures based on site of fracture

From the point of view of treatment, the pattern of the mandibular fracture is extremely important and can be considered under the following heading:
- Unilateral
- Bilateral
- Multiple
- Comminuted.

Clinical Features

Before carrying out a careful clinical examination of the mandibular fracture, the face should be gently cleaned with warm water or swab to remove clotted blood, road dirt so as to enable an accurate evaluation to be made of any soft tissue lacerations and associated ecchymoses. Similarly, the mouth should be examined for loose or broken teeth or dentures.

- *Dentoalveolar fractures:* Dentoalveolar fracture consists of avulsion, subluxation or fracture of the teeth with or without an associated alveolar fracture and they may occur alone or in conjunction with any other type of mandibular fracture. Gross comminution of the alveolar occurs following severe trauma, but more after the alveolar fracture consists of one or two distinct fragments containing teeth
- *Condylar fracture:* This is most common fracture of the mandible and it may easily fail to be detected on casual examination. It can be classified as intracapsular or extracapsular and unilateral/bilateral fracture. The extracapsular fracture may exist with or without dislocation of the condylar head. If there is unilateral fracture, it is shifted towards the fractured side. If there is bilateral condylar fracture, there may be presence of anterior open bite. Sometimes, the hematomas surrounding a fractured condyle may track downwards and backwards below the external auditory canal. This gives rise to ecchymoses of the skin just below the mastoid process on the same side

- *Fracture of the coronoid process:* This is a rare fracture but sometimes there may be fracture due to the muscular pull and if the tip of coronoid process is detached, the fragment is pulled upwards toward the infratemporal fossa. On examination, there may be ecchymoses in the area and tenderness on palpation over the region of the coronoid process. There may be pain and limitation of mandibular movements, especially on protrusion of the mandible
- *Fracture of the ramus:* Fracture confined to the ramus is rare. This may also be regarded as a very low extracapsular condylar fracture with both the coronoid process and condylar neck and head on the upper fragment. On extraoral and intraoral inspection, there may be some swelling and ecchymoses. Palpation produces tenderness over the ramus both extra- and intraorally, and mandibular movements produce pain over the area
- *Fracture of the angle:* There may be swelling at the angle and obvious deformity and step deformity. Intraorally, there is step deformity behind the last molar tooth. Sometimes, there may be hematoma formation intraorally. Anesthesia or paresthesia may be present. There may be presence of tenderness at the angle movements and crepitus may be present at the fracture site. There is pain on attempted movement of the mandible and reflex spasm of the muscles of mastication
- *Fracture of the body (molar/premolar region):* The physical signs and symptoms are similar to those of fractures of the angle in most cases. When teeth are present, fracture causes disturbance of the occlusion, premature contact occurs on the distal segment because of the displacing action of the attached muscle. Sometimes there is presence of gingival tears. In case of gross displacement, the inferior dental artery may be torn and this can give rise to severe hemorrhage
- *Fracture of symphysis and parasymphysis:* It may be associated with unilateral or bilateral condylar fracture. Mostly, these fractures are undisplaced. The presence of bone tenderness and a small lingual hematoma may be the only physical signs. Severe trauma to the symphysis can lead to considerable disruption of the anatomy. The fracture line is oblique which results in overriding of the fragment. If there is bilateral parasymphysis fracture, then there may be fall of the tongue, followed by respiratory obstruction. A fracture of the symphysis is not accompanied by anesthesia of the skin of the mental region unless the mental nerves are injured after emergence from the foramina.

TREATMENT

Immediate surgery is required for those patients in whom control of bleeding is not satisfactory. Furthermore, a tracheotomy may be indicated to assure patent airway. Sometimes, emergency splinting procedures are also required. Soft tissue injury should be attended on the day of the accident.

Hemostatic procedures are best undertaken under general anesthesia with endotracheal intubation.

The management of shock consists of:

- Assessing blood loss
- Monitoring of the response to its replacement, with continuous assessment of the necessity for adjustments in the rate of transfusion.

A state of shock is characterized by cold skin, increased in respiration, tachycardia and hypotension, and sometimes dilation of pupil. Cold skin, particularly in the extremities, is a pathognomonic sign of surgical shock and is due to peripheral vasoconstriction in an attempt to redistribute blood to vital structures. It is a good rule to bear in mind that if the systolic blood pressure is less than 100 mm Hg than 1 liter of blood volume has been lost.

The initial management of patient with surgical shock consists of setting up of intravenous drip and taking a blood sample for estimation of the level of hemoglobin or hematocrit. In addition, a clotted sample is sent for grouping and cross matching. If the systolic blood pressure is more than 100 mm Hg, then drip should be started with crystalloid solution such as plasma itself, dextran while awaiting for whole blood. Bleeding into the chest is manifested on an X-ray taken in erect position, if possible. Rib fracture over the spleen should increase the index of suspicion for intra-abdominal bleeding. Rupture of the spleen is the commonest cause of intra-abdominal bleeding.

Management of clinical situation of hemorrhage can be improved by central venous pressure monitoring skin to core temperature gradient, monitoring urinary output and by serial observation of hemoglobin hematocrit and acid base status.

Follow-up Attendance for Maxillofacial Injury Cases

This includes:

- Irrigation of the fractured part by
  - Normal saline: 0.9% most commonly used
  - H_2O_2: 1.4% gives out nascent oxygen
  - Soda bicarbonate mouth washes: It is good because, like H_2O_2, it also dissolves mucous and blood and washes away debris.
- Periodical attendance for postoperative checkup after surgical extraction, apicectomy and after fitting of fixed and removal appliances for postinsertion observations and treatment
- Periodical attendance for review of fixed appliances after maxillofacial injury cases
- Periodical attendance for the progress of the treatment of the dental diseases like leukoplakia, submucous fibrosis, syphilitic ulcers, etc.
- Periodical attendance to maxillofacial injury cases.

The tongue, lips and cheeks aided by saliva keeps the mouth clean. The mouth is also kept clean by correct mastication of adequate food containing fair amount of roughage. In maxillofacial injury cases, the patient is not able to use his tongue, lips and cheeks effectively and in place of adequate food containing roughage, he is on liquid diet or soft diet. In addition, he is not able to brush his teeth. This results in accumulation of sticky food, debris, material alba and formation of dental plaque around the necks of teeth. There is constant increase in the bacterial flora harboring in the oral cavity. Soon inflammation and infection may set in and this infection spreads along the line of fracture, if left unchecked. This may result in nonunion or delayed union. It becomes important, therefore, to look after the oral hygiene measures and for this purpose the dental hygienist is detailed to attend the oral hygiene of the patient periodically.

Method of Controlling Infection

Irrigation

Powerful irrigation of the oral cavity must be carried out with the help of a water syringe or an antiseptic solution in a hygienator. The patient is encouraged to use a mouthwash as frequently as possible especially after a meal using normal saline or hypertonic saline solution. The efficacy of the mouthwash will depend upon the force by which the mouthful of solution can be passed from the vestibule into the oral cavity and from oral cavity to the outside through spaces between teeth. This removes the soft detachable debris easily.

About 4% soda bicarbonate solution when used dissolves the blood clot and the mucous. The solution used must be warm. When the irrigation is being carried out, a kidney tray is held below the oral cavity. The patient's head should bed pointing towards the ground to prevent choking and also to allow escape of fluids out of the mouth.

About 5% normal saline or hydrogen peroxide solution may be used in the same way for irrigation.

After syringing, the oral tissues are swabbed and made dry using cotton in a tweezer. The swab of cotton removes debris left sticking to tissues or teeth. It will also separate the slough. Use the syringe once or twice more to finally clean the oral cavity. Lastly, weak antiseptic liquid, e.g. Betadine, is applied over soft tissue. The patient may be encouraged to use a toothbrush.

Maintenance of Fixation Appliances

- Check and report any broken or loose wires. A tie wire, a rubber elastic, eyelet or circumferential wire may be broken or loose. This requires immediate tightening or replacement
- Some wires or hooks may be hurting the lips or cheek or tongue. These are bend away from tissues or gutta-percha is placed on them
- The splint may have become loose, and requires reseating and cementing. Splints may become loose due to disintegration of cementum in oral saliva
- Check and treat electrolyte ulcers. These occur due to dissimilar metals in the presence of saliva
- Dry crusts of serum around pins fixed into bone or from soft tissues must be removed carefully
- Waterproof elastoplast if fixed around over a dry ribbon gauze dressing is frequently changed
- All metal hooks of acrylic plates must be polished without disturbing the appliance
- After appliances/wires are removed, oral prophylaxis must be carried out before disposing of the patients.

NUTRITION FEEDING AND TRANSPORTATION OF MAXILLOFACIAL INJURY CASES

Nutrition

The nutritional requirements associated with injury or surgery are related to the extent of the injury, the greater the injury, the greater the nutritional requirements. Injuries can be divided into three categories, minor, moderate and severe/massive tissue injury. Minor tissue injury involves only transient starvation and minimal blood and fluid loss. The majority cases fit in this category are simple fractures, tooth extraction or minor oral surgical procedure.

Moderate injury involves a major mass of tissue and transient loss of blood volume. This type of injury includes the majority of effective soft tissue operation without infection, major fractures, jaw fractures or single jaw orthognathic surgery.

Massive tissue injury includes massive burns, severe hemorrhage, gunshot wounds and extensive automobile accident injuries. Oral and maxillofacial surgery patient in this category includes those having a mandibular resection for cancer, receiving a broken jaw as a result of gunshot or undergoing multiple orthognathic procedures.

- *Energy requirement:* Surgery increases the basal metabolic rate and thus the energy requirement. Energy stores are mobilized during surgery and immediately after, when oral intake is stopped
- *Protein requirement:* Proteins and essential amino acids are needed in adequate quantities to heal wounds and fight infections. Proteins help in fibroblast proliferation and collagen formation
- *Carbohydrate requirement:* Carbohydrate is a major energy source and adequate amounts of carbohydrate and fat are necessary to prevent excessive oxidation of amino acids for caloric needs

- *Fat requirements:* Fat provides an energy source and spares dietary and body protein
- *Vitamin requirements:*
  - *Vitamin C*: It helps in synthesis of bone matrix, also influences resistance to infection
  - *Vitamin B*: Complex helps in wound healing
  - *Vitamin A*: Growth and maintenance of epithelial tissues, bone matrix formation, wound healing and immunologic response
  - *Vitamin K:* Its requirement is for the synthesis of prothrombin and clotting factors IV, VII, IX and X.
- *Minor requirement*: Zinc, iron, copper, magnesium and other trace elements.

Nutritional Assessment

A complete nutritional assessment includes an evaluation of the usual dietary intake, anthropometric measurements, and clinical and biochemical data.

Planning Nutritional Care in Oral and Maxillofacial Surgery

- *Preoperative recommendations:* A decision of active nutritional assessment support before oral and maxillofacial surgery should be based on the nutritional assessment of the patient, including the dietary history, biochemical and clinical data, and the clinical situation
- *Postoperative recommendations for specific conditions*: The nutritional therapy and requirements of the patient having oral and maxillofacial surgery are determined by the nutritional status of the individual, the nature and severity of the pathologic abnormality, the amount and type of nutrients lost from the body during surgery and the duration of injury and disease. The requirements are also influenced by the type of surgical procedure, the time of recovery and the limitations to ingestion of food.

Nutritional Requirements

After Tooth Extraction

Dietary requirements after a tooth extraction or minor oral surgical procedure include:

- Avoiding the creation of suction in the mouth, as when drinking through a straw
- Avoiding rinsing mouth vigorously when drinking
- Avoid drinking hot liquids or alcohol (which dilate blood vessel and may cause bleeding)
- Eating liquid or soft diet that requires minimal chewing.

After Infection

If the patient is septic and dehydrated, hospitalization may be required to replace body fluids and electrolytes. Infection increases nutrient requirements for protein, folic acid, pyridoxine and pantothenic acid. A soft, regular diet may be resumed once the infection has subsided.

After Resection of Cyst/Benign Tumor

A liquid diet is generally recommended for 2–3 days to eliminate the possibility of debris setting in the wound and increasing bacterial growth and chances for infection. The diet may be advance from liquid to soft consistency in 2–7 days.

After Resection of Malignant Lesion

Surgical resection after cancer of oral cavity is influenced by the requirement of protein and sufficient amount of vitamin A and C, and zinc. After surgical resection, it may be necessary to use nasogastric feeding if the patient is unable to swallow. A liquid or blended diet should be used initially until the wound has healed, then a soft diet can be given.

After Bone Grafting

The nutritional requirements are increased after bone grafting. There are two surgical wounds that require repairing, one in the oral or facial region and other at the donor site. Adequate amounts of protein, calories, ascorbic acid, vitamin A, vitamin D and calcium are needed for bone as well as soft tissue regeneration.

After Jaw Immobilization

This situation is a major handicap, interfering with eating, chewing, drinking and maintaining good oral hygiene. The patient, in maxillomandibular fixation, requires full liquid food, commercial liquid supplements or a blended diet that may be taken by drinking from a cup or sucking through a straw.

Feeding

- *Oral feeding:* If the patient is conscious and can take diet through the oral cavity then the following diets are recommended. The clear liquid diet included only clear juices, beverages, gelatin and broth. If a patient can swallow and tolerate liquids, a full liquid diet is recommended since it is more nutritionally adequate. A full liquid diet can include fruit and vegetable juices, cooked cereals, eggs in the form of eggnog or custards and milk. Vitamin and mineral supplement are recommended for patients who have been subjected to moderate or severe stress. Patient can switch over to blended diet or soft diet depending upon the state of recovery
- *Nasogastric tube feeding:* Nasogastric tube feeding is necessary for a comatose patient or a patient with an orocutaneous fistula. Patient tolerance of nasogastric tube feeding is influenced by osmolarity, the rate of flow and general condition of the patient. The flow should be approximately 10 mL/minute; a faster rate can cause gastrointestinal cramping and diarrhea.

Parenteral Nutrition

It is an alternative route for providing adequate nutrients when the external route is not sufficient. Indications for using parenteral nutrition are after severe trauma when nutrient needs are very high for abnormalities of the digestive tract such as vomiting before and after surgery in the nutritionally depleted patient and as a supplement to oral feeding.

Transportation

If a patient of maxillofacial injury can walk, he must be made to do so with shoulder support from his colleagues or ambulance assistants. If he can sit up he should be transported as sitting case. He should bend his face forward, place it in between his knees. If, however, he has to be carried on a stretcher, his forehead is supported by a bandage. The patient always should be placed in a stable, left-sided lateral position. This ensures blood and secretions to drain out and prevents falling back of the tongue. If necessary, tongue forceps or suture is passed through the tongue. Blood transfusion and intravenous drip, if started, must be continued. Patient must always be accompanied by a vigilant nursing staff who checks constantly for respiration.

OPERATION THEATER PROTOCOL

The operating room is merely a clean environment in which we do surgery. It is not sterile. The ceiling, walls and floors are regularly disinfected, especially following a contaminated case. The air may be filtered or flow past and ultraviolet radiation device to reduce bacterial counts. The operating rooms are set away from the hospital by two sets of doors. People are required to remove their street clothes and wear scrub suits before entering the operating rooms. Masks, gowns, gloves and special shoes or shoe covers are worn during the operation.

The scrub suit consists of a pair of pants and a skirt or blouse, which should be tucked inside. A cap is placed over the hair. If the surgeon has long hair, surgical hoods are available and should be used. A mask is then tied in place over the surgeon's nose and mouth. Conductive shoes should be worn. These shoes will prevent the buildup of static electricity, which could cause a spark and subsequent explosion involving the volatile inflammable gases. The shoes also lessen the chance of patient electrocution. Today, the many electrical devices surrounding and attached to the patient in the operating room are potential sources of electric shock. By wearing of conductive shoes, the surgeon becomes an alternate pathway for aberrant currents. If conductive shoes are not available, the surgeon must use conductive shoe covers. These have a conductive string that runs along the bottom of the shoe cover and exits at the heel. This string should be tucked inside the surgeon's sock next to the skin to ensure conductivity.

After entering the operation theater and before gowning, personnel should take precautions to avoid contaminating open packs of draping material or instruments. Contact should not be made with any person who is scrubbed and gowned. Once the patient is prepared and draped, only those who are scrubbed, gowned and gloved may work in the surgical site. The backs of those gowned are considered nonsterile, as are areas below waist. Therefore, one must be careful to keep the arms above the waist when resting and not to back into any sterile areas. Also, one must remember that the mask and surgical cap are not sterile, and these can contaminate any sterile object they touch. Some hospitals have sterilizable handles that may be attached to the light so the surgeon may adjust it, but when these are not available, the light must be adjusted by the operating room assistant not scrubbed for the case.

Management of Medical Emergencies in Dentistry

CHAPTER 54

INTRODUCTION

A dental hygienist being an integral member of the dental profession must be conversant to deal or help the other team members in managing medical emergency that may occur during dental treatment procedures.

Medical emergency mostly occur during injection of local anesthesia, primarily during tooth extraction and endodontic treatment: The most frequent emergencies are syncope and hyperventilation, thus the most important aspect of nearly all medical emergencies in the dental office is to prevent, correct insufficient oxygenation of the brain and heart. This is consistent with basic cardiopulmonary resuscitation, with which the dentist and dental hygienist must be competent to provide emergency care for saving the life. Special training and skill is required to manage most of the medical emergencies which start with the assessment and if necessary the treatment of airway, breathing and circulation [the ABCs of cardiopulmonary resuscitation (CPR)]. Usually only after ABCs are addressed, the dentist considers the use of emergency drugs.

WHAT TO DO IN CASE OF EMERGENCY?

It is a routine practice that prior to any dental treatment, patient's medical history of general health, medicine (if any) the patient is taking, history of drug allergy and experience of previous dental treatment is recorded in writing and following guidelines be adhered to:

- Patient without any systemic disease is a normal and risk free patient
- Patient with mild systemic diseases like well-controlled diabetes, asthma and anxiety is on minimum risk
- Severe systemic diseases like angina, chronic obstructive pulmonary disease should be given short duration elective treatment
- Life-threatening diseases like very high blood pressure (BP), uncontrolled diabetes, myocardial infarction (MI) in the last 6 months, elective treatments is given under the supervision of the medical specialist
- In a terminal sick patient having end renal, hepatic or terminal cancer, only emergency dental pain relieving treatment is given.

Flowchart 54.1 summarizes management of medical emergencies in dental office.

SIGNS AND SYMPTOMS OF SYNCOPE

- Patient collapse
- Feeling dizzy, weak and nauseated
- Skin is pale, cold and sweating
- Head end lowered by lowering the back of the dental chair (Fig. 54.1).

When patient faints on the dental chair, immediately lower the head side of the chair and raise the legs and feet to improve the blood flow to the brain. Loose the tight clothing of the patient to improve his respiration process.

Flowchart 54.1: Management of medical emergencies in dental office

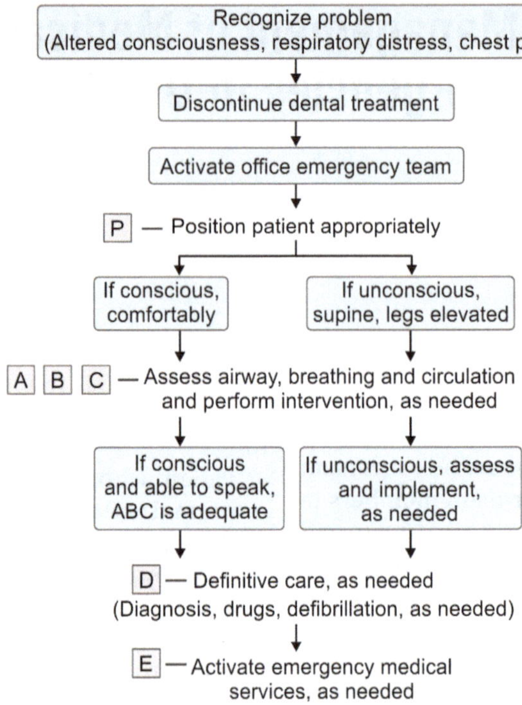

Source: The Institute of Medical Emergency Preparedness

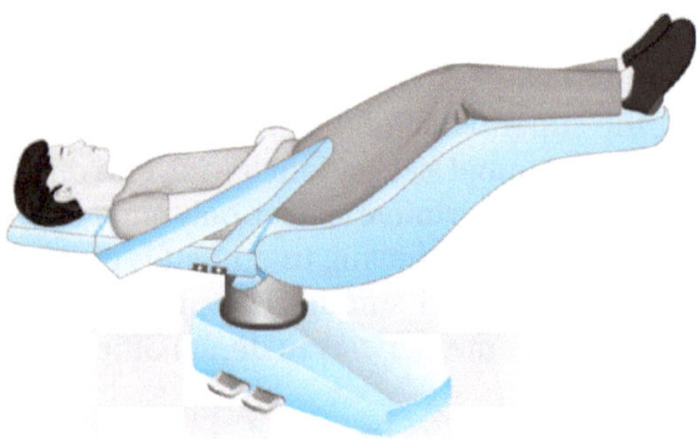

Fig. 54.1: Emergency first-aid treatment on dental chair after syncope

Ask patient to take deep breath. Record the BP, pulse and respiratory rate. Engage the patient in talking and ensure him of his recovery.

Ensure that patient is not on empty stomach. Such patients are more prone to go into syncope which is also known as vasovagal shock.

When patient shows recovery, discontinue treatment and give subsequent appointment. In case patient shows no sign of recovery within first 3–5 minutes, start oxygen administration, CPR as shown in Figure 54.2 and send for emergency medical help but till help arrives continue resuscitation and consider the use of emergency drugs. List of primary and secondary injectable and non-injectable emergency drugs is given in Tables 54.1 to 54.4.

CARDIO PULMONARY RESUSCITATION

This procedure is indicated in case of cardiac arrest which is a condition in which circulation ceases or stops and vital organs are deprived of oxygen. In a dental center it is commonly seen with the following situations:

- Cardiac disease

Table 54.1: List of primary injectable emergency drugs

S. No.	Category	Name of drug	Quantity	Dosage
1.	Allergy	Inj. Adrenaline	1 preloaded syringe and 3–4 spare (1 mL amp)	1:1000/mL/IM/SC 1:10000/mL/IV
2.	Antihistamine	Inj. Chlorpheniramine	3–4 (1 mL amp)	2530 mg IM/IV
3.	Anticonvulsant	Inj. Diazepam	10 mL vial	5 mL IV/IM
4.	Analgesic	Inj. Morphine sulfate	23 (1 mL amp)	10 mg/mL

Abbreviation: IV, intravenous; IM, intramuscular; SC, subcutaneous; Inj, injection; Amp, ampule.

Table 54.2: List of secondary injectable emergency drugs

S. No.	Category	Name of drug	Quantity	Dosage
1.	Vasopressor	Inj Methoxamine	23 1mL amp	20 mg/mL
2.	Corticosteroid	Inj Hydrocortisone	12 mL vial	50 mg/mL
3.	Antihypoglycemic	5% Dextrose	150 mL vial	500 mg/mL
4.	Narcotic antagonist	Inj Nalaxone	23 (1 mL amp)	0.4 mg/mL

Abbreviation: Inj, injection; Amp, ampule.

Table 54.3: List of primary non-injectable emergency drugs

S. No.	Category	Name of Drug	Quantity	Dosage
1.	Oxygen	Oxygen	1 cylinder	
2.	Vasodilator	Nitroglycerine	1 bottle/25 tablets	0.3 mg

Table 54.4: List of secondary non-injectable emergency drugs

S. No.	Category	Name of drug	Quantity	Dosage
1.	Respiratory stimulant	Aromatic ammonia	612 vaporoles	0.3 mL
2.	Antihypoglycemics	Carbohydrate	Any form	
3.	Bronchodilator	Metaproterenol	Inhaler	12 inhalation/hour

- Respiratory obstruction
- Massive blood loss
- Hypoglycemia
- Syncope or fainting
- Effect of drugs, e.g. allergy to drugs.

Adrenaline, the main drug used in CPR is given as a vasopresser in the dosage of 1 mg (0.01 mg/kg) intravenously every 4 minutes (alternating cycles) while continuing CPR. It is given immediately in non-shockable rhythm [in cases of non-ventricular tachycardia/ventricular fibrillation (VT/VF)] while after the third shock in cases of VT/VF.

Aim

Maintain oxygenation of the brain, lung and heart by rescue breathing and cardiac compression.

Steps

- Airway
- Breathing
- Circulation.

Airway

Open the mouth and clear the airway, tilt the head and lift the chin, clear the mouth of foreign bodies like vomitus, loose dentures, etc.

Breathing

Ascertain presence or absence of breathing by looking at the chest movements, placing the ear near the victim's nose and auscultation of the chest. If breathing is absent then it can be supported in the following ways:

- Mouth to mouth
- Mouth to nose
- Mouth to airway.

Circulation

Check for the carotid artery pulse along with other pulses, if absent or weak/irregular, external cardiac compression should be started to establish circulation, which can be done as follows:

- Position the patient supine on firm surface
- Locate the lower margin of the victim's rib cage
- Locate the lower part of the sternum (central part of rib cage)

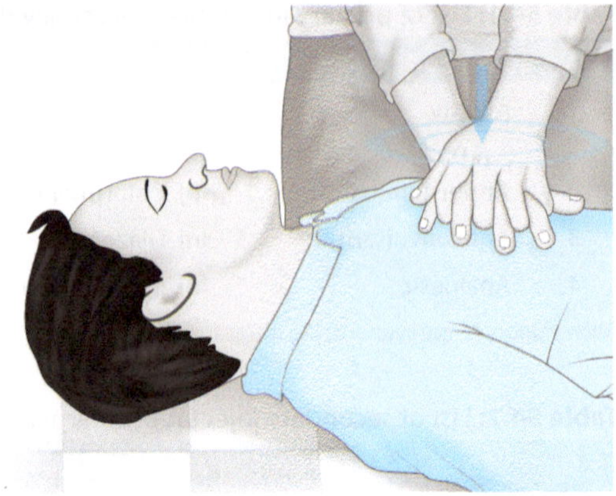

Fig. 54.2: Cardiopulmonary resuscitation

- Place hand on top of the fist, with long axis of the rescuer's hand perpendicular to the long axis of the sternum
- Fingers are interlocked
- Rescuer's elbow locked so that the arms are straight
- Start compression to depress the chest by ½ to 1½ inches
- Feel for carotid pulse, optimal compression would generate a carotid pulse (Fig 54.2).

When two rescuers are available, the compression ventilation ratio should be 5:1 and when a single rescuer is available then the ratio should be 15:1.

CHAPTER 55

Dental Materials

INTRODUCTION

A wide variety of materials are used in dentistry and the dental hygienist and other paradental personnel should be familiar with the general structure, composition, properties and uses of these materials. Some of these materials are used for registering the impressions and are called impression materials. Some materials are used for restoring teeth of the patient in the surgery. Still other materials are used as part of restorative fabrication procedures used in the plaster room and in the laboratory. One should know how these materials will behave under laboratory and clinical conditions.

FILLING MATERIALS

These can be divided into two types as described below.

Temporary Filling Materials

These are soothing or quickly applied materials.

- Zinc oxide eugenol (ZOE) (sedative)
- Zinc oxide - carbolized resin
- Zinc phosphate cements (longer lasting cements)
- Gutta percha (rubber-like and is heat-softened).

These temporary filling materials are also used as cavity lining materials. Other lining materials used are:

- Calcium hydroxide
- Cavity varnishes are resins in solvents like acetone, chloroform or ether.

A relatively new lining material, cementing material and a permanent material in children's dentistry is the polycarboxylate cement. It is zinc oxide mixed with polycarboxylic acid. It adheres to tooth substance, stainless steel and unpolished gold. It is nonirritant and fairly strong (compressive and tensile strength is good, if not exposed to moisture). The bonding to tooth substance is good. However, shear strength of zinc phosphate is better for purposes of cementing inlays and crowns.

Permanent Filling Materials

These are classified as:

- Dental amalgams, e.g. Silver amalgams are alloys whose one of the constituents is Mercury. Silver alloy has silver 69%, Tin 26%, Copper 4%, and zinc 1%
- *Tooth-colored filling materials:*
  - Silicate cements as a permanent or semipermanent filling material for anterior teeth, consists of SiO_2 (45%) AI_2O_3 (30%), Ca (10%) and fluorides (15%) and liquid phosphorus acid (42%) with aluminum and zinc phosphate (18%) and water (40%). It sets to a hard mass.
  - Phosphate cements.
- Composite resins are composed of organic phase (acrylic resin) and inorganic phase (small particles of inert substance like glass and ceramics). Also catalyst and bonding agents are added. This gives them high

strength less toxicity to pulp, less setting shrinkage but caries resistance is slight as compared to silicates
- Dental porcelain in which powder and liquid is mixed and then baked by firing
- Dental gold are cohesive gold foil and casting gold alloys. For casting work, solders, fluxes and investment materials are used. Investment materials make the molds into which the molten metal can be forced
- Dental waxes and base plate materials are used in denture work, for making casting patterns, as temporary cementing materials and even as impression materials.

- *Denture base materials:* These are of two types:
  1. *Metallic:* Gold alloys, chromium cobalt alloys, stainless steel, and aluminum.
  2. *Nonmetallic:* Acrylic resin-heat cured.
     - ◊ Tooth materials: Acrylic and porcelain
     - ◊ Abrasive and polishing materials.

IMPRESSION MATERIALS

To produce a dental impression, the impression material is placed in the mouth in a special tray when it is in proper plastic or pliable or moldable state and held in position until the materials set or firm. The tray together with thin material is removed from the mouth. From this negative reproduction is then made a positive model in stone plaster. This model is the positive duplication of oral tissues.

The impression materials should have the following desirable properties:

- Accuracy
  - Accuracy of surface detail
  - Accuracy of reproduction of recorded details on to the casts
  - Recording of undercut areas, e.g. an impression may be plastic or brittle, if it is to give accurate reproduction of undercuts, e.g. compound, plaster of Paris (POP) are unsuitable.
- Reasonably quick to set or harden
- Harmless to the oral tissues
- Pleasant tasting
- Easy manipulation, i.e. easy to use
- Dimensionally stable after setting
- Compression or favorable placement of soft tissues by the impression materials.

Classification

These are of following types:

- Those materials that set or harden by physical changes are called as thermoplastic materials
  - Modeling plastic or impression compound
  - Impression waxes and resins
  - Reversible hydrocolloids.
- Those materials that set by chemical reaction
  - Rigid materials:
    - ◊ Plaster of Paris (POP)
    - ◊ Zinc oxide eugenol paste.
  - Elastic impression materials:
    - ◊ Irreversible hydrocolloid
    - ◊ Rubber base impression materials.

Thermoplastic Materials

- *Modeling plastic or impression compound:* This is a resinous material used for taking the impressions usually of edentulous mouths. It is hard and rigid at room temperature and is softened by heat. It is available in three forms: (1) in cake form—used for taking the initial impression, (2) in the form of sticks called tracing sticks—this is lower fusing compound and is used for border molding of the special tray for final impression, (3) in the form of cones for crown and bridge work—used with copper bands and is low fusing material
  - *Composition:*
    - ◊ Thermoplastic material and waxes, e.g. Resins, shellac, paraffin wax, carnauba wax, etc. - 45-65%
    - ◊ French chalk - 30% (filler and prevents stickiness)

◊ Glycerin - 2.5% (for easy softening)
◊ Fatty acids - hardener
◊ Coloring agents.

- *Softening*: Whenever possible, compounds should be softened with "dry and heat", e.g. in an oven or flame, but it should not ignite. But large quantities are conveniently softened in a water bath at 55–65° C. Prolonged heating in a water bath makes it brittle and grainy. On the other hand, if water is incorporated during manipulation the plasticity of the compound is increased and its flow may be doubled resulting in move distortion on setting or cooling
- *Advantages:*
  ◊ Surface can be corrected, and impressions retrieved
  ◊ Can be used for border molding of tissue for peripheral seal
  ◊ Can be used in combination with other materials.
- *Disadvantages:*
  ◊ It distorts easily and gives drag
  ◊ It is unhygienic.
- *Uses:*
  ◊ It is used as a base for washing impressions
  ◊ It is used to develop peripheral seal
  ◊ It is used as an initial impression to make special tray.

• *Impression waxes and resins:* Low-fusing impression waxes are not sufficiently accurate for final impression for complete dentures. These can be used as a corrective material for a small area or as a border refining material. Example is correcting wax which is being used for registering impressions for extension base partial dentures
• *Reversible hydrocolloids:* It is agar-agar 8–15% by weight, rest water. When agar is dissolved in water, its particles attract water and swell up in size thus forming hydrocolloid. The hydrocolloid solutions pass the property of changing into gel which can support considerable shear stress (Skinner). They give accurate impressions but require special cooling trays, which is a disadvantage. It can be used for impressions for dentures, splints, crown and bridge work. The main use is duplicating the models.

Chemical Materials

• *Rigid materials:*
  - *Plaster of paris (POP):* It is beta-hemihydrates of calcium sulfate, i.e. $(CaSO_2)_2.H_2O$
    ◊ *Composition*: Other constituents are:
      ▸ Potassium sulfate: 4%
      ▸ Borax: 0.4%
      ▸ Alizarin (pink color): 0.4%
      ▸ Starch (renders impressions soluble)
      ▸ Fluorescent agents.

    Potassium sulfate reduces setting expansion from 0.2% to 0.05%. It accelerates the setting time so that the impression plaster sets faster. Borax is a retarder and increases the setting time to the desired 2–3 minutes (It reduces setting expansion). This quick setting plaster is therefore used as a very thin mix in contrast to plaster for making casts which is mixed as thick as possible. High W/P ratio of 60 parts water to 100 parts of plaster (weigh) (thin mix) is used to reduce strength and the exothermic heat. Increased spatulation causes rapid set. Increased temperature up to 30° C accelerates the setting time.
  - *Uses of plaster:*
    ◊ It is used for taking the final impressions of knife-edge ridges covered by flabby tissues
    ◊ It is used for corrective wash impressions
    ◊ It is used for making transfer registration of crown positions in crown and bridge work.

- *Zinc oxide eugenol (ZOE):* It is metallic oxide impression paste used as corrective wash impressions of completely edentulous mouths. It is used to temporarily reline the dentures to stabilize base plates in bite registration in dentures work and in crown and bridge work. It is also used as a temporary filling material, as a root canal filling material and as a dressing material
  - ◊ *Composition:* In two tubes, zinc oxide tube (base material) and the second tube (accelerator) contain eugenol in paste form. It contains other ingredients:
    - ▸ Resin or gum
    - ▸ Talc as filler
    - ▸ Mineral oil and olive oil (plasticizer)
    - ▸ Magnesium or calcium chloride (accelerator).
  - ◊ *Manipulation*: Setting time is accelerated by:
    - ▸ Increase in temperature
    - ▸ It is hygienic
    - ▸ Reduces nausea to minimum
    - ▸ Adheres well (no flaking)
    - ▸ Can be added, readapted and rechecked.

- *Elastic impression materials*
  - *Irreversible hydrocolloids alginate*: The alginate base impression materials are used for impressions of the dental arches in which the natural teeth are present and for the preparation of study models for diagnostic facts. This material shows elastic recovery. Therefore it is used to record undercut areas
    - ◊ *Composition:*
      - ▸ Sodium alginate or potassium alginate: 20%
      - ▸ Calcium sulfate (dehydrate) (retarder): 16%
      - ▸ Sodium phosphate: 1–18%
      - ▸ Zinc oxide or magnesium oxide (modifier): 7% or good setting
      - ▸ Special diatomaceous earth (filler): 44–50%
      - ▸ Potassium titanium fluoride (as modifier to accelerate setting of stone plaster): 60% as coloring and flavoring agents.
    - ◊ *Mixing:* The powder is mixed quickly but thoroughly with specified amount of water within one minute or form a homogeneous paste. The tray should be perforated properly and uniformly spaced for enough thickness of the material. The impression material requires to be properly locked in the tray by forcing the material through the perforations. Adhesive plaster can be applied on the periphery ion sticky wax or chloroform can use with cotton fibers or adhesive. The paste gels chemically in 3–5 minutes forming a strong elastic gel which may then be removed at a jerk, setting time can be altered by:
      - ▸ Temperature of the water-cooler water will increase the setting time and warm water will decrease setting time
      - ▸ Water and powder ratio will also alter the setting time but it should not be used against the manufactures instructions.
    - ◊ The impressions made from alginate base material should be poured immediately because the material undergoes dimensional changes in storing.

- *Rubber base impression materials:* It is modern material for registering the impression for partial dentures, crowns and bridge work and for inlays
  - *Composition*: Basic composition is polysulfide rubber. It comes in two tubes.
    - ◊ White paste
      - ▸ Polysulfide rubber 80%
      - ▸ Zinc oxide (filler) 4.89%
      - ▸ Calcium sulfate (filler) 15%.

- ◊ Brown paste
  - Lead peroxide 70% (main accelerator)
  - Sulfur (accelerator) 3%
  - Castor oil 19%.
- *Mixing*: Equal parts of two pastes. Mix for one minute. Undermixing to be avoided
- *Setting*: By polymerization of polysulfide rubber. Setting time 5–8 minutes. It is safer to wait longer up to 10 minutes or even longer up to 12 minutes, accuracy is excellent. It is most accurate of all materials.

CHAPTER 56

Dentists (Code of Ethics)

HISTORY OF DENTISTRY

The ancient Hebrews stressed the importance of the dental apparatus as a prime element of mental and physical force and vigor. They used therapeutic remedies in treatment of dental disorder. In addition to gold and silver shell crown, they made bridgework and pivot teeth.

In ancient Chinese practice of dentistry, they used chewsticks. The modern toothbrush was invented by the Chinese in 1498. Their therapeutic method of acupuncture included 388 points puncturing of these, 26 were used as a remedy for the toothache and 6 others for curing pain in the gums.

The authentic history of dentistry began with the writings of Hippocrates (460–377 BC). The following subjects are among the many of dental interests discussed in the collection: formation of the teeth, relation of the teeth to speaking, erosion, mouthwashes and dentifrices, relations between the malformation of the skull and palate and irregularities of the teeth, scorbutus, necrosis of the jaw, influence of atmospheric conditions on the occurrence of oral maladies, dental or gingival symptoms originating in different maladies, ulcers caused by broken sharp teeth, complete and incomplete fracture of the jaw and fractures of symphysis.

The earliest record of orthodontic treatment by finger pressure is mentioned in "Demedicina" by Cornelius Celsus of Rome in the year 25 BC - AD 50. Archigenus in Rome AD 100 surmised that toothache often results from a disease of the interior part of the tooth. He perforated the tooth with a small drill of his own invention. The Arabians while making important progress in chemistry and pharmacology, made very little progress in the healing arts. Rhazes (Ninth century), earliest of the important Arabian physicians, recommended filling the carious cavity with cement composed of mastic and alum. The Arabian book "De chirurgia" was the first book to include illustrations of dental instruments. The Arabians also made rules for the extraction of teeth called the rules of Abulcasis Giovanni Plateario introduced the sitting position for operations on the teeth in the Fifteenth century. His predecessors had made the patient lie in a horizontal position or held his head between their knees.

In Italy during the year 1563, Eustachius presented in several tables the number of roots of molar teeth and all the variation occurring in their number and in their length and form.

Shushratha Samhita (1000 BC) gives numerous descriptions of severe periodontal disease with the loose teeth and purulent discharge. In 1723, Pierre Fauchard, a French Surgeon was credited as "Father of Modern Dentistry" while Dr. R Ahmed (1890-1965) is referred as the "Father of modern Indian Dentistry".

Alfred Fones (1869-1938), an American dentist from Bridgeport, Connecticut is called as the founder of the profession of dental hygiene, starting in 1906. He created the term "Dental Hygienist " and established the first school of dental hygiene in 1913.

DENTAL ETHICS

Dental hygienists are governed by the dentists (Code of Ethics) Notified by Dental Council of India (No-DE-97-2014) dated the 27th June 2014. A dental hygienist has to follow all the provisions laid down in the notification. Briefly, it constitutes the implementation of following aspects:

- Provide oral health care using the highest levels of professional knowledge, judgment and ability
- Serve all patients without discrimination
- Hold professional relationships in confidence
- Use every opportunity to increase public understanding of oral health practices
- Generate public confidence in members of the dental health professions
- Cooperate with all health professions in meeting the health needs of the public
- Participate in the professional association and uphold its purposes
- Maintain professional competence through governing this profession
- Recognize and uphold the laws and regulations governing this profession
- Exchange professional knowledge with other health profession
- Represent dental hygienist with high standards of personal conduct.

LEGAL ISSUES

Legal issues include:

Professional Duties

- Professional's duties to:
  - Possess the skill and expected knowledge
  - Exercise the skill and knowledge in the community.
- Duty to refer to a specialist, when indicated, who possess and exercise the standard of care
- Duty to render treatment only to patients already accepted for treatment
- Duty to continue or complete treatment started within a reasonable time or to arrange alternative sources of treatment for patients already accepted for treatment
- Duty to obtain informed consent from responsible parties before treatment; informed consent must be based on:
  - Adequate maturity of the patient or guardian
  - Complete information presented to the patient regarding the risk, costs and benefits of the proposed treatment.

Malpractice—Professional Negligence

Criteria for Malpractice

- Health professional owes a duty to the client; relationship between the client and health care provider establishes a duty
- Duty breached by the health care provider
- Client sustained injury or damage
- Injury or damage is the direct result of the breach of duty.

Common Grounds for Malpractice

- Poor results when success is guaranteed
- Failure to exercise proper techniques in:
  - Sterilization
  - Radiographs.
- Failure to adequately inform the patient regarding treatment procedures, outcomes and risks
- Failure to obtain permission
  - Technical assault—touching or treating without consent
  - Invasion of privacy—divulging private information without consent.

Defence Against Malpractice

- Exercise due care, using reasonable skill and care
- Keep accurate and complete records of each case
- Contributory negligence by the patient relieves the health professional of liability

- Statute of limitations limits the length of time in which a suit may be brought
  - In adults this is usually 2 years after the injury or damage has been recognized or discovered
  - For children this is a reasonable time period after the child reaches the age of maturation
  - Question of proximate cause; if there are possible intervening causes or contributory negligence, these may relieve the health professional from liability
  - Types of damages or redress:
    - ◊ *Nominal damages:* Monetary compensation for the loss
    - ◊ *Compensatory damages:* Actual costs to cover repairs or treatment plus general damages to cover pain and suffering
    - ◊ *Punitive damages:* Additional monetary compensation to punish the defendant usually awarded in cases where professional acted with recklessness or indifference.

DENTIST ACT, 1948 AND DENTAL COUNCIL OF INDIA

Dental Council of India (DCI) came into being in 1949 following the passing of dentist's act in 1948 by Indian parliament in March 1948. Before this, there was no laid downregulation for the dental profession. The main purpose of this act was to formulate the DCI and establish a standard for dental education in aid to establish the profession of dentistry on the scientific, moral and ethical basis.

The Dental Act 1948, Section 6 of 1948 means an act to regulate the profession of dentistry by constituting DCI under the class-B dental hygienist are covered, whereas under Section 6-A dental surgeon are covered.

Constitution of DCI

This is composed of:

- Two representatives from each state out of which one is elected and other nominated
- Four elected representatives from dental institutions
- One representative from Medical Council of India
- One representative from each University
- Six members nominated by central Government with the Director General of Health Service as an ex-officio member.

Functions of DCI

- To accord recognition to the dental qualifications granted by Indian Universities
- To accord recognition to foreign dental qualifications obtained by Indian citizens
- To accord recognition to dental hygienist, dental assistant and dental mechanic diploma courses.

To appoint inspectors at regular intervals to inspect all the dental institutions and report on the adequacy of courses and facilities existing for teaching the various course.

- The council at any given time can withdraw the recognition if observes a failure in the standard
- Prepare an all India dentist register
- To prescribe the standard curriculum for the training of dentist and dental hygienist and the conditions for admission to courses of such training
- To prescribe standards at the examination and other requirements to satisfied to secure required registration for a qualification under dentist's act 1948.

PREVENTIVE DENTISTRY APPROACH

The physician's task should be care of the healthy, not care of the sick. This extreme way of stating the old saying about prevention being better than cure implies that ultimately, there should be no sickness and preventive sciences will control the disease. Why not? Medical, Surgical and Dental research is proceeding towards this. As the etiologies of more diseases, morbidity and mortality statistics drop.

In general terms, preventive dentistry is at present approached from three directions:

1. *Dental research:* More information about the causes of dental disease comes to light with each issue of the dental journals. A complete understanding in biochemical terms cannot be far away.
2. *Integration of preventive dentistry into dental curriculum:* The subject has to fight for time in curriculum becoming increasingly crowded by restorative techniques, and hygienists are people who have manual dexterity, and who are used to working on their own. Positive attitudes towards prevention must not be submerged by the pressures of the job.
3. *Environmental control:* The fight against devoutly held moral attitudes (when promoting the fluoridation of public water supplies) is a up-hill task. With respect to fluoridation, it is a sad fact that more than one-third of the US children are still not protected against caries by this simple measure. Fluoridation originated in the USA a generation ago.

TEST YOURSELF

Expected Theory Questions

- Write in detail about impression materials.
- Write a note on the role of a dental hygienist in tobacco cessation.
- Explain in detail about CPR used in medical emergencies.
- Write in detail about classification of mandibular fractures along with their clinical features.
- What are the various symptoms of deficiency or excess of vitamin A, D, K, C, E and B complex?

Expected Viva Questions

- What are the calcium requirements for an adult?
- In which year Dental Council of India was established?
- What is the chemical composition of Plaster of Paris?
- What is malpractice and professional negligence in dentistry?
- What are the typical clinical features of bilateral fracture of maxilla in Lefort II and Lefort III?

Annexure

SAMPLE QUESTION PAPERS FOR DENTAL HYGIENIST EXAMINATION

ARMED FORCES MEDICAL COLLEGE
Department of Medical Surgery
Paper - I
(Anatomy, Physiology, History, Dental Hygiene and Oral Prophylaxis)

Time - 3 hours **MM 75**

All Questions are Compulsory

1. Discuss the anatomy of temporomandibular joint and draw a neat labeled diagram. 12
2. Name various brushing techniques. Describe one of these in detail. 14
3. (a) Write the time of eruption of deciduous and permanent dentitions. 7
   (b) Write the functions of saliva. 7
4. (a) Write the role of dental hygienist in armed forces. 7
   (b) Draw labeled diagrams of mandible to show insertion of various muscles of mastication. 8
5. Write short notes on any four (4) of the following: 20
   (a) Periodontal ligament.
   (b) Periodic dental inspection.
   (c) Histology of gingiva.
   (d) Care of inter proximal areas.
   (e) Principles of periodontal instrumentation.

Paper - II

(Material Medical, Pathology and Bacteriology, Dental Health Education, Social and Public Health Dentistry, Preventive dentistry)

Time - 3 hours **MM 75**

All Questions are Compulsory

1. Discuss what will you perform to treat the cases of AIDS and Hepatitis B? 12
2. How will you differentiate between: 15
   (a) Attrition, abrasion and erosion.
   (b) Gingival and periodontal abscess.
   (c) Degeneration and necrosis.
3. Define sterilization and disinfection. Discuss step-by-step, the process of autoclaving dental equipment. 20
4. Discuss signs and symptoms of acute necrotizing ulcerative gingivitis. How will you differentiate this condition from acute herpetic gingivostomatitis? 8
5. Write short notes on any four (4) of the following: 20
   (a) Halitosis.
   (b) Audio visual aids.
   (c) Intrinsic stains.
   (d) Fluorosis of teeth.
   (e) Astringents.

Paper–III

(Operating Room Technique, Chairside Assistance of Dental Materials. Dental Ethics and Jurisprudence, Dental Radiology, Food and Nutrition)

Time - 3 hours **MM 75**

All Questions are Compulsory

1. (a) Classify impression materials. Write the properties of an ideal impression material. 7
   (b) Write the composition of silver alloy and the function of each constituent. 7
2. (a) Write the limitations of X-ray in dentistry. 6
   (b) What are the hazards of radiation? 7
3. (a) Write briefly the role of vitamin C and vitamin D for oral health of tissues and teeth. 7
   (b) Write the properties of ideal cement. 7
4. (a) What is a dentifrice? Write the composition of one dentifrice. 7
   (b) Draw a labeled diagram to show the organs that take part in digestion of food. 7
5. Write short notes on any four (4) of the following: 20
   (a) Dental Council of India.
   (b) Use of computers in dentistry.
   (c) Syncope.
   (d) Chlorhexidine.
   (e) Dental ethics.

Paper–IV

(Anatomy, Physiology, Histology, Dental Hygiene and Oral Prophylaxis)

Time - 3 hours **MM 75**

All Questions are Compulsory

1. (a) Define and classify impression materials. Write properties of an ideal impression material.
   (b) Draw and label diagram of external carotid artery. 20
2. (a) Name muscles of mastication. Write origin, insertion and function of each. Describe masseter muscle.
   (b) Draw a diagram of histological structure of normal gingiva. 20
3. State whether the following statements are true or false: 15
   i. The mentalis muscle inserts into lower lip.
   ii. All gingiva of the upper jaw is supplied by branches of the maxillary nerve.
   iii. All gingiva of the lower jaw is innervated by branches of the mandibular nerve.
   iv. Calcium is not necessary for coagulation of blood.
   v. Proteins are formed in the tissue by the chemical union of amino acids.
   vi. Plaque control may be expected to have greater impact on prevention of gingivitis than dental caries.
   vii. Dentifrices are not essential for removal of plaque by tooth brushing.
   viii. Stippling is normally seen on the marginal gingiva.
   ix. Microorganisms are the major component of dental plaque.
   x. The alveolar process and the teeth divide the oral cavity into the oral vestibule and the oral cavity process.
4. Write short notes on any four (4) of the following: 8
   (a) Bacterial plaque.
   (b) Use of interdental stimulators.
   (c) Disclosing solutions.
   (d) Dental caries.
   (e) Syncope.
5. How will you differentiate between the following: 12
   (a) Gingival and periodontal abscess.
   (b) Gingivitis and periodontitis.
   (c) Attrition, abrasion and erosion.
   (d) Degeneration and necrosis.

Paper - V

(Material Medical, Pathology and Bacteriology, Dental Health Education, Social and Public Health Dentistry, Preventive dentistry)

Time - 3 hours **MM 75**

All Questions are Compulsory

1. Write signs and symptoms of acute necrotizing ulcerative gingivitis. How will you differentiate it from acute herpetic gingivitis? 10
2. (a) Describe the role of dental hygienist in armed forces.
   (b) Write sequence wise the instruments that you will lay on trolley to operate a case of gingivectomy. 10
3. How will you protect yourself and your patients from cross infection of hepatitis B and HIV? 10
4. Write short notes on any three (3) of the following: 15
   (a) Hemostatics.
   (b) Caustics.
   (c) Vasoconstrictors.
   (d) Gum paint.
   (e) Counter irritants.
5. Write in brief about any three (3) the following subjects: 30
   (a) Inflammation.
   (b) Public health dentistry.
   (c) Oral physiotherapy.
   (d) Role of fluoride.

Paper–VI

(Operating Room Technique, Chairside Assistance of Dental Materials. Dental Ethics and Jurisprudence, Dental Radiology, Food and Nutrition)

Time - 3 hours **MM 75**

All Questions are Compulsory

1. What is balanced diet? Give its composition. What should be the diet of a pregnant woman? 15
2. Discuss the principles of sharpening instruments. 8
3. (a) Discuss the role of radiographs in the diagnosis of diseases. 8
   (b) What are the hazards of radiation? 8
   (c) How will you protect yourself and your patient from such side effects? 7
4. (a) What is the composition of silver alloy? Write in brief the role of each constituent. 7
   (b) Name various materials which can be used for periodontal dressings. 7
   (c) What are the advantages and disadvantages of periodontal dressings? 8
5. Write in brief or any three (3) of the following: 15
   (a) Dentist's Act 1948.
   (b) Autoclaving.
   (c) Dentifrices.
   (d) Dental ethics.
   (e) Home care instructions to periodontal patients.

REGULATIONS AND SYLLABUS FOR DENTAL HYGIENIST COURSE

DENTAL COUNCIL OF INDIA

Notification

New Delhi, 19th August, 2008, No.DE542007. In exercise of powers conferred by clause (1) and subclause (g) and (h) of clause (2) of section 20 of the Dentists Act, 1948 (XVI of 1948), the Dental Council of India, after consultations with the State Governments and with the previous approval of the Central Government hereby make the following Dental Hygienists Course Regulations, 2008.

- Short title and commencement (i) these regulations may be called the Dental Council of India Dental Hygienists Course Regulations, 2008.
- They shall come into force on the date of their publication in the Official Gazette.

REGULATIONS FOR THE MAINTENANCE OF MINIMUM EDUCATIONAL STANDARD FOR DENTAL HYGIENISTS

Dental Hygienists Course Regulations

"Dental Hygienist" means a person, not being a dentist or a medical practitioner, who scales, cleans or polishes teeth, or gives instructions on dental hygiene. He shall work under the supervision of the registered dental surgeon.

In order to regularize and standardize the conferment of the qualification for dental hygienists, it is prescribed that:

1. The Dental Hygienists Diploma Course can be started by a recognized dental college or a dental college, which got the permission from the Central Government for 3rd year Bachelor of Dental Surgery (BDS) course onwards with maximum of 20 seats.
2. The institutions wishing to start courses for dental hygienists should obtain essentiality certificate from the concerned state government and obtain prior approval of the Dental Council of India.
3. The course of studies should extend over a period of two academic years and lead to the qualification of Dental Hygienist Diploma.
4. A separate course shall be arranged for the training of dental hygienists by the institutions.
5. For the purpose of establishment of uniformity in dental education in this course throughout India, it is necessary that the course of instructions to be pursued in all the institutions should be standardized. To achieve this:
    a. A candidate should be at least 17 years of age at the time of admission or within 3 months of it and should be medically fit to pursue the course.
    b. The candidate must have passed 10+2 or two years intermediate or equivalent course there of with science subjects, i.e. physics, chemistry and biology from a recognized Indian University or Pre-university or Intermediate Board.
6. The medium of instruction shall be in English and the course of studies and regulations for the diploma examinations and syllabus to be followed in each subject has been drawn up and appended.

I. MINIMUM REQUIREMNTS FOR INSTITUTIONS IMPARTING TRAINING FOR DENTAL HYGIENISTS

1. The minimum hours devoted to the under mentioned subjects shall be as follows:

	Subject	*Lectures*	*Practical/ Demonstrations/ Clinical*	*Total*
Primary				
1.	Anatomy, General and Dental	50	100	150
2.	Physiology and Histology, General and Dental	20	40	60
3.	Pharmacology General and Dental	15	10	25
4.	Pathology and Microbiology	30	70	100
5.	Dental Radiology.	10	40	50
6.	Food and Nutrition	25	30	55
7.	Dental Hygiene and Oral Prophylaxis	50	280	330
8.	Basic knowledge of Computers	20	50	70
			Total	840
Final				
1.	Dental Hygiene and Oral Prophylaxis	25	350	375
2.	(i) Dental Health Education (ii) Community Public Health Dentistry (iii) Preventive Dentistry	50	200	250
3.	Dental Ethics and Jurisprudence; Orientation in Dentistry	15		15
4.	Dental Materials	10	10	20
			Total	660

2. The classes in different subjects of the curriculum should be taught exclusively for this course.
3. There should be at least one instructor for every 10 students working in the clinics at any given time.
4. For the teaching dental subjects no persons except those holding recognized dental qualification shall be employed as instructors. For clinical and practical/demonstrations persons holding recognized dental hygiene qualification shall be eligible.
5. The institutions imparting training in this course must possess of the following minimum requirements:
    a. One histopathological laboratory equipped with as many number of microscopes as is required by half of the admission strength for demonstration purposes.
    b. At least two class room, i.e. one each for 1st and 2nd year students, one of which must be equipped with a liquid crystal display (LCD) projector and overhead projector (OHP).
    c. Specific/subject wise technical laboratories so that each student of a class is provided with suitable facilities required for the course.

   d. A dental hygienist clinic fitted with one dental chair, one dental unit with ultrasonic autoclave for every 5 students for sterilization.
   e. A library should be available to the students.
6. Teaching Staff: In addition to the requirement of BDS and MDS Staff, exclusive teaching staff will be as under:
   a. Reader MDS (Periodontics)...........................One.
   b. Lecture MDS (Periodontics).........................One.
   c. Tutor Dental Hygienist.........................One.
   d. Other Staff: As per requirement of the syllabus from the Dental Institution.

   Note: Department to teach the Dental Hygienist Course: That in view of the difficulties experienced by the dental departments and dental teachers of dental colleges, the teaching of dental hygienist course is entrusted to the Department of Periodontics.

II. EXAMINATIONS

1. An examination for the grant of Diploma of Dental Hygienists shall be conducted by a board of three examiners imparting training for qualification of Dental Hygienists Course approved by the Dental Council of India. One of the examiners must be external from outside that institution.

   Note: Qualifications/eligibility to appointment as examiners for dental hygienist examinations:
   i. Out of 3 members of examining board, the external and one internal examiner should be a reader in Periodontics (MDS) and third could be tutor (Dental Hygienist Course) involved in teaching of the course.
   ii. That medical persons teaching medical subjects may be appointed as examiners for medical subjects even though they are not registered under the Dentists Act 1948.
   iii. He should be an active teacher of the concerned course of in the concerned subject/s at a recognized dental or medical institution.
2. The examination shall be held twice a year, on such dates as may be fixed. The examination shall consist of two parts (1) Primary and (2) Final Diploma Examination.

The Primary Examination (First Year)

3. The Examination shall be open to any student who:
   i. Has been enrolled during one academic year preceding the examination in an institution approved or recognized by the Dental Council of India for this purpose.
   ii. The candidate must have passed 10+2 or two years intermediate or equivalent course there of with science subjects, i.e. physics, chemistry and biology from a recognized Indian University, Pre-university or Intermediate Board.
   iii. Has his/her name, submitted to the board of examiners, by the head of the institution in which he/she is enrolled.
   iv. Produces the following certificates signed by the head of the institutions:
      a. Good character;
      b. Having attended not less than 75% of the full course of lectures delivered and practical or demonstrations clinical conducted in each of the subjects of examinations.
4. Every candidate shall forward his/her application to the examining body by a date fixed by that body, accompanied by the prescribed fee. A candidate who fails to pass or present himself/herself for examination shall not be entitled to claim a refund of the fee.
5. Every candidate shall be examined in the following subjects comprising of three theory papers as follows:
   i. Paper I: Anatomy, Physiology and Histology

ii. Paper II: Pharmacology, Pathology and Microbiology
iii. Paper III: Food, Nutrition and Radiology.

Marks for each of the papers shall be as under:

Written	:	75
Oral	:	25
Practical	:	100
Total	:	200

Each written paper shall be of three hours.

6. Every candidate shall be required to take up all subjects of the examination. A candidate failing in any paper or papers of this examination before being permitted to reappear at the subsequent examination shall produce evidence of having pursued such a course of training as the head of the institution may determine.

   A candidate, who passes in any one or more papers of the examination shall be exempted from appearing in which he/she has passed and shall be allowed to reappear in the rest in which he/she has failed in any subsequent examination within a period of two years. After two years the candidate will have to appear in all the papers of this examination.

7. The minimum number of marks required to pass the examination shall be 50% in each paper both in the (i) written with oral and (ii) practical parts of the examination.

   Candidates who obtain minimum of 75% marks in any paper under examination and passes in all three subjects in first attempt shall be declared to have passed with distinction in a particular subject/s. Candidates who do not pass in all the papers in the first attempt and later passes with distinction marks, shall be declared as passed but without distinction.

   As soon as possible after the examination the board of examiners shall publish a list of the candidates who have passed. Each successful candidate shall be granted a "Primary Diploma".

The Final Diploma Examination

8. This examination shall be open to any student who:
   i. Has been enrolled for primary academic year preceding the examination in an institution approved by the Dental Council of India for the purpose.
   ii. Has previously passed the primary examination for the Diploma of Dental Hygienists:
   iii. Has his/her name submitted to the board of examiners by head of the institution in which he/she is enrolled.
   iv. Produces the following certificates signed by the Head of the Institution:
      a. Good character.
      b. Having attended not less than 75% of the full course of lectures delivered and practical/demonstration/clinical conducted in each of the papers of the examination.
      c. Having passed the primary examination in all papers.
      d. There shall not be a gap of more than two academic years between primary and final diploma exams.
9. Every candidate shall forward his/her application to the examining body by a date fixed by that body, accompanied by the prescribed fee. A candidate who fails to pass or present himself/herself for examination shall not be entitled to claim a refund of the fee.
10. Every candidate shall be examined in the following subjects comprising of three papers as follows:
   i. Paper I: Dental Hygiene and Oral Prophylaxis
   ii. Paper II: Dental Health Education, community or Public Health Dentistry Preventive Dentistry
   iii. Paper III: Dental Materials, Dental Ethics and Jurisprudence, Orientation in Dentistry

Marks for each of the papers shall be as under:

Written	:	75
Oral	:	25
Practical	:	100
Total	:	200

Each written paper shall be of three hours.

11. Every candidate shall be required to take up all papers of the examination. A candidate failing in any paper or papers of this examination before being permitted to reappear at the subsequent examination shall produce evidence of having pursued such a course of training as the head of the institution may determine.

    A candidate, who passes in any one or more papers under examination shall be exempted from appearing in which he/she has passed and shall be allowed to reappear in the rest in which he/she has failed in any subsequent examination within a period of two years. After two years the candidate will have to appear in all the papers of this examination.
12. The minimum number of marks required to pass the examination shall be 50% in each paper both in (i) written with oral and (ii) practical parts of the examination. Candidates who obtain minimum of 75% marks in any paper under examination shall be declared to have passed with distinction in a particular subject provided he/she passed all subjects of examination in first attempt. Candidates who do not pass in all the papers of the "Final Examination" at one and the same time shall not be declared to have passed with distinction.
13. The college authority will apply two months in advance along with practical examination date sheet to the Dental Council of India for recognition of the diploma course.
14. As soon as possible after the examination, the board of examiners shall publish a list of those candidates who have passed. Each successful candidate shall be granted a diploma subject to the approval by the Dental Council of India.

III. SYLLABUS FOR THE DENTAL HYGIENISTS COURSE PRIMARY (1ST YEAR)

1. Anatomy, General and Dental

Lectures

- General structure of mucous membrane (tongue, pharynx, lips), bones, muscles, blood vessels, lymphatics, glands and nerves. Blood and nerve supply in relation to face in general and teeth and associated structures in particular
- Elementary knowledge of development of the jaws and teeth
- Relationship of teeth with investing tissues
- Muscles of mastication and facial expression
- Temporomandibular articulation
- Course and distribution of Vth and VIIth cranial nerves.

Practical

- Osteology of head and neck in general and face including jaws in particular
- Morphology of teeth
- Alveolar process of jaw bones
- Section of tooth in situ.

2. Physiology and Histology, General and Dental

Lectures

- Cell structure of the human body
- Brief description of the histology and function of various dental and oral tissues, e.g. Gingiva, periodontal membrane, alveolar process, cementum, enamel, dentin, nasmyth's membrane, pulp, etc.
- Salivary glands, ducts and their functions
- Composition and function of saliva
- Blood: Composition and functions
- Mastication, deglutition and phonation
- General outlines of the physiological processes of the human body particularly circulatory.

Practical

- Study of prepared histological slides of oral and dental tissues, sections of a tooth
- Routine blood examination.

3. Pharmacology, General and Dental

Lectures

- Brief description, nomenclature, derivation, dosage, pharmacological action and therapeutic uses of drugs commonly used in dentistry (Obtundent, astringent, mouth wash, antiseptics).

Practical

- Preparation of gun paints, mouth washes and dentifrices.

4. Pathology and Microbiology, General and Dental

Lectures

- General principles of pathology
- Inflammation, degeneration and repair
- Application of general principles of pathology to tooth and surrounding tissues
- Dental anomalies
- Attrition, abrasion and erosion
- Oral manifestation of systemic diseases like diabetes, syphilis, anemia vitamin deficiencies and infectious diseases like AIDS and hepatitis B
- Infection control in dental operatory and biomedical waste management and handling
- Neoplasm with reference to oral cavity
- Elementary knowledge of bacteriology, asepsis, infection, immunity, brief description of pathology and bacteriology of dental caries and gingival infections.

Practical

- Study of prepared pathological and bacteriological sides relating to oral and dental conditions
- Clinical demonstration of oral and dental manifestation of systemic disorders.

5. Dental Radiology

Lectures

- Fundamental and elementary principle of dental radiology including X-ray machine, its components and maintenance
- Basic knowledge of radiovisiography technique and extra oral radiographs including panoramic (orthopantographs and cephalostats)
- Automatic film processing
- Cataloging and indexing of intraoral periapical (IOPA) films
- Knowledge of occlusal, bitewing and digital radiography
- Technical aspects of dental radiographs, i.e. the taking processing and mounting of dental radiographs
- Characteristics of acceptable image, factors that influence finished radiographs, rules of radiation protection, radiation hazards.

Practical

- Taking processing and mounting of intra and extraoral radiographs.

6. Food and Nutrition

Lecture and Practical

- Basic "food chemistry" in relation to general and oral health
- Physical nature of diet in prevention of dental diseases
- Carbohydrates, fats, proteins, vitamins, minerals and water in relation to dental and oral health
- General food requirements for growth, maintenance and repair of the body
- Assessment and charting of individual diet and counseling
- Special diet and its administration in maxillofacial injury cases.

7. Dental Hygiene and Oral Prophylaxis (Primary and Final)

Lecture

- Definition of hygiene
- Objectives of dental hygiene
- Oral prophylaxis: Various methods
- Oral prophylaxis: Treatment system
- Stains on teeth: Extrinsic, intrinsic and their management
- Dental calculus
- Technical knowledge of ultrasonic scaling
- Brief description and the role of oral prophylaxis in gingivitis, periodontitis, periodontal and alveolar abscess.

Clinical

- Instruments, technique of oral prophylaxis
- Destaining and polishing of teeth
- Topical application of fluorides
- Care of oral cavity and appliances during treatment of maxillofacial cases.

IV. SYLLABUS FOR THE DENTAL HYGIENISTS COURSE FINAL (2ND YEAR)

1. Dental Hygiene and Oral Prophylaxis

- Combined courses at para 7 above [as mentioned in 1st year (primary) above].

2. Dental Health Education, Community Public Health Dentistry and Preventive Dentistry

Lectures

- Definition of health and dental health
- Aims and objectives of dental health education
- Dental health and children
- Steps in preventive program, patient counseling
- Dental health education parents, mothers (anti and postnatal), infants preschool
- Children and grown up handicapped children
- Dental caries prevalence and prevention
- Prevention by fluoridation
- Periodontal diseases
- Saliva in relation to dental health and disease
- Dietary habits and dental health
- Habits and malocclusion
- Oral cancer
- Brief outline of historical background of public health, history of dentistry and public health services
- Dental health team in relation to community health
- Technical knowledge of topical fluoride application.

Practical

- Preparation of models of jaws and teeth normal and pathological dental conditions
- Designing, drawing and painting of posters on dental health education
- Procedure for arranging short talks, skits and features on dental and oral health, visual aids
- Collection of oral health related statistics by conducting a small survey of an area.

3. Dental Ethics, Jurisprudence and Orientation in Dentistry

Lectures and Practical

- Difference between ethics and law, types of law
- Legal impositions in relation to dental practice, code of ethics
- Unlicensed practice of dentistry
- Regulatory and professional organization
- Place and function of dental profession in the society and discussion of economic problems involved therein
- Social factors in dental progress, income and living standard of people
- Objective and scope of dentistry.

4. Basic Knowledge of Computer

- General office routine economics, record-keeping services, professional referrals and computing skill.

5. Dental Materials

Lectures and Practical

- General knowledge of various material used in dentistry such as impression material gypsum products, waxes, investing materials and various filling materials, temporary and permanent cements, orthodontic material and implant materials, materials used in maxillofacial and surgical prosthesis
- Recognition and knowledge of various dental equipment and stores used in dental establishment
- Organization of dental stores, storage and accounting, handling and maintenance of dental items, assembly and minor repair of dental equipment.

Index

Page numbers followed by *b* refer to box, *f* refer to figure, *fc* refer to flow chart, and *t* refer to table.

G

M

Q

R

S

U

V

W

X

Z